Statistics for Biology and Health

Series Editors
M. Gail, K. Krickeberg, J. Samet, A. Tsiatis, W. Wong

Tomasz Burzykowski
Geert Molenberghs
Marc Buyse
Editors

The Evaluation of Surrogate Endpoints

With 57 Illustrations

Springer

Tomasz Burzykowski
Center for Statistics
Limburgs Universitair Centrum
3590 Diepenbeek
Belgium
tomasz.burzykowski@luc.ac.be

Geert Molenberghs
Center for Statistics
Limburgs Universitair Centrum
3590 Diepenbeek
Belgium
geert.molenberghs@luc.ac.be

Marc Buyse
International Drug Development Institute
1050 Brussels
Belgium
marc.buyse@iddi.com

Library of Congress Cataloging-in-Publication Data
The evaluation of surrogate endpoints / [edited by] Tomasz Burzykowski, Geert Molenberghs, Marc Buyse.
p. cm. — (Statistics for biology and health)
Includes bibliographical references and index.

1. Clinical trials. 2. Drugs—Testing. I. Molenberghs, Geert. II. Buyse, Marc E. III. Burzykowski, Tomasz. IV. Series.
R853.C55E935 2005
610′.72′4—dc22

ISBN 978-1-4419-1906-9 e-ISBN 978-0-387-27080-7

Softcover reprint of the hardcover 1st edition 2005

9 8 7 6 5 4 3 2 1

springeronline.com

Bożenie i Mikołajowi

Voor Conny, An en Jasper

A Monique, Céline et Mathieu

Preface

More than ever is there a strong drive to search for and evaluate potential surrogate markers and surrogate endpoints for randomized clinical trials. A successful surrogate endpoint is able to reduce follow-up trial time and/or to reduce the number of patients needed to establish a certain treatment effect. From a statistical perspective, Prentice's framework (1989), amplified by Freedman, Graubard, and Schatzkin (1992), was instrumental to start the debate as to how statistical validation or, more modestly formulated, statistical evaluation, of a potential surrogate endpoint could be undertaken. Much debate ensued, also in the light of the historic "accidents" with surrogates not carefully evaluated, and it is fair to say the surrogate marker debate has since been laden with a certain amount of skepticism.

Connected to his involvement in clinical trial methodology, Marc Buyse has always had a strong interest in the surrogate marker validation debate. In April 1994, Marc and Geert met at a *Drug Information Association* meeting in Bruges, at the time where Marc was thinking about the *relative effect* as a measure to supplement the *proportion explained.* One thing led to another and soon an LUC-based research team was formed, headed by the three of us, that, over the years, has encompassed fifteen members from various research institutes. The team has investigated a number of aspects of surrogate marker validation. A move was soon made from the so-called single-trial framework to a meta-analytic or hierarchical one, in line with ideas developed by Michael Hughes and Michael Daniels, and also by Mitch Gail and his co-workers. A lot of subsequent activity focused on finding appropriate hierarchical statistical models for various types of surrogate and true outcomes. Formulating such models is not always straightforward, let alone fitting them, and consequently the need arose to explore simplified modeling and fitting strategies, and the Bayesian framework was considered as a potential alternative. Also, as different models incorporate different association parameters, the need arose to try and unify the surrogate marker evaluation measures.

While doing this, an eye had to be kept on several important application areas, such as oncology, HIV, and mental health. Even though there is a common basis for surrogate marker validation across these areas, a good number of aspects are area specific. For example, it is fair to say that the speed of the developments in HIV is tremendous, compared to other therapeutic areas. In mental health, the delineation between true and surrogate endpoints is not as clear as it would be in other areas. Finally, because surrogate marker evaluation takes place, to a large extent, in the development of medicinal product arena, the perspectives of the pharmaceutical industry and the regulatory authorities have to be taken into account in a proper fashion.

This text hopes to give an accessible synthetic account of the developments just sketched, giving proper credit to historical developments, providing a balance between statistical considerations of a modeling and computation nature, scientific considerations coming from the various therapeutic areas, and the positions taken by the pharmaceutical industry and the regulatory authorities. As in any scientific debate, different people approach surrogate marker evaluation with various degrees of comfort. We hope the current text does proper justice to all views, not just the editors' views.

Although a variety of authors have contributed to this book, we have chosen a strongly edited form to achieve a smooth flow. As far as possible, a common set of notations has been used by all authors. Ample cross-references between chapters are provided. The book should be suitable either to read a selected number of chapters or the integral text.

Tomasz Burzykowski (LUC, Diepenbeek)

Geert Molenberghs (LUC, Diepenbeek)

Marc Buyse (IDDI, Brussels, and LUC, Diepenbeek)

Acknowledgments

Over the years, our research team has published several papers on the subject, has communicated at conferences and has taught short courses and held workshops in a wide variety of locations worldwide. This has been done for various audiences, including statistical and biopharmaceutical audiences. We are sure that not only preparing for the various communications, but also the numerous discussions have had a beneficial impact on this book.

Aloka Chakravarty, author of Chapter 3, would like to express appreciation for the support and encouragement received from Drs. R.T. O'Neill, C. Anello, M.F. Huque, G.Y.H. Chi, S. Machado, H.M. Hung, G. Chen, G. Soon, R. Sridhara, and P.L. Yang.

Ross L. Prentice, author of Chapter 19, expresses gratitude for support from National Institutes of Health grant CA53996.

Michael D. Hughes, author of Chapter 17, gratefully acknowledges support from National Institutes of Health grants AI24643, AI38855, and AI41110.

Tomasz Burzykowski and Geert Molenberghs gratefully acknowledge support from Belgian IUAP/PAI network "Statistical Techniques and Modeling for Complex Substantive Questions with Complex Data."

Tomasz, Geert, and Marc

Diepenbeek, September 2004

Chapter Authors

Ariel Alonso Abad
Limburgs Universitair Centrum, Diepenbeek, Belgium

Tomasz Burzykowski
Limburgs Universitair Centrum, Diepenbeek, Belgium

Marc Buyse
International Drug Development Institute, Brussels, Belgium
Limburgs Universitair Centrum, Diepenbeek, Belgium

Aloka Chakravarty
Food and Drug Administration, Rockville, MD, U.S.A.

José Cortiñas Abrahantes
Limburgs Universitair Centrum, Diepenbeek, Belgium

Laurence Freedman
Bar-Ilan University, Ramat Gan, Israel

Mitch Gail
National Cancer Institute, National Institutes of Health, Bethesda, MD, U.S.A.

Helena Geys
Limburgs Universitair Centrum, Diepenbeek, Belgium

Michael D. Hughes
Harvard School of Public Health, Boston, MA, U.S.A.

Annouschka Laenen
Limburgs Universitair Centrum, Diepenbeek, Belgium

Geert Molenberghs
Limburgs Universitair Centrum, Diepenbeek, Belgium

Ross L. Prentice
University of Washington, Seattle, WA, U.S.A.

Didier Renard
Eli Lilly & Company, Mont Saint Guibert, Belgium

Arthur Schatzkin
National Cancer Institute, National Institutes of Health, Bethesda, MD, U.S.A.

Ziv Shkedy
Limburgs Universitair Centrum, Diepenbeek, Belgium

Franz Torres Barbosa
Limburgs Universitair Centrum, Diepenbeek, Belgium

Tony Vangeneugden
Tibotec, Mechelen, Belgium

Contents

1

Introduction

Geert Molenberghs, Marc Buyse, and Tomasz Burzykowski

1.1 The Concept of a Surrogate Endpoint

One of the most important factors influencing the duration and complexity of the process of developing new treatments is the choice of the endpoint, which will be used to assess the efficacy of the treatment. Two main criteria to select the endpoint are its sensitivity to detect treatment effects and its clinical relevance to goals of the study (Fleming 1996). The relevance depends on, for example, whether evidence for biological activity of a drug is sought (as in Phase II trials) or whether a definitive evaluation of clinical benefit to patients has to be made (as in Phase III trials). For instance, in life-threatening diseases, such as cardiovascular diseases or cancer, the endpoint relevant for definitive evaluation of a treatment typically is survival.

It often appears, however, that the most sensitive and relevant clinical endpoint, which will be called the "true" endpoint throughout this text, might be difficult to use in a clinical trial. This can happen if the measurement of the true endpoint:

- is costly (for example, to diagnose "cachexia," a condition associated with malnutrition and involving loss of muscle and fat tissue, expensive equipment measuring content of nitrogen, potassium, and water in patient's body is required);
- is difficult (for example, involving compound measures such as typically is the case in quality of life or pain assessment);
- requires a long follow-up time (for example, survival in early-stage cancers);
- requires a large sample size due to a low incidence of the event (for

example, short-term mortality in patients with suspected acute myocardial infarction).

In such cases, use of the true endpoint increases the complexity and/or the duration of research. To overcome these problems, a seemingly attractive solution is to replace the true endpoint by another one, which is measured earlier, more conveniently, or more frequently. Such "replacement" endpoints are termed "surrogate" endpoints (Ellenberg and Hamilton 1989).

Note that several related but somewhat distinct terms are in use, such as surrogate endpoint, surrogate marker, or biomarker. *Surrogate endpoint* has the connotation of replacement of the true endpoint in a clinical study by another one. A *marker* on the other hand is an outcome, a measurement, or a set of measurements that is indicative for a variable or a general concept. For example, a number of blood, urine, and other measurements can be used to detect environmental stress in living organisms. Although there are common aspects in the evaluation of surrogate endpoints and markers, the contexts are different. In this book, we will largely focus on surrogate endpoints, with a lot of emphasis on randomized clinical trials.

1.2 Why Is There Reservation Toward the Use of Surrogate Endpoints?

Because of the possible benefits for the duration of a clinical trial, surrogate endpoints have been used in medical research for a long time (Ellenberg and Hamilton 1989, Fleming and DeMets 1996). Table 1.1 presents several examples. The use of the surrogate endpoints presented in Table 1.1 was based on an established *association* between them on the one hand and the corresponding true endpoints on the other hand. However, the mere existence of an association between a candidate surrogate endpoint and the true endpoint is not sufficient for using the former as a surrogate. As Fleming and DeMets (1996) put it, "a correlate does not make a surrogate." What is required is that the effect of the treatment on the surrogate endpoint reliably predicts the effect on the true endpoint. Unfortunately, partly due to the lack of appropriate methodology, this condition was not checked in the early attempts to use surrogates. Consequently, for most of the surrogates mentioned in Table 1.1, it was found that their use, at least in some applications, led to erroneous, or even harmful, conclusions. A review of several such examples is given by Fleming and DeMets (1996). Probably the best known case is the approval by the Food and Drug Administration (FDA) in the United States of the use of three drugs: encainide, flecainide, and moricizine. The drugs were approved based on the fact that

TABLE 1.1. *Examples of surrogate endpoints used in medical research.*

Disease	Endpoints	
	Surrogate	True
Early stage cancer	Time to progression	Survival time
Advanced cancer	Tumor response	Survival time
Osteoporosis	Bone mineral density	Bone fracture
Ophthalmology (glaucoma)	Intraocular pressure	Long-term visual acuity
Chronic granulomatous disease	Superoxide production	Serious infection
	Ability to kill bacteria	Serious infection
Cardiovascular disease	Ejection fraction	Myocardial infarction
	Blood pressure	Stroke, survival time
	Arrythmias	Survival time
HIV infection	CD4 counts; viral load	Development of AIDS, survival time

they were shown to effectively suppress arrythmias. It was believed that, because arrythmia is associated with an almost fourfold increase in the rate of cardiac-complication-related death, the drugs would reduce the death rate. However, a clinical trial conducted after the drugs had been approved by the FDA and introduced into clinical practice showed that in fact the death rate among patients treated with encainide and flecainide was more than twice the one among patients treated with placebo (The Cardiac Arrhythmia Suppression Trial (CAST) Investigators 1989). An increase of the risk was also detected for moricizine.

This and other examples of unsuccessful replacement of true endpoints led to the scepticism about usefulness of surrogate endpoints. Consequently, negative opinions about the use of surrogates in the evaluation of treatment efficacy have been voiced (Fleming 1996, Fleming and DeMets 1996, DeGruttola *et al.* 1997).

1.3 Why the Use of Surrogate Endpoints Is Still Being Considered?

It will be clear from the previous section that the very mention of surrogate endpoints has always been very controversial. However, not all early applications were failures. For example, the dramatic surge of the AIDS epidemic, the impressive therapeutic results obtained early on with zidovudine, and the pressure for an accelerated evaluation of new therapies have all led to, first, the use of CD4 blood count and then, with the advent of highly active antiretroviral therapy (HAART), viral load as endpoints that replaced time to clinical events and overall survival (DeGruttola *et al.*

1995), in spite of some concerns about their limitations as surrogates for clinically relevant endpoints (Lagakos and Hoth 1992).

Generally, before a new drug can be accepted for the use in clinical practice, its efficacy and safety needs to be rigorously assessed in a series of clinical trials. This process of testing a new therapy can (and, in fact, does) take many years. At the same time, the number of candidate biomarkers and ultimately the number of surrogate endpoints based upon them is increasing dramatically. Indeed, an increasing number of new drugs have a well-defined mechanism of action at the molecular level, allowing drug developers to measure the effect of these drugs on the relevant biomarkers (Ferentz 2002). There is also increasing public pressure for new, promising drugs to be approved for marketing as rapidly as possible, and such approval will have to be based on biomarkers rather than on some long-term clinical endpoint (Lesko and Atkinson 2001). The pressure can become especially high in a situation where rapidly increasing incidence of a disease can become a serious threat to public health. As an illustration of this trend toward early decision-making, recently proposed clinical trial designs use treatment effects on a surrogate endpoint to screen for treatments that show insufficient promise to have a sizeable impact on survival (Royston, Parmar, and Qian 2003). Last but not least, if the approval process is shortened, there will be a corresponding need for earlier detection of safety signals that could point to toxic problems with new drugs. It is a safe bet, therefore, that the evaluation of tomorrow's drugs will be based primarily on biomarkers, rather than on the longer-term, harder clinical endpoints that have dominated the development of new drugs until now.

In conclusion, because surrogate endpoints can shorten the duration of the process, their use does constitute an attractive option. Thus, although many would like to avoid surrogate endpoints altogether, sometimes surrogates will be the only reasonable alternative, especially when the true endpoint is rare and/or distant in time.

Another reason to shorten the duration of the process of testing new therapies may be related to new discoveries in medicine and biology, which create a possibility for development of many potentially effective treatments for a particular disease. In such a situation, a need to cope with a large number of new promising treatments that should be quickly evaluated with respect to their efficacy might appear. As a matter of fact, this can already be observed happening in oncology, as the increased knowledge about the genetic mechanisms operating in cancer cells led to the proposal of qualitatively new approaches to treat cancer. An example is found in the use of a genetically modified virus that selectively attacks p53-deficient cells, sparing normal cells (Heise *et al.* 1997). It is known that for several cancers, mutations of the p53 gene are quite common. For instance, in head and neck tumors they are detected in 45-70% of the cases (Khuri *et al.* 2000), whereas in pancreatic tumors, this is about 60% of the cases (Barton *et al.* 1991). Consequently, in these cancers the injection of the virus in the tumor might result in the eradication of the cancer cells without affecting normal cells. In fact, clinical trials investigating the efficacy of such a treatment have already been started, showing promising results (Von Hoff *et al.* 1998, Khuri *et al.* 2000, Lamont *et al.* 2000, Nemunaitis *et al.* 2001). With the results of the human genome mapping now available (International Human Genome Sequencing Consortium 2001, Venter *et al.* 2001), development of even a larger spectrum of treatments aimed at disease mechanisms present at the gene level might be expected.

From a practical point of view, shortening the duration of a clinical trial also limits possible problems with non-compliance and missing data, which are more likely in longer studies, and therefore increases effectiveness and reliability of the research.

Finally, an important area of potential application of surrogate endpoints is the assessment of safety of new treatments. Duration and sample size of clinical trials aimed at development of new drugs are usually insufficient to detect rare or late adverse effects of the treatment (Dunn and Mann 1999, Jones 2001). The use of surrogate endpoints (for toxicity-related clinical endpoints) might allow one to obtain information about such effects even during the clinical testing phase.

All of these reasons apply to the current state of research on novel treatments. Despite the failed past attempts, it is therefore difficult to abandon the idea of using surrogate endpoints altogether.

1.4 Validation of Surrogate Endpoints

Nevertheless, the failed past attempts to use surrogate endpoints do make it clear that, before deciding on the use of a candidate surrogate endpoint, it is of the utmost importance to investigate its validity. (The term validity is used here in a broad sense, and not in the narrow, well-defined psychometric sense, even though there is a relationship between both, see also Chapter 16.) Consequently, formal methods allowing for validation are required. Such methods have become the subject of intensive research over the past decades. In this volume, the results of this research, as well as some novel concepts and techniques, will be presented.

2

Setting the Scene

Geert Molenberghs, Marc Buyse, and Tomasz Burzykowski

2.1 Historical Perspective

Often, the most clinically relevant endpoint, that is, the "true" endpoint, is difficult to use in a clinical trial. In cancer trials, for instance, survival is still regarded as the ultimate endpoint of interest, but it may lack sensitivity to true therapeutic advances, it may be confounded by competing risks and second-line treatments, and it is observed late, which results in long delays before new drugs can be approved. In such cases, a seemingly attractive solution is to replace the true endpoint by another one, which might be measured earlier, more conveniently, or more frequently. As stated in Chapter 1, such "replacement" endpoints are termed "surrogate" endpoints.

Before a surrogate can replace a true endpoint, it should be *validated* or *evaluated*. Merely establishing a correlation between both endpoints is not sufficient (Baker and Kramer 2003). Several formal methods for this purpose have already been proposed (Prentice 1989, Freedman, Graubard, and Schatzkin 1992, Daniels and Hughes 1997, Buyse and Molenberghs 1998, Buyse *et al.* 2000a, Gail *et al.* 2000). With the statistical methods available, it ought to be possible to conduct a formal investigation on the quality of various endpoints used as surrogates in clinical practice. Such an investigation can shed light on the feasibility of the use of these endpoints and guide the regulatory agencies, for example, in the choice of the endpoints that can be used for accelerated approval of investigational drugs. Of course, as stated earlier, a quantitative evaluation is important but is by no means the only component in the decision process leading to the replacement of the true endpoint by the surrogate one. Several parties are involved, including the regulatory agencies (Section 2.2) and the industry developing a medicinal product.

2.2 A Regulatory Agencies Perspective

The need to develop new drugs and treatments as quickly as possible has become acute nowadays. Regulatory agencies from around the globe, in particular in the United States, in Europe, and in Japan, have reacted to this challenge through various provisions and policies.

In the United States, there are mechanisms available for accelerated approval based on surrogate endpoints, in order to reduce the time to review an application for indications with no known effective therapy and for providing access to patients for unapproved drugs. Accelerated approval (sometimes referred to as "conditional approval" or "Subpart H") refers to an acceleration of the overall development plan by allowing submission of an application, and if approved, marketing of a drug on the basis of surrogate endpoints while further studies demonstrating direct patient benefit are underway. Accelerated approval is limited to diseases where no effective therapies exist and is based on a surrogate endpoint likely to predict clinical benefit.

The recent recommendation of the Food and Drug Administration (FDA) for accelerated approval of investigational cancer treatments states that

> "FDA believes that for many cancer therapies it is appropriate to utilize objective evidence of tumor shrinkage as a basis for approval, allowing additional evidence of increased survival and/or improved quality of life associated with that therapy to be demonstrated later"

(Food and Drug Administration 1996). This marks a departure from the traditional requirements for new cancer treatments to show survival or disease-free survival benefits prior to being granted market approval (Fleming *et al.* 1994, Cocchetto and Jones 1998). If the achievement of a complete remission has indeed a major impact on prognosis in hematological malignancies (Armitage 1993, The International Non-Hodgkin's Lymphoma Prognostic Factors Project 1993, Kantarjian *et al.* 1995), the relationship between tumor response and survival duration is far less clear in solid tumors, even though the shrinkage of metastatic measurable masses has long been the cornerstone of the development of cytotoxic therapies (Oye and Shapiro 1984). In the United States, response rate has been used as a surrogate for patient benefit for accelerated approval and as a component of full approval for some hormonal and biological products. Among them are docetaxel for second-line metastatic breast cancer, irinotecan for second-line metastatic colorectal cancer, capecitabine for refractory metastatic breast cancer, liposomal cytarabine for lymphomatous meningitis, and temozolomide for second-line anaplastic astrocytoma. Two drugs received accelerated approval for supplemental indications: liposomal doxorubicin for refractory ovarian cancer and celecoxib for polyp reduction in familial adenomatous polyposis.

In the European Union, there is a different "accelerated approval" mechanism. The European legislation allows for granting a marketing authorization under "exceptional circumstances" where comprehensive data cannot be provided at the time of submission (e.g., because of the rarity of the disease) and provided that the applicant agrees to a further program of studies that will be the basis for post-authorizations review of the benefit/risk profile of the drug. Although this primarily refers to situations where randomized clinical trials are lacking, it applies equally well to absence of data on a particular endpoint. According to the European Agency for the Evaluation of Medicinal Products (EMEA) guideline for the evaluation of anticancer agents, the choice of endpoints should be guided by the clinical relevance of the endpoint and should take into account methodological considerations. Possible endpoints for phase III trials in oncology include progression-free survival, overall survival, response rate (and duration), and symptom control/quality of life. The guideline also states that if objective response rate is used as the primary endpoint, compelling justifications are needed and normally additional supportive evidence of efficacy in terms of, for example, symptom control is necessary (Committee for Proprietary Medicinal Products 2001). Thus, where justified, the use of surrogate endpoints in oncology is possible although it may require confirmation of efficacy in the post-authorization phase, e.g., by confirming an effect on the true endpoint or in confirmatory trials. The initial EMEA experience with antineoplastic and endocrine therapy agents has shown that in the majority of cases, approval was indeed obtained based on a surrogate endpoint such as objective response rate. This was the case, e.g., for docetaxel in second-line (monotherapy) metastatic breast cancer, liposomal doxorubicin in AIDS-Kaposi sarcoma, and paclitaxel in second-line AIDS-Kaposi sarcoma. Topotecan was approved in second-line metastatic ovarian cancer based on response rate and progression-free survival, and temozolomide was approved in recurrent glioblastoma and recurrent anaplastic astrocytoma based on progression-free survival. Thus, the European system is coming close to an accelerated approval system like in the United States perhaps with more flexibility.

The situation is somewhat different in Japan. Objective response rate has played there the central role for oncology drug approvals where cytotoxic drugs can be approved based on tumor shrinkage in phase II studies, as defined in the guideline issued in 1991. The initial approval of a drug is considered to be conditional on a subsequent re-examination of the safety and efficacy of the drug at something like four to ten years after marketing authorization. At least two independent randomized trials with survival as an endpoint need to be conducted in a post-marketing setting and results need to be made available at the time of re-examination.

At the international level, the International Conference on Harmonization (ICH) Guidelines on Statistical Principles for Clinical Trials state that

> "In practice, the strength of the evidence for surrogacy depends upon (i) the biological plausibility of the relationship, (ii) the demonstration in epidemiological studies of the prognostic value of the surrogate for the clinical outcome and (iii) evidence from clinical trials that treatment effects on the surrogate correspond to effects on the clinical outcome"

(ICH Guidelines 1998). As such, it is close in spirit to the procedures proposed by the U.S., European, and Japanese regulatory authorities.

A detailed regulatory perspective is provided in Chapter 3.

2.3 Main Issues

Taking into account the arguments developed in the Introduction and earlier in this chapter, it is difficult to abandon the idea of using surrogate endpoints altogether, in spite of the failed attempts, described in the Introduction. However, it has also been stated, and this is in line with the regulatory authorities' policies, that there is a need for formal evaluation as an important component of the decision whether or not a surrogate endpoint can be used. Prentice (1989) formulated a definition of surrogate endpoints, as well as operational criteria for validating a surrogate endpoint. Freedman, Graubard, and Schatzkin (1992) introduced the concept of *proportion explained*, which was meant to indicate the proportion of the treatment effect mediated by the surrogate. Buyse and Molenberghs (1998) decomposed the proportion explained further into the *relative effect* and *adjusted association*, and argued in favor of using these quantities instead. The aforementioned proposals, reviewed in Chapter 5, were formulated under the assumption that the validation of a surrogate is based on data from a single randomized clinical trial.

This leads to problems with untestable assumptions and too low statistical power. To overcome these problems, the combination of information from several groups of patients (multi-center trials or meta-analyses) was suggested by Albert *et al.* (1998). It was subsequently implemented by Daniels

TABLE 2.1. *Examples of possible surrogate endpoints in various diseases (Abbreviations: AIDS = acquired immune deficiency syndrome; ARMD = age-related macular degeneration; HIV = human immunodeficiency virus).*

Disease	Surrogate endpoint	Type	Final endpoint	Type
Resectable solid tumor	Time to recurrence	Censored	Survival	Censored
Advanced cancer	Tumor response	Binary	Time to progression	Censored
Osteoporosis	Bone mineral density	Longitudinal	Fracture	Binary
Cardiovascular disease	Ejection fraction	Continuous	Myocardial infraction	Binary
Hypertension	Blood pressure	Longitudinal	Coronary heart disease	Binary
Arrhythmia	Arrhythmic episodes	Longitudinal	Survival	Censored
ARMD	6-month visual acuity	Continuous	24-month visual acuity	Continuous
Glaucoma	Intraoccular pressure	Continuous	Vision loss	Censored
Depression	Biomarkers	Multivariate	Depression scale	Continuous
HIV infection	CD4 counts + viral load	Multivariate	Progression to AIDS	Censored

and Hughes (1997), Buyse *et al.* (2000a) and Gail *et al.* (2000), among others. The meta-analytic framework is introduced in Chapter 7.

Statistically speaking, the surrogate endpoint and the clinical endpoint are realizations of random variables. As will be clear from the formalisms developed in Chapter 7, interest needs to focus on the joint distribution of these variables. The easiest situation is where both are Gaussian random variables. This is, however, seldom the case, because the surrogate endpoint and/or the clinical endpoint are often realizations of non-Gaussian random variables. Table 2.1 shows a number of settings that can occur in practice. Thus, grouped by type of endpoint, one can encounter:

- Binary (dichotomous): biomarker value below or above a certain threshold (e.g., CD4+ counts over 500/mm3) or clinical "success" (e.g., tumor shrinkage).
- Categorical (polychotomous): biomarker value falling in successive, ordered classes (e.g., cholesterol levels <200 mg/dl, 200–299 mg/dl, 300+ mg/dl) or clinical response (e.g., complete response, partial response, stable disease, progressive disease).
- Continuous (Gaussian): biomarker (e.g., log-PSA level) or clinical measurement (e.g., diastolic blood pressure).

- Censored continuous: time to biomarker below or above a certain threshold (e.g., time to undetectable viral load) or time to clinical event (e.g., time to cardiovascular death).
- Longitudinal or repeated measures: biomarker (e.g., CD4+ counts over time) or clinical outcome (e.g., blood pressure over time).
- Multivariate longitudinal: several biomarkers (e.g., CD4+ and viral load over time) or several clinical measurements (e.g., dimensions of quality of life over time).

The models used to validate a surrogate for a clinical endpoint will depend on the type of variables observed in the problem at hand. Chapters following Chapter 7 are dedicated to a variety of settings.

3

Regulatory Aspects in Using Surrogate Markers in Clinical Trials

Aloka Chakravarty

3.1 Introduction and Motivation

Surrogate marker plays an important role in the regulatory decision processes in drug approval. The possibility of reduced sample size or trial duration when a distal clinical endpoint is replaced by a more proximal one hold real benefit in terms of reaching the intended patient population faster, cheaper, and safer as well as a better characterization of the efficacy profile. In situations where endpoint measurements have competing risks or are invasive in nature, certain latitude in measurement error can be accepted by deliberately choosing an alternate endpoint in compensation for a better quality of life or for ease of measurement.

3.1.1 Definitions and Their Regulatory Ramifications

Over the years, many authors have given various definitions for a surrogate marker. Some of the operational ramifications of these definitions will be examined in their relationship to drug development.

Wittes, Lakatos, and Probstfield (1989) defined surrogate endpoint simply as "an endpoint measured in lieu of some so-called 'true' endpoint." While it provides the core, this definition does not provide any operational motivation. Ellenberg and Hamilton (1989) provides this basis by stating: "investigators use surrogate endpoints when the endpoint of interest is too difficult and/or expensive to measure routinely and when they can define some other, more readily measurable endpoint, which is sufficiently well correlated with the first to justify its use as a substitute." This paved the way to a statistical definition of a surrogate endpoint by Prentice (1989):

"a response variable for which a test of null hypothesis of no relationship to the treatment groups under comparison is also a valid test of the corresponding null hypothesis based on the true endpoint." This definition, also known as the Prentice Criteria, is often very hard to verify in real-life clinical trials. An operating definition given by Temple (1999) states: "a laboratory or physical sign that is used in therapeutic trials as a substitute for a clinically meaningful endpoint that is a direct measure of how a patient feels, functions, or survives and that is expected to predict the effect of the therapy." This definition has been used as the operational definition of surrogate endpoints in a regulatory setting.

International Conference on Harmonization (ICH) document E8 states: "a validated surrogate endpoint is an endpoint which allows prediction of a clinically important outcome but in itself does not measure a clinical benefit. When appropriate, surrogate outcomes may be used as primary endpoints." It further states that the "methods used to make the measurements of the endpoints, both subjective and objective, should meet accepted standards for accuracy, precision, reproducibility, reliability, validity and responsiveness (sensitivity to change over time)," thus providing a valid premise to use it in multinational trials.

A well-validated surrogate will predict the clinical benefit of an intervention both quantitatively and qualitatively with consistent results in several settings. According to Temple (1999), a surrogate endpoint is a laboratory measurement or physical sign used in therapeutic trials as a substitute for a clinically meaningful endpoint that is expected to predict the effect of the therapy. The U.S. Food and Drug Administration (FDA) is able to rely on validated surrogates for accelerated approval of drugs that provide meaningful benefit over existing therapies for serious or life-threatening illnesses (e.g., acquired immunodeficiency syndrome). In these cases, the surrogates should be reasonably likely to predict clinical benefit based on epidemiological, therapeutic, pathophysiologic, or other scientific evidence. However, in general, trials examining surrogate endpoints, even where the endpoint is well correlated with a clinical outcome, surrogates will be unable to evaluate clinically relevant effects of the drug not related to the surrogate, whether these are beneficial or adverse.

3.1.2 Support for Surrogates

Next, we examine what are the motivations for using a surrogate endpoint. The motivation to use a surrogate can be judged by its biological plausibility, its expected success in clinical trials, and its risk-benefit ratio or public health considerations. We summarize these issues in Table 3.1.

TABLE 3.1. *Support for surrogates.*

Factor	Favors surrogates	Does not favor surrogates
Biological plausibility	Epidemiological evidence extensive and consistent	Inconsistent epidemiology
	Quantitative epidemiological relationship	No quantitative epidemiological relationship
	Credible animal model shows drug response	No animal model
	Well-understood disease pathogenesis	Pathogenesis not clear
	Drug mechanism of action well-understood	Novel actions not previously studied
	Surrogate relatively late in the biological path	Surrogate remote from clinical outcome
Success in clinical trials	Effect of surrogate has predicted outcome with other drugs of same pharmacological class	A negative outcome without clear explanation
	Effect on surrogate had predicted outcome in several classes	Inconsistent results across classes
Risk-benefit, public health considerations	Serious or life-threatening illness and no alternate therapy	Disease not life-threatening and alternate therapy with different pharmacological action known to affect outcome
	Large safety database	Little known about safety
	Short term use	Long-term use
	Difficulty in studying clinical endpoint (rare, delayed)	Easy to study clinical endpoint
		Long-delayed, small effect in healthy people

Thus, a surrogate to be useful has to have unequivocal biological plausibility, be expected to perform consistently in a clinical trial, and possess superior public health benefits.

3.1.3 *Criteria for Surrogate Markers To Be Used in Drug Development*

In epidemiological studies, a useful surrogate marker is a causal factor for the disease of interest, not merely a correlated factor. As Fleming (1996) stated, "a correlate does not a surrogate make." The higher the level of explanatory evidence the surrogate is able to carry, the better it is to explain the disease process. Table 3.2 summarizes the relationships surrogate endpoints (SEP) can have with the "true" clinical endpoints (CE).

Then, *sensitivity* (SE) of the surrogate endpoint for the clinical endpoint

TABLE 3.2. *Relationship of surrogate endpoints with the clinical endpoints.*

	T good	T poor	Total
S good	a	b	$a+b$
S poor	c	d	$c+d$
Total	$a+c$	$b+d$	N

a = number of patients where both S and T provide good disease characterization.
b = number of patients where S is good but T provide poor disease characterization.
c = number of patients where S is poor but T provide good disease characterization.
d = number of patients where both S and T provide poor disease characterization.

is defined by

$$SE = \frac{a}{a+c}. \tag{3.1}$$

Specificity (SP) of the surrogate endpoint for the clinical endpoint is defined by

$$SP = \frac{d}{b+d}. \tag{3.2}$$

For the surrogate to be useful, both sensitivity and specificity have to be numerically close to 1.

The *relative risk* (RR) is defined as

$$RR = \frac{a(c+d)}{c(a+b)} \tag{3.3}$$

and the *attributable proportion* (AP) as

$$AP = \frac{SE}{1 - \frac{1}{RR}}. \tag{3.4}$$

For a surrogate marker to be a successful one, AP has to be numerically close to 1. Schatzkin, Freedman, and colleagues proposed strategies for determining whether a biomarker is a valid surrogate for a disease of interest, for instance whether human papillomavirus infection is a valid surrogate for cervival dysplasia. The attributable proportion is a useful measure of association between the surrogate endpoint and the clinical endpoint, but establishing the causality of the relationship between the surrogate and the clinical endpoint require data from either observational studies or, preferably, intervention studies. Intervention studies would focus on the triplet intervention / biomarker / disease in much the same way as a clinical trial would focus on the triplet treatment / surrogate endpoint / clinical endpoint.

3.1.4 Surrogate Markers and Biomarkers

Definitions and Differences

Biological marker or biomarker, as more commonly known, refers to a variety of physiologic, pathologic, or anatomic measurements that are thought to relate to some aspect of normal or pathological biologic processes (Temple 1995, Lesko and Atkinson 2001). These biomarkers include measurements that suggest the etiology of, the susceptibility to, or the progress of disease; measurements related to the mechanism of response to treatments; and actual clinical responses to therapeutic interventions. Biomarkers differ in their closeness to the intended therapeutic response or clinical benefit endpoints, classified as follows:

1. biomarkers thought to be valid surrogates for clinical benefit (e.g., blood pressure, cholesterol, viral load);
2. biomarkers thought to reflect the pathologic process and be at least candidate surrogates (e.g., brain appearance in Alzheimer's disease, brain infarct size, various radiographic/isotopic function tests);
3. biomarkers reflecting drug action but of uncertain relation to clinical outcome (e.g., inhibition of ADP-dependent platelet aggregation, ACE inhibition);
4. biomarkers that are still more remote from the clinical benefit endpoint (e.g., degree of binding to a receptor or inhibition of an agonist).

From a regulatory perspective, a biomarker is not considered an acceptable surrogate endpoint for a determination of efficacy of a new drug unless it has been empirically shown to function, as a valid indicator of clinical benefit (i.e., a valid surrogate). Theoretical justification alone does not meet the evidentiary standards for market access. Many biomarkers will never undergo the rigorous statistical evaluation that would establish their value as a surrogate endpoint to determine efficacy or safety, but they can still have use in earlier drug development process. Changes in biomarkers typically exhibit a time course that is different from changes in clinical endpoints and often are more directly related to the time course of plasma drug concentrations, possibly with a measurable delay. For this reason, exposure-response relationships based on biomarkers may help establish the dose range for clinical trials intended to establish efficacy that will then be studied more formally, indicate how soon dose titration should occur, examine potential pharmaco-dynamic interactions, and give insight into potential adverse effects.

TABLE 3.3. *Biomarkers as surrogate endpoints – possible relationships.*

Type of relationship	Value of biomarker	Example
Unreliable interaction between biomarker and the treatment intervention	Biomarker is of no value as a surrogate endpoint	Prostate-specific antigen (PSA) is a useful biomarker for prostate cancer detection but unreliable as an indicator of treatment response
The full effect of the intervention is observed through the biomarker assessment	Biomarker is an ideal surrogate endpoint	None known at present
Intervention affects the endpoint and the biomarker independently; only a proportion of the treatment effect is captured by the surrogate endpoint	Biomarker has value as a surrogate endpoint but explains only a part of the treatment effect	Most established surrogate endpoints (e.g., development of opportunistic infections with HIV anti-viral and mortality)
Intervention affects favorably on the biomarker but unfavorably on the well-state and disease	Biomarker is of little practical use as a surrogate endpoint but may have utility in exploratory studies	Suppression of ventricular ectopy as a biomarker of fatal arrhythmia following myocardial infarctions (CAST trial)

Relationship Between Biomarkers and Surrogate Markers

While all surrogate markers are biomarkers, it is likely that only a few single biomarkers will qualify as surrogate endpoints in therapeutic intervention trials, or as surrogate markers in natural history or epidemiological studies. For ease of reference, we use the terms surrogate "markers" and surrogate "endpoints" interchangeably, although we acknowledge that some surrogate endpoints (such as patient self-assessment scales) are not biomarkers. For the concept of a surrogate endpoint to be useful, one must specify the clinical endpoint, class of intervention, and population in which the substitution of the biomarker for a clinical endpoint is considered reasonable. Table 3.3 summarizes the various possible relationships that can exist between a surrogate marker and a biomarker.

Figure 3.1 gives a schematic description of the conceptual model for surrogate endpoints and biomarkers.

It shows that only a small proportion of biomarkers will be useful to be considered as a surrogate endpoint, which will then have to be subjected to a rigorous set of risk-benefit considerations to eventually arrive as an instrument of global intervention assessment.

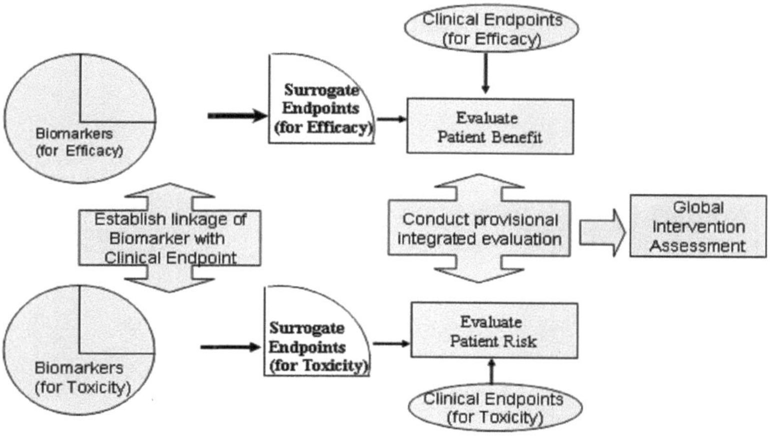

FIGURE 3.1. *A conceptual model between surrogate endpoints and biomarkers.*

3.2 Surrogate Markers in Regulatory Setting

The U.S. Food and Drug Administration has supported the use of surrogate markers when clinically appropriate to bring therapeutic agents through the approval process faster and in a more efficient way. If a surrogate endpoint can be measured more easily or efficiently or with higher precision, then it translates into faster treatment access for the patients. If a surrogate endpoint is less affected by other treatment modalities, then the precision of the trial can also be expected to increase. The FDA has responded to faster approval of promising through various specific regulatory mechanisms, which we will discuss now.

3.2.1 Fast Track Program – A Program for Accelerated Approval

Fast Track programs at the U.S. Food and Drug Administration are designed to facilitate the development and expedite the review of new drugs that meet two criteria: (1) are intended to treat serious or life-threatening conditions and (2) demonstrate the potential to address unmet medical needs for the condition. Whether a condition is serious or not is a matter of judgment, but is generally based on its impact on such factors such as survival, day-to-day functioning, or the likelihood that the disease if left untreated would progress from a less severe condition to a more serious one. When focusing on morbidity, consideration is given to its persistence or recurrence if it is not irreversible (57 Federal Register 13234 dated April 15, 1992). Whether a therapeutic agent is intended to treat a serious condition

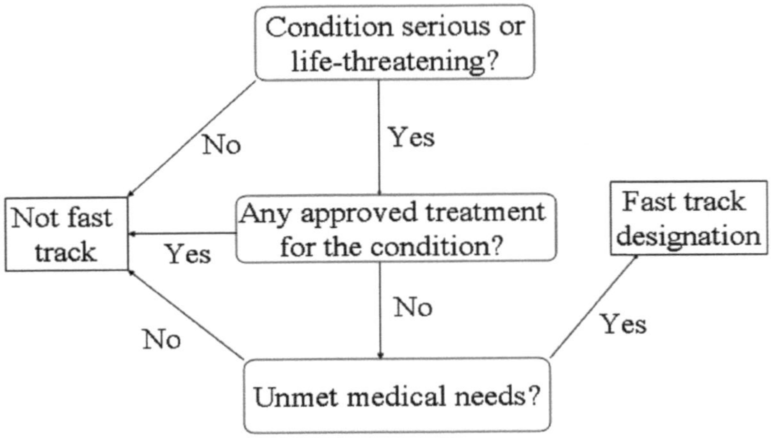

FIGURE 3.2. *Schema to determine Fast Track designation of a product.*

is determined by the following criteria: (1) a therapy directed at serious symptoms or serious manifestations of the condition; (2) a diagnostic evaluated for the impact on a serious aspect of the condition; (3) a preventive intended to prevent a serious aspect; (4) a product that could ameliorate serious side effects of other treatments. Now let us discuss the second criteria. For an agent to demonstrate potential to address unmet medical needs, the following conditions have to be considered: (1) there is no existing therapy for the condition; (2) the new therapy is better; (3) the new therapy is for the patients intolerant or unresponsive to existing therapy; (4) the new therapy is less toxic, but preserves similar benefit; (5) the new therapy improves compliance which is shown to improve effects on serious conditions. Details on the designation, development and application review of a fast track therapy can be found at `http://www.fda.gov/cder/guidance`.

Figure 3.2 summarizes the criteria in a schematic format.

Fast Track emphasizes the critical nature of close early communication between the FDA and the sponsor. It highlights the procedures such as pre-trial (before Investigational New Drug (IND) is initiated) and End-of-Phase I meetings as methods to improve the efficiency of pre-clinical and clinical development. It focuses on efforts by the FDA and the sponsor to reach early agreement on the design and analysis of the major clinical efficacy studies that will be needed to support approval. The requests for Fast Track are expected to be resolved within a designated 60-day period from the initial request. As of June 30, 2002, 151 applications for Fast Track have been submitted. As seen from Table 3.4, there has been a marked increase in fast track designation requests in recent years and most requests have been acted upon within the 60-day period.

TABLE 3.4. *Responses to request for Fast Track designation.*

Fast track requests	Granted	Denied	Pending	Total (%)
Submissions 1998–2002				
Within goal of 60 days	96	30	4	130 (79.3%)
Overdue (>60 days)	13	12	9	34 (20.7%)
Submissions in fiscal year 2004				
Within goal of 60 days	12	7	7	26 (96.0%)
Overdue (>60 days)	1	0	0	1 (4.0%)

NOTE: These figures are for sponsor requests for 'Fast Track' designation for a specific drug product and indication, which is not necessarily the same as a product being granted Approval under Subpart H. Report updated through April 28, 2004.

3.2.2 Subpart H and Its Relevance to Surrogate Markers

So far, from the discussion of the process, it is indicatead that Fast Track can be considered irrespective of whether surrogate endpoints were used or not. For drug development programs specifically utilizing surrogate endpoints, a special regulatory mechanism called Subpart H (refers to the specific code of regulations governing it) is available. Under Subpart H, approval may be based on a surrogate endpoint or on an effect on a clinical endpoint other than survival or irreversible morbidity ("Surrogate") [21 Code of Federal Register (CFR) 314.510 and 21 CFR 601.41], or a product may be approved with restrictions to assure safe use ("Restricted") [21 CFR 314.520]. Note that Subpart H applications are usually candidates for Fast Track also, but not necessarily so.

The FDA may grant marketing approval for a new drug product on the basis of

> "... adequate and well-controlled clinical trials establishing that the drug product has an effect on a surrogate endpoint that is reasonably likely, based on epidemiological, therapeutic, pathophysiologic, or other evidence, to predict clinical benefit or on the basis of an effect on a clinical endpoint other than survival or irreversible morbidity. Approval under this section will be subject to the requirement that the applicant study the drug further, to verify and describe its clinical benefit, where there is uncertainty as to the relation of the surrogate endpoint to clinical benefit, or of the observed clinical benefit to ultimate outcome. Post-marketing studies would usually be studies al-

ready underway. When required to be conducted, such studies must also be adequate and well controlled. The applicant shall carry out any such studies with due diligence."

Tables 3.5–3.7 summarize New Drug Applications (NDAs) that have been approved under Subpart H regulations.

Tables 3.8 and 3.9 summarize already approved drugs that were considered for a different disease indication using surrogate markers. These applications are known in regulatory parlance as NDA Supplements.

Fast Track policies are primarily designed to expedite drug development during the IND stage, whereas Approval Under Subpart H allows for marketing approval of an NDA based on an effect on a surrogate endpoint along with well-controlled post-marketing studies.

A post-approval study will not necessarily be required in the exact population for which approval was granted. For example, where a product was approved to treat patients with refractory malignancy, additional information from that population may not, for example, be as useful as randomized controlled trials in a previously untreated population. In many instances, additional studies would be already under way at the time the accelerated approval is granted. If such studies are adequate and well controlled (either utilizing proper historical controls or randomization), they may fulfill the accelerated approval requirements for post-approval studies. All required post-approval studies should be carried out with due diligence. Failure to do so would constitute grounds to withdraw approval of the product application (21 CFR 314.530(a) or 21 CFR 601.43(a)). FDA may also withdraw approval of the application if studies fail to demonstrate clinical benefit based on the traditional long-term endpoint.

Next, three therapeutic areas where surrogate markers have been used will be discussed – in anti-viral, anti-cancer, and cardiovascular drug products. It is not meant to be an exhaustive treatise; there are several other therapeutic classes where use of surrogate markers is being considered or done. However, the experience is most established in these three areas.

TABLE 3.5. *NDAs approved under Subpart H based on surrogate endpoints. Part I.*

NDA	Trade name	Generic name	Approval date	Indication for treatment
20199	Hivid	Zalcitabine	19-Jun-92	Combination therapy with zidovudine in advanced HIV infection.
50698	Biaxin	Clarithromycin (suspension)	23-Dec-93	Disseminated mycobacterial infections due to Mycobacterium avium and Mycobacterium intracellular.
20412	Zerit	Stavudine	24-Jun-94	Adults with advanced HIV infection – alternative therapy.
20212	Zinecard	Dexrazoxane	26-May-95	To reduce the incidence and severity of cardiomyopathy associated with doxorubicin administration in certain breast cancer patients.
20498	Casodex	Bicalutamide	04-Oct-95	Use in combination therapy with a Luteinizing-Hormone Releasing Hormone (LHRH) analogue for the treatment of advanced prostate cancer.
20564, 20596	Epivir	Lamivudine	17-Nov-95	HIV infection in selected patients.
50718	Doxil	Doxorubicin hydrochloride (liposomal formulation)	17-Nov-95	AIDS-related Kaposi's sarcoma in patients with disease that has progressed on prior combination chemotherapy or in patients who are intolerant to such therapy.
20628	Invirase	Saquinavir mesylate	06-Dec-95	Advanced HIV infection in selected patients in combination with nucleoside analogues.
20659, 20680	Norvir	Ritonavir	01-Mar-96	In combination with nucleoside analogues or as monotherapy for the treatment of HIV infection.
20685	Crixivan	Indinavir sulfate	13-Mar-96	HIV infection in adults.
20449	Taxotere	Docetaxel	14-May-96	Patients with locally advanced or metastatic breast cancer who have progressed or relapsed during anthracycline based therapy.
20571	Camptosar	Irinotecan hydrochloride	14-Jun-96	Refractory colorectal cancer.
20636	Viramune	Nevirapine	21-Jun-96	Combination with nucleoside analogues for the treatment of HIV-1 infected adults who have experienced clinical and/or immunologic deterioration.
20604	Serostim	Somatropin	23-Aug-96	AIDS wasting associated with catabolism loss or cachexia.
19815	ProAmatine	Midodrine hydrochloride	06-Sep-96	Treatment of symptomatic orthostatic hypotension.
20778, 20779	Viracept	Nelfinavir mesylate	14-Mar-97	HIV infection when therapy is warranted.
20705	Rescriptor	Delavirdine mesylate	04-Apr-97	HIV infection in combination with appropriate antiretroviral agents when therapy is warranted.
20896	Xeloda	Capecitabine	30-Apr-98	Patients with metastatic breast cancer resistant to both paclitaxel and an anthracycline-containing chemotherapy regimen or resistant to paclitaxel and for whom further anthracycline therapy may be contraindicated.

Updated through April 30, 2004.

TABLE 3.6. *NDAs approved under Subpart H based on surrogate endpoints. Part II.*

NDA	Trade name	Generic name	Approval date	Indication for treatment
19832	Sulfamylon	Mafenide acetate	05-Jun-98	As an adjunctive topical antimicrobial agent to control bacterial infection when used under moist dressings over meshed autografts on excised burn wounds.
21024	Priftin	Rifapentine	22-Jun-98	Pulmonary tuberculosis (TB).
20933	Viramune	Nevirapine	11-Sep-98	Provides for an oral suspension, which is indicated for use in combination therapy with other antiretroviral agents for the treatment of HIV-1 infection.
20972	Sustiva	Efavirenz	17-Sep-98	In combination with other antiretroviral agents for the treatment of HIV-1 infection.
20977, 20978	Ziagen	Abacavir sulfate	17-Dec-98	In combination with other antiretroviral agents, for the treatment of HIV-1 infection.
21041	Depocyt	Cytarabine liposomal injection	01-Apr-99	Intrathecal treatment of lymphomatous meningitis.
21029	Temodar	Temozolomide (capsules)	11-Aug-99	Adult patients with refractory anaplastic astrocytoma, i.e., patients at first relapse who have experienced disease progression on a drug regimen containing a nitrosourea and procarbazine.
21007, 21039	Agenerase	Amprenavir	15-Apr-99	In combination with other antiretroviral agents, for the treatment of HIV-1 infection.
50747	Synercid	Quinupristin/ dalfopristin I.V.	21-Sep-99	Vancomycin-resistant Enterococcus faecium.
21174	Mylotarg	Gemtuzumab/ ozogamicin	17-May-00	Patients with CD33 positive acute myeloid leukemia in first relapse who are 60 years of age or older and who are not considered candidates for cytotoxic chemotherapy.
21226, 21251	Kaletra	Lopinavir/ ritonavir	15-Sep-00	In combination with other antiretroviral agents for the treatment of HIV-1 infection in adults and pediatric patients age six months and older.
21205	Trizivir	Abacavir sulfate, lamivudine, & zidovudine	14-Nov-00	Either alone or in combination with other antiretroviral agents for the treatment of HIV-1 infection.
21335	Gleevec	Imatinib mesylate	10-May-01	Use of 50 and 100 mg capsules for the treatment of patients with chronic myeloid leukemia (CML) in blast crisis, accelerated phase, or in chronic phase after failure of interferon-alpha therapy.
21356	Viread	Tenofovir disoproxil fumarate	26-Oct-01	In combination with other antiretroviral agents for the treatment of HIV-1 infection in adults.
21272	Remodulin	Treprostinil sodium	21-May-02	Use of 1.0, 2.5, 5.0, and 10.0 mg/ml injection for the treatment of pulmonary arterial hypertension (PAH).

Updated through April 30, 2004.

TABLE 3.7. *NDAs approved under Subpart H based on surrogate endpoints. Part III.*

NDA.	Trade name	Generic name	Approval date	Indication for treatment
21196	Xyrem	Sodium oxybate	17-Jul-02	Provides for the use of Xyrem Oral Solution for the treatment of cataplexy associated with narcolepsy (restricted use, not on surrogate endpoint.)
21492	Eloxatin	Oxaliplatin injection	9-Aug-02	Provides for the use of Eloxatin in combination with infusional fluorouracil/leukovorin (5-FU/LV) for the treatment of patients with metastatic carcinoma of the colon or rectum whose disease has recurred or progressed during or within 6 months of completion of first line therapy with the combination of bolus 5-FU/LV and irinotecan.
21481	Fuzeon	Enfuvirtide injection	13-Mar-03	Provides for the use of Fuzeon in combination with other antiretroviral agents, for the treatment of HIV-1 infection in treatment experienced patients with evidence of HIV-1 replication despite ongoing antiretroviral therapy.
21588	Gleevec	Imatinib mesylate tablets	18-Apr-03	Provides for the use of Gleevec for the treatment of patients with chronic myeloid leukemia (CML) in blast crisis, accelerated phase, or in chronic phase after failure of interferon-alpha therapy.
21399	Iressa	Gefitinib tablets	5-May-03	Provides for the use of IRESSA as monotherapy for the treatment of patients with locally advanced or metastatic non-small cell lung cancer after failure of both platinum-based and docetaxel chemotherapies.
21602	Velcade	Bortezomib injection	13-May-03	Provides for the use of Velcade for the treatment of multiple myeloma patients who have received at least two prior therapies and have demonstrated disease progression on the last therapy.
21320	Plenaxis	Abarelix injectable suspension	25-Nov-03	Provides for the use of Plenaxis for the palliative treatment of men with advanced symptomatic prostate cancer and specific symptoms (restricted use, approval not based on surrogate).

Updated through April 30, 2004.

TABLE 3.8. *NDA Supplements approved under Subpart H based on surrogate endpoints. Part I.*

NDA	Supp	Trade name	Generic name	Approval date	Indication for treatment
50697	N	Biaxin	Clarithromycin (tablets)	23-Dec-93	Disseminated mycobacterial infections due to Mycobacterium avium and Mycobacterium intracellular.
20636	SE1 009	Viramune	Nevirapine	11-Sep-98	Provides for the inclusion of pediatric information into the labeling.
50718	SE1 006	Doxil	Doxorubicin hydrochloride (liposomal formulation)	28-Jun-99	Treatment of metastatic carcinoma of the ovary in patients with disease that is refractory to both paclitaxel- and platinum-based chemotherapy regimens.
21156	N	Celebrex	Celecoxib	23-Dec-99	To reduce the number of adenomatous colorectal polyps in Familial Adenomatous Polyposis (FAP), as an adjunct to usual care.
19537	SE1 038	CIPRO	Ciprofloxacin hydrochloride	30-Aug-00	Inhalational anthrax (post-exposure).
19847	SE1 024	CIPRO	Ciprofloxacin hydrochloride	30-Aug-00	Inhalational anthrax (post-exposure).
19857	SE1 027	CIPRO	Ciprofloxacin hydrochloride	30-Aug-00	Inhalational anthrax (post-exposure).
19858	SE1 021	CIPRO	Ciprofloxacin hydrochloride	30-Aug-00	Inhalational anthrax (post-exposure).
20780	SE1 008	CIPRO	Ciprofloxacin hydrochloride	30-Aug-00	Inhalational anthrax (post-exposure).
21335	SE1 001	Gleevec	Imatinib mesylate	1-Feb-02	Patients with Kit (CD117) positive unresectable and/or metastatic malignant gastrointestinal stromal tumors (GIST).

Updated through April 30, 2004.

TABLE 3.9. *NDA Supplements approved under Subpart H based on surrogate endpoints. Part II.*

NDA	Supp	Trade name	Generic name	Approval date	Indication for treatment
21107	SE8 005	Lotronex	Alosetron hydrochloride	7-Jun-02	Restricted use of Lotronex for women only with severe diarrhea-predominant irritable refractory to conventional therapy (not based on surrogate).
20541	SE1 010	Arimidex	Anastrozole tablets	5-Sep-02	Provides for the use of ARIMIDEX for adjuvant treatment of postmenopausal women with hormone receptor positive early breast cancer.
21335	SE1 004	Gleevec	Imatinib mesylate 100 mg capsules	20-Dec-02	Provides for the use of Gleevec for the treatment of newly diagnosed adult patients with Philadelphia chromosome positive chronic myeloid leukemia (CML). Follow-up is limited.
21335	SE5 003	Gleevec	Imatinib mesylate tablets	20-May-03	Provides for the use of Gleevec for the treatment of pediatric patients with Ph+ chronic phase CML whose disease has recurred after stem cell transplant or who are resistant to interferon alpha therapy.

Updated through April 30, 2004.

3.3 Use of Surrogate Markers in Anti-viral Drug Products

Surrogate markers have been widely used in anti-viral drug therapies. It is one of the first areas that surrogates were used, as a response to the AIDS epidemic and the thrust to bring potential therapies to the market within the earliest time frame.

Various biological markers have been considered during early drug development processes in anti-HIV therapies. They included CD4 count, p24 and ICD p24 antigen level, β_2-microglobulin, neopterin, HIV-1 RNA, HIV-1 DNA among a few. The cumulative evidence base suggests that both CD4 count and HIV-1 RNA provide important prognostic factor for AIDS. Some surrogate markers such as β_2-microglobulin and neopterin have proved to be of limited use in a clinical trial.

It has been indicated that the natural history of HIV-1 infection can be characterized by increased HIV-1 RNA level leading to CD4 count depletion which in turn leads to AIDS and eventually death. Following the initial HIV-1 infection, there is a latency period of up to 7 years where little virus is detected in the blood but there is still virus particles being produced on a daily basis. It was thought that if virus replication can be completely blocked by potent anti-retroviral drug combinations, it would take between two and three years of treatment to completely eradicate the virus from the infected host.

HIV-1 RNA as a surrogate endpoint has several unique properties. First, HIV-1 RNA is a marker of the severity of the disease – the higher it is, the more severe the infection. Second, it has been shown repeatedly that AIDS-defining illness is much less frequent when HIV-1 RNA is below a certain threshold, e.g., 5000 copies/ml. Third, HIV-1 RNA is usually high at the time of initial HIV-1 infection, and often increases near the time of an AIDS-defining illness such as an opportunistic infection. Following the 1997 NIH workshop and the subsequent publication of two guidance documents by the Department of Health and Human Services, the consensus was to monitor HIV-1 viral load and CD4 count of HIV-infected patients on a routine basis to make treatment decisions.

In August 1999, FDA issued a draft Guidance for Industry discussing Clinical Considerations for Accelerated and Traditional Approval of Anti-Retroviral Drugs Using Plasma HIV RNA (`http://www.fda.gov/cder/guidance/index.htm`). Although accelerated approvals are routinely based on changes in endpoints such as CD4 cell counts and plasma HIV RNA levels, clinical endpoint trials assessing effects on mortality and/or disease progression had been a requirement for traditional approvals prior to July

1997. With the availability of potent anti-retroviral drug regimens and sensitive assays for assessing plasma HIV RNA, the standards of clinical practice evolved to a paradigm emphasizing maximal and durable HIV RNA suppression.

To evaluate feasibility of using HIV-1 RNA as a study endpoint, a collaborative group of pharmaceutical, academic and government scientists investigated relationships between treatment-induced changes in HIV-1 RNA and clinical endpoints from ongoing and completed anti-retroviral trials. In several analyses of multiple trials involving more than 5000 patients, a clear association was seen between initial decreases in plasma HIV-1 RNA within first 24 weeks, and a reduction in the risk of clinical progression and death. This relationship was observed across a range of patient characteristics including pretreatment CD4 counts and HIV-1 RNA levels, prior drug experience, and treatment regimen. Based on these data, it was proposed that the accelerated approvals could be based on studies that show a drug's contribution toward shorter-term reductions in HIV-1 RNA (e.g., 24 weeks), whereas traditional approvals could be based on trials that show a drug's contribution toward durability of HIV-1 RNA suppression (e.g., at least 48 weeks). In addition, the changes in CD4 cell counts need to be consistent with observed HIV-1 RNA changes (Hughes *et al.* 2000).

According to the 1999 Guidance, studies in a broad range of patient populations (gender, age, and race) and a range of pre-treatment characteristics (e.g., advanced and early disease, heavily pre-treated and treatment naïve) are recommended to characterize the activity of the drug in at least two adequate and well-controlled trials with a minimum of 24 weeks duration to support accelerated approval. In combination therapies, analyses at some earlier time points (e.g., 16 weeks) have proven to be less discriminatory. Every attempt is to be made to design randomized, blinded, controlled trials that provide all study patients with treatment regimens according to a standard clinical practice. If the studies are designed as superiority trials, add-on or substitution comparisons can be included, where the regimen with the experimental drug should show superiority to the control regimen. If equivalence trials using substitution comparisons are to be designed, it is important that the contribution of the substituted drug to the regimen's overall activity be previously characterized in the population of interest.

Historically, zidovudine (ZDV) was approved in 1987 based on 17 weeks survival. The next product, didanosine (ddI) was approved in 1991 based on surrogate endpoint of CD4 counts with a limited indication in patients refractory to AZT failures. It was not until 1992 that the accelerated approval mechanism was used in the approval of dideoxycytidine (ddC). Since then many other HIV drugs have been approved under this regulation. For approvals prior to 1995, the accelerated approval was based on either change

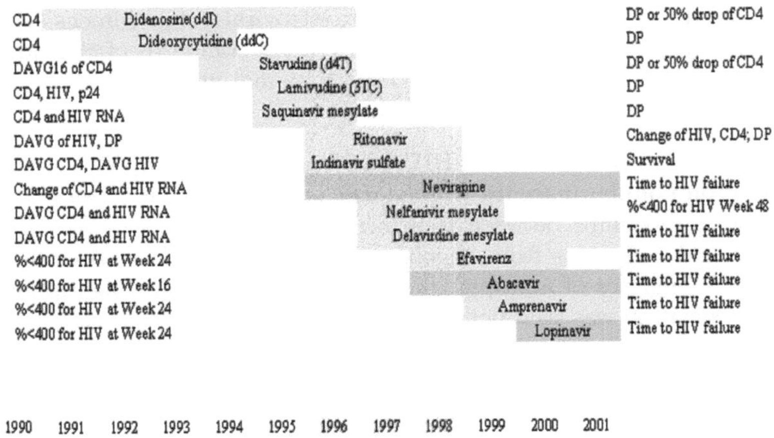

FIGURE 3.3. *Endpoints used in approval of anti-HIV drug products.*

in CD4 count or time-averaged change in CD4 count (DAVG). Between 1995–1998, HIV-1 RNA load was gradually being more frequently used. The metric used for HIV-1 RNA included change from baseline, DAVG or the percentage of patients below a certain threshold. After 1998, most of the accelerated approvals have been based on the criteria of having HIV-1 RNA <400 and/or 50 copies/ml. The endpoints used in traditional approvals of anti-HIV agents were primarily based on disease progression (DP) prior to 1997. From 1997 onwards, the traditional approvals are mostly based on HIV-1 RNA, either as percentage of patients having less than 400 copies/ml or the time to virologic failure.

According to Gilbert *et al.* (2001), the selection of primary endpoints for AIDS trials is complicated by the long clinical course of the disease, the frequent onset of anti-viral drug resistance, and the limitations in data for validating surrogate endpoints. However, increasing the objectivity of the selection process in the future requires expansion of available information for the elucidation of the complex relationship between various surrogate endpoints and clinical endpoints. Only through vigilant collection of clinical outcomes data (e.g., through routine collection of death event data from national death records) and data from long-term studies that monitor virologic, immunologic, and clinical information throughout sequences of regimens can this goal be achieved.

Figure 3.3 summarizes the endpoints traditionally used in accelerated and traditional approval of anti-HIV drugs. The endpoints on the left axis refer to the surrogate endpoints used for accelerated approval; endpoints on the right axis refer to the clinical endpoints used for traditional approval. The horizontal axis gives the approval timelines.

TABLE 3.10. *Crixivan. Basis for accelerated approval (CD4 count: comparison of MK-containing arms to ZDV).*

Statistic	Crixivan (MK) vs. zidovudine (ZDV)	MK+ZDV vs. ZDV
Study 028		
Difference	66	69
p-value	<0.0001	<0.0001
95% CI	42-89	45-93
Study 033		
Difference	62	47
p-value	<0.0001	<0.0001
95% CI	40-84	25-69

Next, we discuss two examples of therapeutic agents that have undergone the accelerated approval and eventually went through the traditional approval.

3.3.1 Crixivan: A Case Study

Crixivan (indinavir sulfate), also referred to as MK-639 or simply MK or IDV, was submitted in 1996 for accelerated approval based upon change from baseline in CD4 cell counts. Change from baseline of HIV-1 RNA was also considered as a secondary endpoint.

Two Phase III studies (Study 028 and 033) were examined for this review, (see Table 3.10), and the regulatory decision was based on the interim analyses of the surrogate markers. Study 028 was a double-blind study in 224 patients with no prior nucleoside analogue experience. The patients were randomized to receive one of the three treatment regimens — the test drug (MK)+Zidovudine (ZDV)+ddI, MK monotherapy or ZDV+ddI. The comparisons of each arm containing MK versus the control arm were conducted using ANOVA adjusting for center and CD4 strata at baseline.

Study 033 was performed in 266 subjects with prior ZDV experience and was randomized to one of the three regimens — MK+ZDV+lamivudine (also known as 3TC), MK monotherapy and ZDV+3TC. Analysis plans were similar to Study 028.

Two short term (24-week) Phase II studies were also examined in order to provide preliminary efficacy information regarding triple combination therapy. It was seen that the results were convincing enough to warrant accelerated approval.

Crixivan was submitted for traditional approval following completion of the pivotal trials (see Table 3.11). The clinical endpoint was defined as the first occurrence of death from any cause or the diagnosis of AIDS as predefined in the protocol. The comparisons were to be based on time-to-first failure methods, including Kaplan-Meier, log-rank test and Cox proportional hazards regression models. Study 033, later conducted as AIDS Cooperative Trial Group (ACTG) 320, used the area under the response-time curve for each patient divided by the time from randomization to the last available evaluation of the patient minus the baseline value (AUCMB). The ACTG Data and Safety Monitoring Board (DSMB) monitored the course and conduct of this study. One interim look was planned after 250 events or one year, and the Peto and Pike stopping boundary was used. The trial was to be considered for early stopping if the nominal p-value <0.001. The trial was indeed stopped early by DSMB after 1156 patients were enrolled.

When considered in the light of the results of Trial 028 and the patterns seen over time in ACTG 320, it appeared that the failure to reach the traditional 0.05 level is the result of the premature discontinuation of ACTG 320. The achieved significance level was still felt to be sufficient to support the results of study 028 that Crixivan is associated with a reduction in rate of progression or death due to HIV.

3.3.2 *Viramune: A Case Study*

Accelerated Approval

Viramune (nevirapine, or NVP) belongs to a new class of anti-retroviral agents called non-nucleoside reverse transcriptase inhibitor (NNRTI). The accelerated approval of this drug was sought in patients with advanced HIV-1 infection whose current anti-retroviral therapy is no longer deemed adequate. Three studies, two in nucleoside experienced population and one in nucleoside naive population, were submitted under accelerated approval to support the claim that the addition of nevirapine to one or more nucleoside drugs provides an improvement in surrogate markers for HIV disease (see Table 3.12). For each study, the surrogate endpoints were CD4 cell count and HIV-1 RNA level in an eight-week window of time at the end of the studies.

Study 1037 was a randomized, double blind, placebo-controlled study comparing ZDV/NVP to NVP monotherapy in 60 patients with prior ZDV experience for 3–24 months and CD4 cell counts between 200 and 500. Subjects were followed for 28 weeks with scheduled visit every 2 weeks in

TABLE 3.11. *Crixivan. Basis for traditional approval (time to first clinical event analysis – treatment comparison).*

Study	Treatment comparison	Stratified log-rank test (two-sided p-value) for time to first clinical event	Stratification factor
Study 028	MK+ZDV vs ZDV	0.0001	Site and CD4
	MK vs ZDV	0.0001	
	MK+ZDV vs MK	0.22	
ACTG 320	MK+3TC+ZDV vs 3TC+ZDV	0.0021*	CD4

* From randomization-based test, required 0.001 to achieve 5% level.

the beginning and every 4 weeks after the fourth week.

Study 1031 (ACTG 241) was a randomized, double blind, placebo-controlled study in 400 patients comparing ZDV/ddI/NVP to ZDV/NVP with similar schedule as Study 1037. Eight of the 16 participating centers, with 200 patients, were to be included in a virology substudy, in which HIV-1 RNA were to be collected in addition. The subjects were to be followed for 48 weeks on CD4 count.

Study 1046 was an international randomized, double blind placebo-controlled trial in 120 patients comparing ZDV/ddI/NVP to ZDV/NVP and ZDV/ddI with same dosing regimen for 52 weeks after the start of therapy.

The studies were analyzed using ANOVA models with baseline CD4 strata and center as covariates.

It is seen that addition of nevirapine to one or nucleosides has been shown to produce an increase in CD4 cell counts and a small decrease in HIV-1 RNA levels. The lack of significance in Study 1046 may be attributed to the much smaller sample size (50/arm versus 200/arm).

Traditional Approval

For traditional approval, the sponsor submitted five randomized, controlled clinical trials. Study 1090, the Atlantic trial, and another trial with the acronym INCAS, were planned pivotal trials: trials ACTG 193a and ACTG 241 were provided as supportive evidence.

Trial 1090 was a placebo-controlled study designed to compare efficacy of

TABLE 3.12. *Viramune. Basis for accelerated approval.*

Endpoint	Metric	N	Treatment		Control	p-value	
Study 1031			Z/D/N*		Z/D		
CD4	Mean change week 20-28	328	26		-5	.001	
	Mean change week 40-48	328	6		-16	.002	
	AUCMB week 28	392	23		6	.001	
	AUCMB week 48	392	20		0	.001	
RNA	Mean change week 20-28	155	-.27		-.08	.137	
	Mean change week 40-48	149	-.14		.11	.024	
	AUCMB week 28	188	-.57		-.27	.001	
	AUCMB week 48	188	-.43		-.17	.003	
Study 1037			Z/N		Z		
CD4	Mean change week 12-16	55	53		-31	.001	
	Mean change week 20-28	55	14		-31	.009	
	AUCMB week 16	60	44		-11	.001	
	AUCMB week 28	60	22		-24	.001	
RNA	Mean change week 12-16	55	.03		.01	.525	
	Mean change week 20-28	55	.16		.12	.590	
	AUCMB week 16	60	-.38		-.01	.001	
	AUCMB week 28	60	-.16		.04	.001	
Study 1046		Z/D/N	Z/D	Z/N	p-values		
					ZDN-ZD	ZD-ZN	ZDN-ZN
CD4	Mean change week 12-16	117	95	44	.44	.08	.01
	Mean change week 20-28	113	78	22	.18	.05	.001
	AUCMB week 16	72	62	57	.58	.77	.39
	AUCMB week 28	87	67	47	.23	.28	.02
RNA	Mean change week 12-16	-1.76	-1.55	-.56	.35	.001	.001
	Mean change week 20-28	-1.72	-1.43	-.55	.14	.001	.001
	AUCMB week 16	-1.61	-1.44	-.99	.24	.002	.001
	AUCMB week 28	-1.63	-1.41	-.85	.15	.001	.001

* Z = ZDV; D = ddI; N = NVP.

NVP when used in combination with 3TC and other anti-retroviral therapies in NNRTI naïve patients with CD4 counts $\leq$200 cells/mm^3. The primary efficacy endpoint was time to clinical disease progression, subsequently changed to time to virologic failure as defined as increase in HIV-1 RNA above limit of quantitation (BLQ). The planned primary analysis, a stratified Fisher's exact test on percentage of subjects without virologic failure at Week 48, stratified by prior anti-retroviral therapy, HIV disease status, baseline CD4 count, and baseline HIV-1 RNA found nevirapine to be superior to placebo with a p-value <0.001.

The INCAS trial was designed to compare one triple-drug regimen, indicated by NVP+ddI+ZDV, to two dual-drug regimens (ddI+ZDV, NVP+ZDV). The primary endpoint was percent BLQ by 48 weeks in HIV-1 infected anti-retroviral naive patients with CD4 cell counts of 200–600 cells/mm^3 without AIDS-defining illness or active invasive infection or malignancy. The primary analysis found adding nevirapine to ddI+ZDV background gave a significant increase in sustained viral suppression from 19% to 45% (log-rank p-value <0.001). It was also found that ddI+ZDV was statistically significantly superior to NVP+ZDV (log-rank p-value <0.001), indicating that nevirapine should not be used with only one NNTI.

The Atlantic trial was designed to compare efficacy of three different triple–drug regimens comparing NVP with indinavir (IDV) and NNTI 3TC when used in conjunction with ddI and stavudine (also known as d4T). The primary efficacy endpoint is percent BLQ at 48 weeks. This trial was conducted in asymptomatic NNTI naive patients with CD4 counts >200 cells/mm^3 and HIV-1 RNA $\geq$500 copies/ml. The primary analysis used 95% two-sided confidence intervals for the difference in success rates, using normal approximation to the binomial. The trial was felt to have too small sample size and the confidence intervals were too wide to support a firm conclusion that nevirapine is no less than 10% worse than indinavir or lamivudine (3TC).

Unlike the previous case study, this example highlights a regulatory decision that was less straightforward. However, it was flexible enough to keep the totality of the drug experience in order to meet the demand for newer treatment regimens faster.

3.4 Use of Surrogate Markers in Anti-cancer Drug Products

Traditionally, therapies for cancer patients have been approved on the basis of objective response to the agent (tumor shrinkage) together with direct evidence that the therapy produces measurable clinical benefit. Typical approval endpoints have been included, such as response rate together with increased patient survival, decreased recurrence rate, increased disease-free interval, and/or improved quality of life. It has been assumed that durable, complete clinical response (complete disappearance of detectable tumor) is a valid surrogate for such clinical benefit, but it is only infrequently achieved. Much more commonly, partial tumor shrinkages are induced, and evidence has accumulated that such responses are often directly linked to longer or better patient survival. In fact, for some new agents, the FDA began to rely on a reasonable high rate of verifiable objective partial response to the therapy as a basis for approval of agents to treat refractory malignancies without requiring evidence of improved survival or quality of life even prior to 1996. Subsequently, additional trials have been conducted to confirm or expand the product's indication. Although the predictive value of partial responses may still be a matter of discussion and study for all types of cancer patients, the FDA had concluded that for patients with refractory malignant diseases or for those who have no adequate alternative, clear evidence of anti-tumor activity is a reasonable basis for approving the drug. In these cases, studies confirming a clinical benefit may be appropriately completed after approval.

In March 1996, U.S. President Bill Clinton and Vice President Al Gore issued a National Performance Review as a part of reinventing the government initiative. This document discussed accelerating approval as well as expanding access to anti-cancer agents. In the introduction, it stated "The Food and Drug Administration has demonstrated a longstanding commitment to the prompt consideration and, when appropriate, early approval of new therapies for cancer patients." To speed up the entire process further, the FDA is adopting a uniform policy that will permit accelerated approval of a significant number of new cancer therapeutics. In the past, the FDA has approved cancer therapies on the basis of an agent's ability to produce an effect on the well-established and long-recognized criteria such as survival, improved quality of life, and relief of symptoms, as well as objective disease regression. When partial response of disease (measurable but incomplete tumor shrinkage) has been noted in patients who have extensive or metastatic cancer, it is often correlated with other approval criteria. Because of this experience, it is believed that for many cancer therapies it is appropriate to utilize objective evidence of tumor shrinkage as a basis for approval, allowing additional evidence of increased survival and/or improved quality of life associated with that therapy to be demonstrated later. By utilizing objective response as a surrogate endpoint in clinical trials, the FDA will decrease the total time needed for marketing approval in many situations.

Although the accelerated approval provisions have been applicable to promising treatments for cancer patients who do not benefit from or cannot tolerate available therapy, this approval mechanism had not been frequently utilized prior to 1996, largely because general agreement on reasonable surrogate endpoints had been lacking.

Under the 1996 initiative, the FDA substantially expanded the use of accelerated approval process based upon verified and recognized demonstration of objective tumor shrinkage. For approval, potential effectiveness of the treatment should outweigh its toxicities and post-approval studies will usually be required to further define the utility of the new agent for the approved and/or other indications, either alone or in combination with other agents. The FDA can also apply accelerated approval provisions to certain products intended to remove a serious or life-threatening toxicity of cancer treatment based on post-approval studies that demonstrate that surrogate measures correspond to clinical benefit and/or effect of therapy on survival.

The greater utilization of the accelerated approval provisions for cancer treatment not only has an important impact on the original applications but also on supplemental application for secondary indications. The actual use of cancer agents may be far broader than the approved indications. Because of the nature of cancer therapy, the approved label does not necessarily convey all the medical conditions for which the agent is used or may be useful. Nonetheless, the FDA-approved label should accurately convey as many as agent's uses as are properly supported by data.

The greater utilization of the accelerated approval provisions for cancer treatment not only has an important impact on the original applications but also on supplemental application for secondary indications. The actual use of cancer agents may be far broader than the approved indications, and because of the nature of cancer therapy, the approved label does not necessarily convey all the medical conditions for which the agent is used and may be useful. Nonetheless, the FDA-approved label should accurately convey as many as agent's uses as are properly supported by data.

The type and quantity of clinical data that is required will vary depending on the cancer indication under study, the availability and acceptability of other therapies, and the specific observations in the studies. According to the Guidance to the Industry document dated December 1998 (`http://www.fda.gov/cder/guidance/index.htm`), there is flexibility regarding the data requirements. In the refractory cancer setting, for example, where therapies with meaningful benefit are unavailable, non-randomized studies showing that a new treatment provides a significant objective response rate with tolerable treatment toxicity may be adequate to support approval under the accelerated approval regulations. In this setting, objective response rates are considered a surrogate endpoint reasonably likely to predict a clinical benefit. Evidence to confirm that clinical benefit can be obtained after approval. In those cases where durable complete responses can be attained, non-randomized studies showing a significant rate of durable complete responses can be persuasive evidence of effectiveness.

During 1992–2002, 15 NDAs involving 13 drugs have been submitted to the Division of Oncologic Drug Products in Center for Drug Evaluation and Research (CDER). Of them, 10 were based on single-arm phase II studies and used objective response as a surrogate endpoint. Only 5 were based on randomized trials. The details are given in Tables 3.13 and 3.14.

This brings up several important trial design issues about optimal accrual of patients in the trials and the extent to which the changing circumstances can impede the conduct of planned studies. Consider the following case study where this scenario has been brought to bear.

3.4.1 Doxil: A Case Study

Doxil (doxorubicin HCl liposome injection) was approved under the accelerated approval mechanism for "the treatment of metastatic carcinoma

TABLE 3.13. *Single-arm trials with no concurrent comparator in the Division of Oncologic Drug Products.*

Drug	Year	Indication	Sample size	Trial details
Liposomal doxorubicin (Doxil)	1995	Kaposi's sarcoma second line	383	77 of 383 identified refractory
Amifostine (Ethyol)	1996	To decrease cisplatin toxicity in NSCLC	100	Two trials, 50 patients each
Docetaxel (Taxotere)	1996	Breast cancer second line	483	6 US trials total 309; 3 Japanese trials 174
Irinotecan (Camptosar)	1996	Colon cancer	132	Single-arm trial
Capecitabine (Xeloda)	1998	Breast cancer refractory	162	Single trial in patients in stage IV disease
Liposomal doxorubicin (Doxil)	1999	Ovarian cancer refractory	145	3 studies
Temozolomide (Temodar)	1999	Anaplastic astrocytoma refractory	162	
Gemtuzumab ozogomycin (Mylotarg)	2000	AML	142	3 studies
Imatinib mesylate (Gleevec)	2001	CML in BC, AC, or CP after interferon failure	1027	3 studies
Imatinib mesylate (Gleevec)	2001	GIST	147	Single 2-arm study

of the ovary in patients with disease that is refractory to both paclitaxel and platinum-based chemotherapy regimens. Refractory disease is defined as disease that has progressed while on treatment, or within 6 months of completing treatment." In November 1998, the drug was assigned an orphan drug designation, given that no drug has been approved for the treatment of ovarian cancer refractory to platinum compounds and paclitaxel. In December 1998, a supplemental NDA was submitted for the above indication containing data from three Phase II non-comparative studies in relapse or refractory ovarian cancer. The primary analysis was based on the surrogate endpoint of response rate on 176 patients. This application also submitted data from an interim analysis of an ongoing Phase III study (Study 30–49) comparing Doxil with Topotecan. The accelerated approval was granted in June 1999. The traditional approval was to be based on the timely completion and final results of Study 30–49.

Study 30–49 (performed May 1997–March 1999) was designed to show safety and efficacy in patients with relapsed ovarian cancer following failure with platinum based chemotherapy in 474 patients. The study was stratified by platinum sensitivity and bulky disease and designed to show superiority of Doxil to Topotecan in either time to progression (TTP) or survival, with a supporting trend demonstrated for the other endpoint. The secondary

TABLE 3.14. *Approvals based on randomized trials in the Division of Oncologic Drug Products.*

Drug	Indication	Year	Endpoint
Dexrazoxane (Zinecard)	Reduction of doxorubicin cardiomyopathy	1995	LVEF, Cardiac heart failure
Liposomal cytarabine (Depocyte)	Lymphomatous meningitis	1999	Cytologic response
Celecoxib (Celebrex)	Reduction of adenomatous polyps	1999	Number of polyps
Oxaliplatin (Eloxatin)	Second-line colorectal cancer	2002	Objective response, Time to progression
Anastrozole (Arimidex)	Adjuvant post-menopausal ER+	2002	Disease-free survival

outcomes were objective response rate (ORR), response duration, survival and safety. If Study 30–49 did not demonstrate the clinical benefit of Doxil, the sponsor would have to perform another study to show clinical benefit of the drug in ovarian cancer.

In June 2000, the sponsor informed the FDA that the planned treatment analysis for Study 30–49 did not demonstrate superiority in TTP, but showed significant survival advantage of Doxil over Topotecan in the platinum-sensitive group, with approximately 50% of the patients still alive. However, in the platinum-refractory subset, the patient population for which it is to be indicated, the results were marginally in favor of the control (hazard ratio $= 1.01$ $[0.78, 1.31]$) (Gordon 2003). This made regulatory decision significantly harder, and accelerated approval was granted after recommendation from a panel of external experts in an Oncology Advisory Committee (ODAC) meeting. Results presented at the ODAC are summarized in Table 3.15 (Hamburger 2003). Based on this scenario, it was agreed that a final survival analysis is to be performed on Study 30–49 when a 90% of the patients (planned size is 474) died or were lost to follow up. The final survival result of Study 30–49 is currently undergoing regulatory review.

A second protocol to prove clinical benefit was required. This Phase IV protocol (SO200), initiated in 2000 and currently enrolling, was an open-label inter-group study between Doxil and carboplatin versus carboplatin in 900 platinum-sensitive patients with recurrent epithelial ovarian carcinoma after failure of initial, platinum-based chemotherapy, to be performed jointly with an oncology group, SWOG. The primary endpoint is overall survival and the secondary endpoints are progression-free survival (PFS), confirmed complete response (CR), time to failure (TTF), and toxicity. It is currently enrolling patients.

This experience brings forth some of the challenges surrounding Phase IV

TABLE 3.15. *Doxil. Median time to progression (TTP) and overall survival (OS) time in weeks at the end of planned treatment.*

Population	Doxil (N)	Topotecan (N)	p-value
		TTP	
All patients	18.4 (239)	18.3 (235)	0.632
Platinum-sensitive	29.9 (109)	26.7 (111)	0.387
Platinum-refractory	9.1 (130)	14.3 (124)	0.941
		OS	
All patients	58.7 (239)	56.7 (235)	0.964
Platinum-sensitive	110.7 (109)	84.7 (111)	0.027
Platinum-refractory	34.6 (130)	41.4 (124)	0.126

commitment trials in oncology, highlighted by the case study.

- The times to complete the Phase IV commitments are often longer than anticipated. In the Doxil case study, after the end of the planned treatment analysis, the primary endpoint was modified to become overall survival. Time to reach 90% event endpoint in Study 30–49 took more than 3.5 years.
- Multiple parties are often involved in finalization and implementation of the Phase IV trials. In the Doxil experience, the transfer and clinical responsibilities had to be coordinated between the sponsor, SWOG, other cooperative groups, National Cancer Institute (NCI), and with the FDA.
- The competition for accrual among other ongoing trials is often so fierce that it impedes the progress of the trial.
- After the accelerated approval, a drug can be prescribed to patients with that indication outside of a clinical study, making it harder to accrue patients needed for completion of Phase IV commitment.

3.5 Use of Surrogate Markers in Cardiovascular Drug Products

The use of surrogate markers in cardiovascular drug products has received mixed response – a rising enthusiasm for providing efficacious drugs at the earliest possible time along with experiences tempered with some unexpected results in some products.

Surrogates can be early or late in the causal chain – cholesterol (a biochemical variable), blood pressure (a pathophysiologic variable), coronary vessel diameter (a morphological variable), or left ventricular hypertrophy (a morphological variable). However, some are closer to certain clinical events such as myocardial infarction and heart failure. Some surrogates are not etiologic but are thought to reflect activity of an underlying process that leads to an adverse event.

The risk of reliance on a surrogate is that the pathway connecting surrogate endpoint to the clinical endpoint may not be clear. It is widely accepted that elevated blood pressure is a direct cause of stroke, heart failure, and renal failure and accelerated coronary disease and that reducing blood pressure reduces morbidity and mortality. However, before the controlled outcome studies of hypertensive drugs were performed in 1960s, there was an active debate that blood pressure was an "adaptive" response to the vascular disease and that lowering it would be harmful (Freis 1990). Recent data on the benefits of 3-hydroxy-3-methylglutaryl coenzyme A (HMG-CoA) reductase inhibitors may have partially settled the role of surrogate markers in cholesterol-lowering drugs, but the real value of other surrogate markers in cholesterol-lowering drugs may not be as clear. The safety database needed to characterize adequately the risk-benefit ratio is often not extensive enough in accelerated approval submissions, leading to the common phrase "there is no surrogate for safety" (Temple 1999).

Distinguishing concern about the validity of the surrogate from the more general question of safety is important because it affects the kind of data that can be used to assess the benefits and risks of treatment. If there is doubt about the surrogate itself, only an outcome study in the specific disease can determine the value of the drug. But if the validity of the surrogate is accepted, studies in a variety of settings may be pertinent to assessment of safety. For example, a drug lowering blood pressure may be about as certain to provide clinical benefit, as would be an anti-anginal drug. However, the safety profile of the drug has to be established, probably from a moderate study in hypertension or angina or from another population more vulnerable to cardiovascular toxicity or from pharmacologically related agents in either population. The absence of outcome studies in certain anti-hypertensives (calcium channel blockers and angiotensin-converting enzyme (ACE) inhibitors) has been cited by critics of the use of surrogates. Table 3.16 summarizes the surrogate endpoints used in cardiovascular drugs.

TABLE 3.16. *Surrogate endpoints used in the Division of Cardiovascular Drug Products.*

Condition	Approval endpoint	Postmarketing outcome studies
Hypertension	Change in blood pressure	No
Hyperlipidemia: initial approval	Change in blood lipid level	Yes[1]
Hyperlipidemia: clinical benefit	Survival, rate of myocardial infarction	No[2]
Hyperglycemia	Change in blood sugar levels, glycosylated hemoglobin	No
Heart failure: symptoms	Exercise, symptoms, together with evidence (except for ACE inhibitors) that there is no adverse effect on survival	No
Heart failure: long-term benefit	Survival, hospitalization	No[2]
Angina, effort	Exercise, symptoms	No
Angina, vasospastic	Angina rate	No
Silent ischemia	Outcome (acute myocardial infarction, survival)	No[2]
Ventricular arrhytmia: symptoms	Symptoms, with evidence of no harm	No[2]
Ventricular arrhytmia: life-threatening	Symptoms, with evidence of no harm; survival	No[2]
Atrial arrhytmia	Symptoms, delayed recurrence, evidence of no adverse effect on survival	No[2]
Acute coronary syndrome, postangioplasty/coronary artery bypass graft	Outcome (death, acute myocardial infarction, urgent intervention)	No[2]
Acute myocardial infarction (thrombolysis)	Survival	No[2]
Orthostatic hypotension	Decreased orthostatic blood pressure	Yes[3]

[1] By Agreement, the sponsors voluntarily agreed to conduct post-marketing studies.
[2] Studied pre-marketing.
[3] Required under the FDA Accelerated Approval Rule.

3.5.1 *Anti-hypertensive Drugs*

Effect of blood pressure is the basis for approval of new hypertensive drugs. The most persuasive support for the surrogate endpoint of blood pressure is experience from numerous long-term outcome studies showing a clear effect on stroke and at least favorable trends on cardiovascular events and survival rates. In addition, substantial epidemiological evidence indicates that blood pressure is continuously related to the risk of stroke and coronary heart disease. Few active drugs have shown any other factor to modulate directly hypertensive benefit, but direct comparisons of high-dose diuretics and beta-blockers showed no real difference (Collins *et al.* 1990), even for cardiovascular events for which they are expected to be superior due to post-infarction benefit and lack of hypokalemic effects. Although the FDA emphasized the importance of such comparisons in the past, comparative studies have not been required of individual sponsors. If ongoing large trials demonstrate differences in outcome with drugs approved using same surrogate procedures, that policy will change (Temple 1999).

3.5.2 Anti-platelet Drugs

Currently, platelet aggregation inhibitors or anticoagulants in various settings (post-infarctions or stroke, peripheral vascular disease, acute coronary syndrome, post-angioplasty or post-bypass) are studied using clinical endpoints (death, new infarction, and urgent procedural intervention). As yet, although various anti-platelet treatments have a long and growing record of success in preventing adverse outcomes, there is no effect on a platelet aggregation or coagulation surrogate endpoint that has been convincingly shown to correspond to a clinical benefit and to define the risk of bleeding.

3.5.3 Drugs for Heart Failure

Increased mortality with two classes of inotropic agents and an inotropic vasodilator drug clearly indicates that hemodynamic or symptomatic benefit in heart failure does not predict improved survival. Therefore, for a drug to be approved for heart failure symptom improvement, evidence of a symptomatic benefit needs to be supported by showing that there is no adverse mortality effect. Long before the adverse outcome effects studies of inotropes were observed (Packer *et al.* 1993), the FDA concluded that "there should be reasonable assurance that survival in high-risk patients is not impaired; the controlled trials thus need to be of sufficient size to detect a substantial increase in mortality" (Temple 1987). This conclusion was based in part on early suggestions of rapid deterioration in open studies of inotropes and in part on the known adverse effects of digoxin.

3.5.4 Drugs for Angina and Silent Ischemia

Anti-anginal drugs are approved based on improvement in exercise tolerance or reduction in symptoms of angina; no current treatments have been shown to improve outcome. Safety of anti-anginal drugs is well supported by studies of calcium channel blockers and beta-blockers in post-infarction settings. Silent ischemia, like symptomatic ischemia, predicts an increased rate of death and myocardial infarction, and it has been proposed that a reduced rate of silent episodes should be a basis for approval. As of now, the FDA has not accepted this suggestion (Temple 1990) concluding instead that the drugs for this indication need to show an effect on a clinical end-point, such as survival or rate of new infarction. It did not seem reasonable that the drugs known only to affect ischemia would provide benefit, when the same drugs used to treat symptomatic angina has not been able to show improved outcome. It also seemed at least possible that ischemia stimulated growth of collateral vessel, which could improve outcome (Temple 1988).

3.5.5 Ventricular Arrhythmias

The most controversial example of an erroneous surrogate is the stunning results of the Cardiac Arrhythmia Suppression Trial (CAST). Details of this trial will be discussed in Section 3.5.6. It definitely established that effective suppression of ventricular premature beats (VPB) does not decrease mortality, despite the well-established association between elevated VPB rates and early arrhythmic death. But although the markedly adverse outcome was certainly unexpected, labeling for encainide and flecainide before the CAST study specifically pointed out the absence of known survival benefit from VPB suppression, the lack of information on safety and effectiveness in the post-infarction state, and the drug's ability to cause worsened arrhythmias. The indicated uses for both drugs were limited to patients with documented life-threatening arrhythmias and symptomatic patients with non-sustained ventricular and frequent VPBs. Since the CAST results were reported, approval of drugs for ventricular arrhythmias that are not immediately life-threatening has required showing improved survival benefits and no adverse effect on survival in case of symptomatic claim. At the present time, no drugs have been able to meet this standard.

3.5.6 The CAST Experience: A Case Study in Ventricular Arrhythmia

The occurrence of ventricular premature depolarizations in survivors of myocardial infarction is a risk factor for subsequent sudden death, but whether anti-arrhythmic therapy reduces risk is not clear. CAST was undertaken to evaluate the effect of anti-arrhythmic therapy, such as encainide, flecainide or moricizine, in patients with asymptomatic or mildly symptomatic ventricular arrhythmia after myocardial infarctions.

The purpose of the study was to test the hypothesis that suppression of ventricular ectopy after a myocardial infarction reduces the incidence of sudden death. The design of the study was multicenter, randomized, placebo controlled with a preliminary, open-label titration to ensure that all patients would respond to at least one of the drugs. The primary endpoint was death or cardiac arrest with resuscitation, either of which due to arrhythmia.

The results of this study were unexpected. The flecainide and encainide arms of this trial were stopped early, after a mean follow up of 10 months. Of 89 deaths or cardiac arrests total, 63 patients were on active drugs versus 26 on placebo ($p = 0.0001$) and of death or cardiac arrest due to arrhythmia, 43 patients were on active drugs versus 16 on placebo ($p = 0.0004$). The conclusions were that the results indicate that encainide or flecainide, when used to prevent ventricular arrhytmias post-myocardial infarction, are detrimental to survival. The study continued limited to the arms of moricizine versus placebo.

After the flecainide and encainide arms of the CAST I were discontinued, a continuation of the CAST I, the CAST II used moricizine to determine if suppressing asymptomatic or mildly symptomatic ventricular ectopy post-myocardial infarction (MI) reduces the incidence of sudden death from ventricular arrhythmias. There were 1325 patients with EF greater than or equal to 40%, who were within 4 to 90 days of having an MI, and who had greater than or equal to 6 repetitive ventricular complexes. The CAST II was a multicenter, randomized, placebo-controlled study in which patients received placebo or up to 900 mg/day of moricizine as necessary to suppress arrhythmias. The primary endpoint was sudden death. There was a 14-day exposure phase and a 2-year long-term evaluation phase.

This study was terminated early because in the 14-day exposure period, there was excess mortality in the moricizine arm (17 deaths in 665 patients) as opposed to the no therapy or placebo group (3 deaths in 660 patients). A less than 8% chance of finding a survival benefit was found if the study was completed. It was concluded that the use of moricizine to suppress asymptomatic or mildly symptomatic ventricular premature depolarizations post-MI is ineffective and increases mortality.

These experiences point to an interesting fact that surrogate markers may not always be useful and have to be validated extensively before being used as a regulatory tool.

3.6 Statistical Issues Related to Accelerated Approval

The accelerated approval process is an important tool for therapeutic agents in serious or life-threatening diseases where no existing therapies are expected to be of help. For example, in oncology, survival and improvement in patient-reported symptoms are considered clinical endpoints while objective response rate and time to progression are considered meaningful surrogate markers. There are several unique situations for drugs submitted under accelerated approval process. It is to be noted that none of them have been used in a regulatory setting so far, so implications of these methods on the drug development procedure are not ascertained.

- Because placebo is considered unethical in most clinical settings appropriate for accelerated approval, the trials are usually conducted in single-arm Phase II studies, sometimes not even in randomized trials.
- The accelerated approval is based on a very small sample size, making regulatory decisions about benefit-risk ratio very hard to characterize.
- The safety databases for such approvals are minuscule, posing serious consideration about the safe use of the drug in a widespread clinical setting.
- After accelerated approval, it is often not possible to perform the Phase IV commitments in the original population, and clinical experiences bridging the original population and the enriched population can be hard.

Some specific statistical issues have arisen in the accelerated approval process. Because the accelerated approval is based on a limited database of patients in which the drug has shown a positive finding, there are two stages in which the regulatory decision has to be taken and hence two points where a Type I error (α) has to be controlled. There has been some discussion (Sridhara *et al.* 2001) that instead of considering the two approval processes as independent events, the more appropriate paradigm would be to distribute the α over both events.

If we consider these series of events in clinical trial terms, the accelerated approval can be treated as a decision based on an interim analysis on a pre-specified surrogate endpoint. The full or traditional approval can then be granted based on the clinical endpoint at the conclusion of Phase IV commitments, which can be treated to be the final analysis. Under this situation, there are several possible scenarios after accelerated approval is granted based on a surrogate endpoint:

1. The drug development continues as planned and full approval is granted based on the Phase IV commitments.
2. Based on the Phase IV commitments, the new drug does not demonstrate significant effect with respect to the desired final clinical outcome. This can happen if:

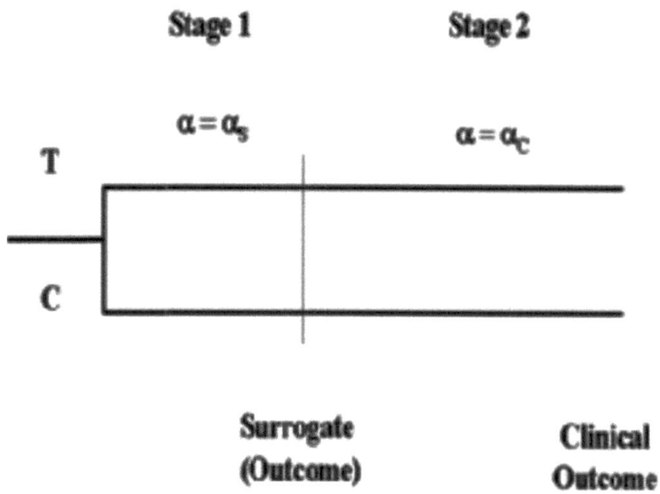

FIGURE 3.4. *Schema showing two-stage approval method.*

- the study conducted for the accelerated approval was a false positive study;
- the surrogate marker used in the accelerated approval study is not predictive of the clinical endpoint;
- the assumptions and/or the design of the accelerated and final approval studies were not appropriate;
- the final clinical risk/benefit ratio is markedly different than what was originally anticipated, e.g., unexpected negative mortality effect.

Under any of the scenarios discussed, the studies have to be designed with sufficient power to detect overall significant difference with respect to the clinical endpoint at the end of the studies. The studies also have to have sufficient assay sensitivity to detect significant difference with respect to the pre-specified surrogate endpoint at the interim analysis stage for the accelerated endpoint.

There have been some methodologies proposed recently for the two-stage design (see Figure 3.4). Two of them will be discussed briefly in the discussion, primarily from a theoretical standpoint.

The first method by Shih *et al.* (2003) proposes a two-stage design with clinical endpoint T and surrogate endpoint S. At the end of the first stage, both S and T are evaluated according to the flowchart in Figure 3.5. At the end of the first stage, the data may support early termination of the trial for clinical benefit based on T or may support accelerated approval based

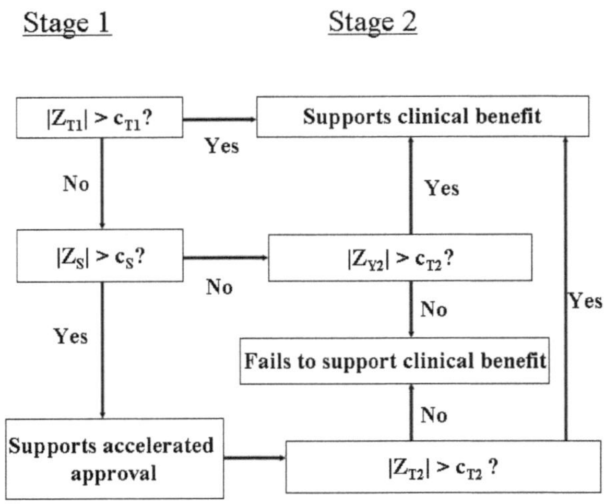

FIGURE 3.5. *Two-stage approval method proposed by Shi* et al. *(2003).*

on the surrogate S. If neither is true, then the trial continues to the second stage. At the end of the second stage, T is evaluated for clinical benefit. This is summarized in Figure 3.5. The "final approval" Type I error rate (α_F) for the clinical endpoint is given by

$$\alpha_F = \alpha_{F1} + \alpha_{F2}, \tag{3.5}$$

where

$$\begin{aligned} \alpha_{F1} &= P(|Z_{T1}| > c_{T1} \mid H_{0T}), \\ \alpha_{F2} &= P(|Z_{T1}| < c_{T1}, |Z_{T2}| > c_{T2} \mid H_{0T}). \end{aligned}$$

H_{0T} is the null hypothesis for T, and Z_{T1} and Z_{T2} are normally distributed test-statistics based on the data available for T at the first and second stages, respectively. If $\alpha_{F1} = 0.001$, then $c_{T1} = 3.29$. If the correlation $\rho(Z_{T1}, Z_{T2}) = \sqrt{0.5}$, then to maintain $\alpha_F = 0.05$ or 0.04, c_{T2} needs to be equal to 1.962 or 2.06, respectively.

The authors raise a question as to what false positive rate, or Type I error, for the surrogate endpoint should we control for. The "accelerated approval" Type I error rate (α_A) is given by

$$\alpha_A = P(|Z_{T1}| < c_{T1} \text{ and } |Z_S| > c_S \mid H_{0S}, H_{0T}), \tag{3.6}$$

where H_{0S} is the null hypothesis for S and Z_S is a normally distributed test-statistic based on the data available for S at the first stage. Some of the choices can be:

- control α_F at the 0.05 level;

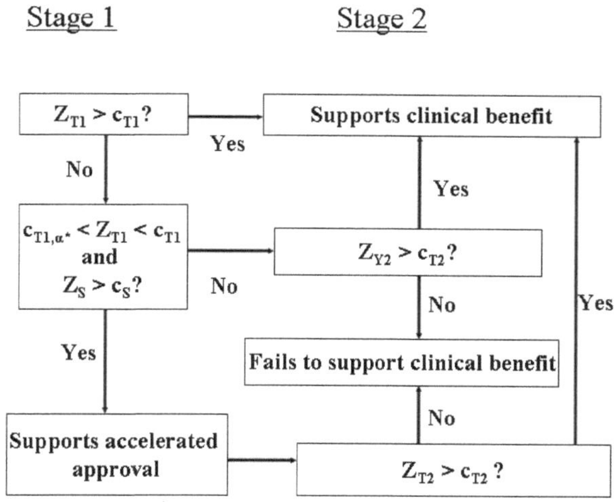

FIGURE 3.6. *Two-stage approval method proposed by Yang* et al. *(2002) and Shridhara* et al. *(2002).*

- control α_F at the 0.05 level and α_A at the 0.01 level;
- control $\alpha_F + \alpha_A$ at the 0.05 level;
- any other appropriate choice.

The second proposed method, due to Yang *et al.* (2002) and Sridhara *et al.* (2002), analogously considers a two-stage design with clinical endpoint T and surrogate endpoint S. At the end of the first stage, both S and T are evaluated according to the flowchart in Figure 3.6. However, unlike Shih's method, there is an additional condition to be satisfied before concluding that the interim data supports accelerated approval. The Type I error rate for the overall clinical endpoint is given again by (3.5) with

$$\begin{aligned} \alpha_{F1} &= P(Z_{T1} > c_{T1}|H_{0T}), \\ \alpha_{F2} &= P(Z_{T1} < c_{T1}, Z_{T2} > c_{T2}|H_{0T}). \end{aligned}$$

But, in addition, it is proposed that the following probability,

$$P(c_{T1,\alpha^*} < Z_{T1} < c_{T1} \text{ and } Z_S > c_S \text{ and } Z_{T2} < c_{T2} \mid H_{0T}), \qquad (3.7)$$

should be controlled at some level γ. The last equation is the joint probability of a positive surrogate outcome and a nominally positive (α^*) clinical benefit at interim, and a non-significant final clinical benefit outcome. If this probability is less than a certain level, say, $\gamma = 0.30$, then the interim positive results on the surrogate endpoint and a nominally positive (α^*) clinical outcome provide a reasonable level of evidence to support the

TABLE 3.17. *Probability of a study to support accelarated approval under an alternative of 80% power to detect a clinical benefit and 90% power for surrogate endpoints. The probabilities are calculated based on the O'Brien-Fleming version of the Lan-DeMets spending function.*

Information fraction	$\text{Corr}(Z_S, Z_T)$	Level of γ		
(t)	(ρ)	0.10	0.20	0.30
1/4	0.1	0.4627	0.5885	0.6618
	0.5	0.4850	0.6082	0.6778
	0.9	0.5087	0.6307	0.6967
1/3	0.1	0.5190	0.6293	0.6887
	0.5	0.5428	0.6478	0.7023
	0.9	0.5696	0.6713	0.7205

drug's accelerated approval (in the absence of other supportive information). With c_{T1} and c_{T2} specified by some spending function, and if we also specify γ, then we can solve for α^*, and thus, c_{T1,α^*}. An example is shown in Table 3.17.

The criterion provides some level of assurance of a clinical benefit in the event that the confirmatory trial may not materialize due to patient crossover, changing standards of care, other available new treatments, etc. The method does require that at the end of the first stage, there should be at least a certain fraction of the expected total events to have occurred.

As a consequence, the submission of evidence based on the surrogate endpoint for an accelerated approval will be slightly delayed until the desired fraction of the expected total events has been achieved. This represents a compromise between the real possibility that the post-marketing trials already underway, or yet to be conducted, to confirm the positive finding on the surrogate endpoint may never materialize.

3.7 Surrogate Markers at Other Phases of Drug Development

At earlier stages of drug development, both positive (efficacy) and negative (safety) effects of a drug can be characterized using a variety of measurements or response endpoints. These effects include clearly clinically pertinent effects (clinical benefit or toxicity), effects on a well-established surrogate (such as blood pressure or QT interval in cardiovascular disease), or effects on a more remote biomarker (such as ACE inhibition or bradykinin levels in cardiovascular disease). All of these measurements can be expected to show exposure-response relationships that can guide therapy, suggest dose/dose intervals, or suggest further study. In many cases, multiple response endpoints are more informative than single endpoints for establishing exposure-response relationships. Methods to combine attributable proportions or relative effects of two or more surrogate markers for the same true clinical endpoint have to be developed. Specifically, less clinically persuasive endpoints (biomarkers, surrogates) can help in choosing doses for the larger and more difficult clinical endpoint trials and can suggest areas of special concern.

In addition, surrogate endpoints can be used to link with external sources of information on the disease or on other treatments. They can be used to integrate the data across all phases to build an evidence base, including validation. This database can be analyzed and mined for the relationship of surrogate endpoints to the disease states, other markers, and patient covariates.

Surrogate marker methodology can play a significant role in drug safety and risk assessment area. The databases can be mined for the signs of potential toxicities. For example, certain liver enzyme tests (ALT, AST, bilirubin) can be considered as surrogate markers for hepatic toxicity. This will enable early detection of potential problems later in the drug development process.

Finally, surrogate markers play an important role in drug development in identifying faster and more focused pathways to bringing a promising drug to patients. However, care needs to be taken in ensuring that the markers are pre-specified, equivocally validated, and predictive of the final clinical benefit to the patients.

4

Notation and Motivating Studies

Geert Molenberghs, Marc Buyse, and Tomasz Burzykowski

In this chapter, we introduce a basic set of notation to be used throughout the book, as well as datasets that will serve as running examples, to illustrate the methods proposed in subsequent chapters.

4.1 Notation

We adopt the following notation: T and S are random variables that denote the true and surrogate endpoints, respectively, and Z is a binary indicator variable for treatment. In general, we will consider settings corresponding to a multi-center trial or a meta-analysis of trials. Thus, the (T, S, Z) notation will be supplemented using indices $i = 1, \ldots, N$ for the ith center or trial, and $j = 1, \ldots, n_i$, to denote the jth subject enrolled in the ith center or trial.

4.2 Key Datasets

Data from randomized clinical trials in different therapeutic areas will be used as running examples throughout many of the chapters.

4.2.1 Ophthalmology: Age-related Macular Degeneration Trial

This example concerns a clinical trial for patients with age-related macular degeneration, a condition in which patients progressively lose vision (Pharmacological Therapy for Macular Degeneration Study Group 1997). Overall, 190 patients from 42 centers participated in the trial. Patients'

V A L I D

A T I O N

O F S U R

R O G A T

E M A R K

E R S I N

R A N D O

M I Z E D

E X P E R

I M E N T

FIGURE 4.1. *Representation of a vision chart.*

visual acuity was assessed using standardized vision charts (see Figure 4.1) displaying lines of five letters of decreasing size, which patients had to read from top (largest letters) to bottom (smallest letters). The visual acuity was measured by the total number of letters correctly read. In this example, the binary indicator for treatment (Z) is set to 0 for placebo and to 1 for interferon-α. The surrogate endpoint S is the change in the visual acuity at 6 months after starting treatment, while the true endpoint T is the change in the visual acuity at 1 year. Various forms (binary, continuous) of the endpoints will be considered. When treated as continuous variables, the endpoints will be assumed to follow a normal distribution. For this case, Figure 4.2 presents the scatterplot of the two endpoints for all patients included in the trial. Overall, there was no statistically significant effect for either the true endpoint (difference of means for $Z = 1$ vs. $Z = 0$ equal to -2.88, $p = 0.218$ for the Student's t-test) or the surrogate (-1.90, $p = 0.314$).

In the analyses, the centers in which the patients were treated will be considered as the units of analysis. Six out of 42 centers participating in the trial enrolled patients only to one of the two treatment arms. These centers were excluded from considerations. A total of 36 centers were thus available for analysis, with a number of individual patients per center ranging from 2 to 18 (183 patients overall).

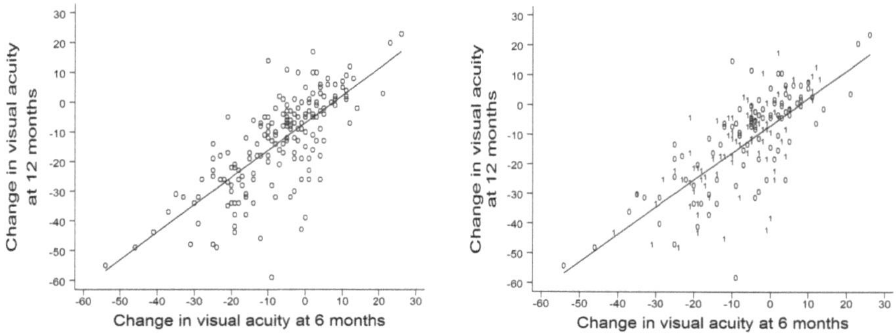

FIGURE 4.2. *Age-related macular degeneration trial. Observed values of the surrogate versus true endpoint (Pharmacological Therapy for Macular Degeneration Study Group 1997). Points in the right plot are marked by the treatment group indicator Z. The straight line contains predictions from a simple linear regression model.*

4.2.2 Advanced Ovarian Cancer: A Meta-analysis of Four Clinical Trials

These data were used in a meta-analysis of four randomized multi-center trials in advanced ovarian cancer (Ovarian Cancer Meta-Analysis Project 1991). Individual patient data are available in these four trials for the comparison of two treatment modalities: cyclophosphamide plus cisplatin (CP) versus cyclophosphamide plus adriamycin plus cisplatin (CAP). The binary indicator for treatment (Z) will be set to 0 for CP and to 1 for CAP. The surrogate endpoint S will be progression-free survival time, defined as the time (in years) from randomization to clinical progression of the disease or death, while the true endpoint T will be survival time, defined as the time (in years) from randomization to death from any cause. The full results of this meta-analysis were published with a minimum follow-up of 5 years in all trials (Ovarian Cancer Meta-Analysis Project 1991). The dataset was subsequently updated to include a minimum follow-up of 10 years in all trials (Ovarian Cancer Meta-Analysis Project 1998). After such long follow-up, most patients have had a disease progression or have died (980 of 1194 patients, i.e., 81.8%). In the majority of cases, death was clearly related to the disease (850 out of 952 deaths, i.e., 89.2%).

Figure 4.3 presents survival and progression-free survival curves by treatment group collapsed over trials. Overall, there was a statistically significant effect in favor of CAP for both survival (relative risk, $RR = 0.84$, $p = 0.008$ for log-rank test stratified by trial) and progression-free survival ($RR = 0.81$, $p = 0.001$).

The ovarian cancer dataset contains four trials. In the two larger trials

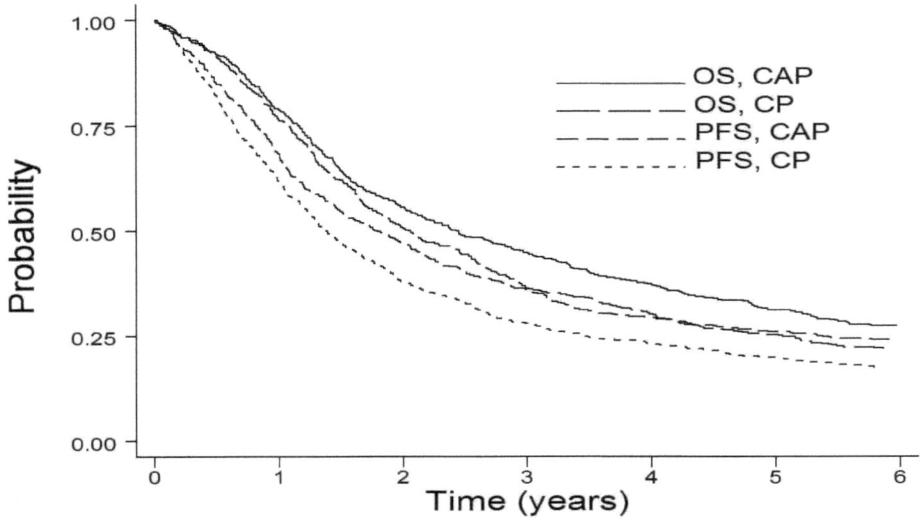

FIGURE 4.3. *Advanced ovarian cancer. Overall survival and progression-free survival curves for the meta-analysis (Ovarian Cancer Meta-Analysis Project 1998).*

of the Gynecologic Oncology Group (GOG, with 412 patients) and the Gruppo Interegionale Cooperativo Oncologico Ginecologia (GICOG, with 383 patients), information is also available on the centers in which the patients had been treated. For the two smaller trials of the Danish Ovarian Cancer Group (DACOVA, with 274 patients) and the Gruppo Oncologico Nord-Ovest (GONO, with 125 patients), the information is not available. According to the clinical investigators, the close collaboration of the members of the corresponding research groups allows to consider the patients treated in these trials as a homogenous group. In the analyses, center will be used as the unit of analysis for the two larger trials, and the trial as the unit of analysis for the two smaller trials. Two centers enrolled only one patient each and were excluded from consideration. A total of 50 "units" are thus available for analysis, with a number of individual patients per unit ranging from 2 to 274.

4.2.3 Corfu Study in Advanced Colorectal Cancer: Two Clinical Trials

These data come from two randomized multicenter trials in advanced colorectal cancer (Corfu-A Study Group 1995, Greco *et al.* 1996). In one trial, treatment with 5FU plus interferon (5FU/IFN) was compared to treatment with 5FU plus folinic acid (5FU/LV) (Corfu-A Study Group 1995). In the

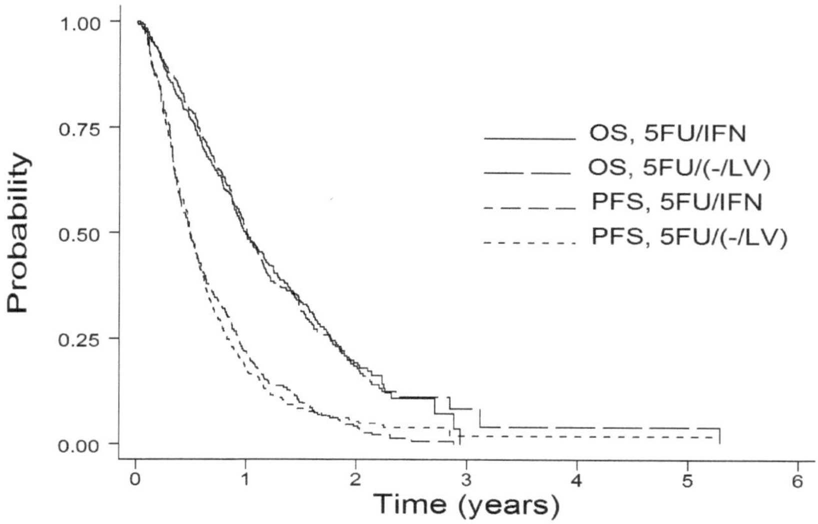

FIGURE 4.4. *Corfu study in advanced colorectal cancer. Overall survival and progression-free survival curves for both randomized clinical trials (Corfu-A Study Group 1995, Greco* et al. *1996).*

other trial, treatment with 5FU/IFN was compared to treatment with 5FU alone (Greco *et al.* 1996). The binary indicator for treatment Z will be set to 0 for 5FU/IFN and to 1 for 5FU/LV or 5FU alone. The surrogate endpoint S will be progression-free survival time, defined as the time (in years) from randomization to clinical progression of the disease or death, while the true endpoint T will be survival time, defined as the time (in years) from randomization to death from any cause. Most patients in the two trials have had a disease progression or have died (694 of 736 patients, i.e., 94.3%). Figure 4.4 presents survival and progression-free survival curves by treatment group collapsed over trials. Overall, there was no statistically significant effect of Z either for survival ($RR = 1.00$, $p = 0.976$ for log-rank test stratified by trial) or progression-free survival ($RR = 1.02$, $p = 0.785$).

Similar to the previous example, center will be considered as the unit of analysis. However, in 8 centers there were no patients accrued to one of the treatment arms. These 8 centers were therefore excluded from the analyses. As a result, a total of 68 "units" were thus available for analysis, with a number of individual patients per unit ranging from 2 to 38 (642 patients overall).

4.2.4 Four Meta-analyses of 28 Clinical Trials in Advanced Colorectal Cancer

We will use data from 28 advanced colorectal cancer trials (Advanced Colorectal Cancer Meta-Analysis Project 1992 and 1994, Meta-Analysis Group In Cancer 1996 and 1998). The individual patient data were collected by the Meta-Analysis Group In Cancer between 1990 and 1996 to obtain an overall quantitative assessment of the value of several experimental treatments in advanced colorectal cancer. In the four meta-analyses, the comparison was between an experimental treatment and a control treatment. The control treatments, referred to hereafter as "FU bolus," were similar across the 4 meta-analyses and consisted of fluoropyrimidines (5FU or FUDR) given as a bolus intravenous injection. The experimental treatments, referred to hereunder as "experimental FU," differed across the four meta-analyses and consisted, respectively, of 5FU modulated by leucovorin (Advanced Colorectal Cancer Meta-Analysis Project 1992), of 5FU modulated by methotrexate (Advanced Colorectal Cancer Meta-Analysis Project 1994), of 5FU given in continuous infusion (Meta-Analysis Group In Cancer 1998), and of hepatic arterial infusion of FUDR for patients with metastasis confined to the liver (Meta-Analysis Group In Cancer 1996). As noted by Daniels and Hughes (1997), the use of an "experimental" treatment that varies among the trials can be defended on the grounds of generalizability of the results of the validation process to future clinical trials and treatments. The "experimental" treatments in our example might be considered as representatives of "the modifications of the standard fluoropyrimidine-based regimen" in advanced colorectal cancer.

Several of the 28 trials were multi-armed. In total, 33 randomized comparisons were considered in the four meta-analyses. Individual-patient data were available for 27 of the comparisons (in 24 studies). From now on, we will refer to each of the comparison as a separate "trial." The total size in the trials ranged from 15 to 382 patients.

The true endpoint T will be survival time, defined as the time (in years) from randomization to death from any cause. Most patients included in the dataset have died (3591 out of 4010 patients, i.e., 89.5%). The surrogate endpoint S will be tumor response. We will define S either as a binary variable indicating complete/partial response, or as a categorical variable with four categories (complete response, partial response, stable disease, progression) (World Health Organization 1979). The binary indicator for treatment (Z) will be set to 0 for FU bolus and to 1 for experimental FU.

Figure 4.5 shows survival curves by treatment within tumor response categories. There is no statistically significant difference between experimental FU and bolus FU in any tumor response category (complete response:

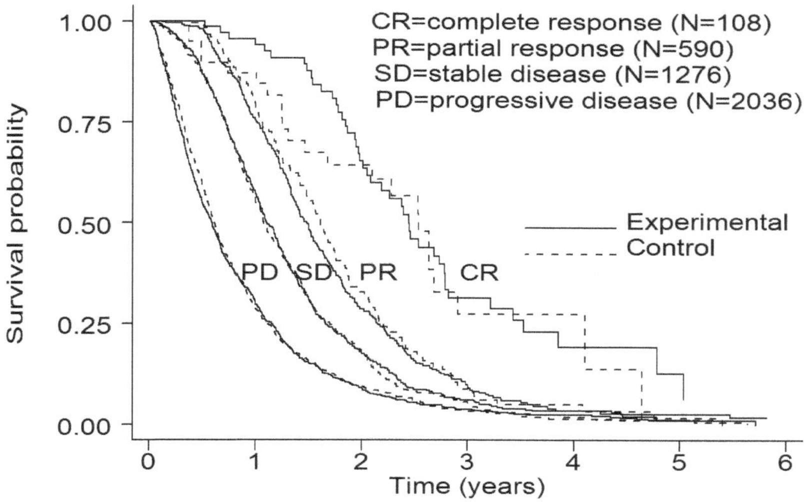

FIGURE 4.5. *Meta-analyses in advanced colorectal cancer. Overall survival curves by tumor response for the four meta-analyses (Advanced Colorectal Cancer Meta-Analysis Project 1992, 1994, Meta-Analysis Group In Cancer 1996, 1998).*

$p = 0.544$; partial response: $p = 0.791$; stable disease: $p = 0.525$; progressive disease: $p = 0.059$ for the log-rank test stratified by trial; three patients with unknown response treated as "progressions"), which suggests that the overall survival benefit in favor of experimental FU ($RR = 0.91$, $p = 0.010$ for log-rank test stratified by trial) is due to the higher tumor response rate obtained with experimental FU as compared to bolus FU. The four meta-analyses showed that the 10%–15% response rate achievable with FU bolus could be increased to over 20% with any of the experimental treatments. Regardless of treatment, though, survival benefits remained modest and naturally doubts were raised as to the usefulness of response as a surrogate for survival.

4.2.5 Advanced Prostate Cancer: Two Clinical Trials

These data come from two open-label clinical trials in which patients with advanced prostate cancer were randomized either to oral liarozole, an experimental retinoic acid metabolism-blocking agent developed by Janssen Research Foundation, or to an antiandrogenic drug: cyproterone acetate (CPA) in the first trial (Debruyne *et al.* 1998) and flutamide in the second. The two trials accrued 312 and 284 patients, respectively. All patients were in relapse after first-line endocrine therapy.

The primary endpoint in each trial was survival time after randomization. Assessments were undertaken before the start of treatment and repeated at 2 weeks, monthly for six months and every three months thereafter, until patients show clinical progression or develop a serious adverse event. All patients were then followed up until death. The assessments included measurement of prostate-specific antigen (PSA) level. PSA is a glycoprotein that is found almost exclusively in normal and neoplastic prostate cells. Serum PSA usually rise in men who have prostate cancer, but also with some infections of the prostate or non-malignant diseases such as benign prostatic hyperplasia. As a consequence, changes in PSA often antedate changes in bone scan, and they have been used as a response indicator in patients with androgen-independent prostate cancer (Kelly *et al.* 1993, Sridhara *et al.* 1995, Smith *et al.* 1998). It is therefore of interest to study more formally to which extent a sequence of PSA measurements can be a valuable surrogate for a patient's survival.

Figure 4.6 shows plots of the individual log-transformed PSA profiles. To avoid overly cluttered plots, profiles were shadowed, and 30 randomly chosen subjects are depicted using darker lines. As can be seen from these plots, the length of the individual sequences of PSA measurements is highly variable across patients, with only a few individuals having very long sequences. Figure 4.7 displays PSA and survival summaries for each trial. The (log-transformed) PSA data were smoothed using the LOESS technique (Cleveland 1979); the survival curves were obtained using the Kaplan-Meier estimator (Kaplan and Meier 1958). Notice the scatter of points in the left-hand plots: most of the subjects had their PSA measurements taken within the first few months after treatment randomization.

In the analyses, country will be used as a grouping unit within each trial in order to have a sufficient number of patients in each unit. This will allow to define 19 groups containing between 3 and 69 patients per group.

4.2.6 Meta-analysis of Five Clinical Trials in Schizophrenia

The data come from a meta-analysis of five double-blind randomized clinical trials, comparing the effects of risperidone to conventional antipsychotic agents for the treatment of chronic schizophrenia. Schizophrenia has long been recognized as a heterogeneous disorder with patients suffering from both "negative" and "positive" symptoms. Negative symptoms are characterized by deficits in cognitive, affective and social functions such as for example poverty of speech, apathy and emotional withdrawal. Positive symptoms entail more florid symptoms such as delusions, hallucinations, and disorganized thinking, which are superimposed on the mental status (Kay, Fiszbein, and Opler 1987).

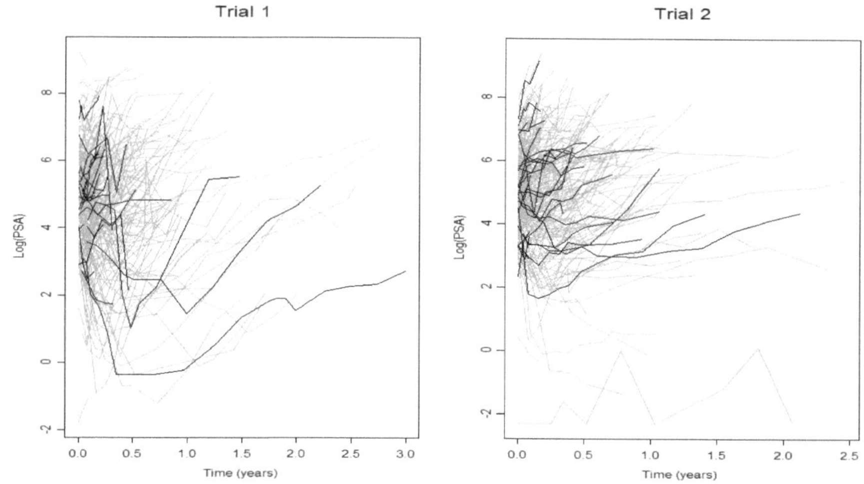

FIGURE 4.6. *Advanced prostate cancer. Individual log-transformed PSA profiles for the liarozole trials (30 randomly chosen subjects are plotted using darker lines).*

Several measures can be considered to assess a patient's global condition. The Clinician's Global Impression (CGI) is generally accepted as a subjective clinical measure of change. Here the CGI overall change versus baseline will be considered. This is a 7-grade scale used by the treating physician to characterize how well a subject has improved since baseline. Other useful and sufficiently sensitive assessment scales are the Positive and Negative Syndrome Scale (PANSS) (Kay, Opler, and Lindenmayer 1988) and the Brief Psychiatric Rating Scale (BPRS) (Overall and Gorham 1962). The PANSS consists of 30 items that provide an operationalized, drug-sensitive instrument, which is highly useful for both typological and dimensional assessment of schizophrenia (Kay, Fiszbein, and Opler 1987). The BPRS is a 19-item scale, essentially derived from the PANSS. Note that both PANSS and CGI are well established scales in psychiatric clinical trials and related research.

Because the package insert in most countries recommends that risperidone is most effective at doses ranging from 4 to 6 mg/day, only patients that received either these doses of risperidone or an active control (haloperidol, levomepromazine, perphenazine, zuclopenthixol) are included in the dataset. Depending on the trial, treatment was administered for a duration of 4 to 8 weeks. For example, in the international trials (INT-2 by Peuskens and the Risperidone Study Group 1995, INT-3 by Chounard, Jones and Remington 1993 and Marder and Meibach 1994, and INT-7 by Hoyberg *et al.* 1993) patients received treatment for 8 weeks; in the study FRA-3 by Blin, Azorin, and Bouhours (1996) patients received treatment

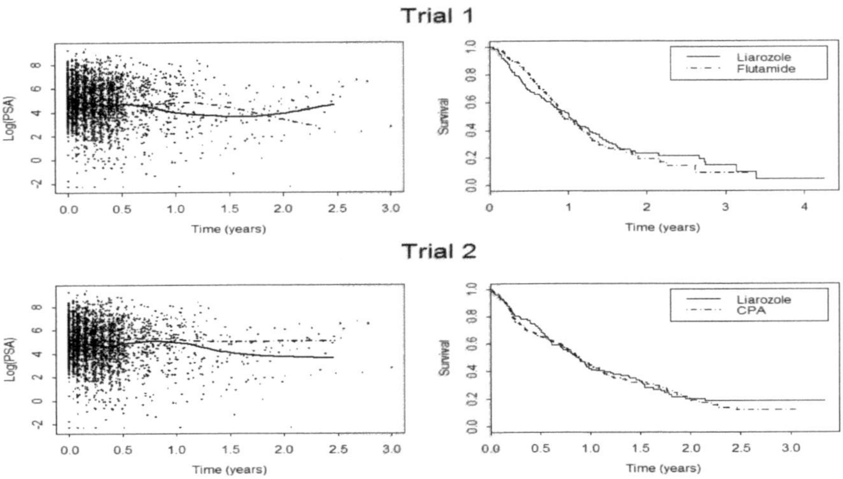

FIGURE 4.7. *Advanced prostate cancer. Longitudinal and event time summaries for the liarozole trials (left: smoothed PSA profiles; right: survival curves).*

TABLE 4.1. *Meta-analysis in Schizophrenia. Number of patients per country.*

Country Id	1	2	3	4	5	6	7	8	9	10
No. patients	31	29	26	44	44	9	37	32	68	49
Country Id	11	12	13	14	15	16	17	18	19	20
No. patients	43	21	25	39	36	17	33	69	30	128

for 4 weeks, while in the study FIN-1 by Huttunen *et al.* (1995) patients were treated over a period of 6 weeks. The sample sizes were 453, 176, 74, 49, and 71, respectively. Measurements were taken at weeks 1, 2, 3, 4, 6, and 8. Our attention will be restricted to the last observed scores during treatment.

Table 4.1 shows the distribution of the number of patients over the 20 country units.

Pooled data from the five trials are presented in Table 4.2. The table shows the binary indicator of global improvement relative to baseline, as measured by CGI (i.e., a CGI score equal to 1 (="very much improved"), 2 (="much improved") or 3 (="minimally improved")), and the binary indicator of a 20% or higher reduction in PANSS score versus baseline. The latter corresponds to a commonly accepted criterion for defining a clinical response (Kay *et al.* 1988). One can observe a strong relationship between both binary indicators (odds ratio, $OR = 31.5$, $\chi^2 = 261.4$, $p < 0.0001$). Note that patients were rated by the same treating physicians on both

TABLE 4.2. *Meta-analysis in Schizophrenia. Pooled data.*

Treatment	PANSS response	CGI-improvement 0	CGI-improvement 1
Active control	0	151 (72%)	58 (28%)
	1	15 (6%)	220 (94%)
Risperidone	0	91 (71%)	37 (29%)
	1	20 (9%)	213 (91%)

scales, thereby bringing some possible contamination bias.

The data contain five trials. In all trials, information is available on the countries where patients were treated, and on the investigators that treated the patients. Depending on the analysis, this information will be used to define groups of patients that will become the units of analysis.

The choice of the unit is an important issue and it is not free of controversy. It can depend on practical considerations, such as the information available in the data set at hand and also on experts' considerations about the most suitable unit for a specific problem. In general, the choice of the unit should be made considering different aspects like physician's opinion, statistical ideas, information available in the data, and so on. Ideally, both the number of units and the number of patients per unit should be sufficiently large to avoid numerical problems (Buyse *et al.* 2000a). For the specific context of schizophrenia, Molenberghs *et al.* (2002) reported a particular instance where choice of units (investigator versus main investigator) has a mild impact only. These authors also compare results from two different trials. Of course, this is only evidence from a particular, though important, example. Cortiñas *et al.* (2004) study a three-level hierarchy (e.g., country, trial, and patient) and the impact on the assessment of surrogacy when either all three levels are used for analysis or when one of the levels is ignored instead.

4.2.7 An Equivalence Trial in Schizophrenia

These data come from an international equivalence trial (INT-10) on schizophrenic patients, described by Nair and the Risperidone Study Group (1998). The trial included 206 schizophrenic patients. All patients received an equal daily amount of risperidone during 8 weeks, but 103 patients were randomized to a one-time daily intake (O.D.), while the remaining 103 patients were randomized to receive risperidone twice a day (B.I.D.). Like

TABLE 4.3. *Equivalence Trial in Schizophrenia. Summary statistics.*

	PANSS		CGI	
	Mean	Median	Mean	Median
Treatment	(s.d.)	(range)	(s.d.)	(range)
One-time daily	−27.55 (31.18)	−27 (177)	2.94 (1.42)	3 (6)
Twice a day	−26.49 (26.79)	−23 (163)	2.90 (1.25)	3 (5)

TABLE 4.4. *Lipid Research Clinics Coronary Primary Prevention Trial. Definite CHD mortality or myocardial infarction according to cholesterol level at 1 year and randomized treatment group (P = Placebo, T = treatment, cholestyramine).*

	At risk* (N)		Events (N)		Events (%)	
Cholesterol (mg/dl)	P	T	P	T	P	T
<180	7	106	0	9	0.0	8.5
[180; 230)	91	675	8	34	8.8	5.0
[230; 280)	1069	742	78	54	7.3	7.3
[280; 330)	636	304	64	23	10.1	7.6
≥330	115	61	18	10	15.7	16.4
Total	1918	1888	168	130	8.8	6.9

* Adjusted for person-years follow-up.

in the previous example, the endpoints of interest will be CGI, PANSS, and BPRS. Similarly, the investigator will be considered as the unit of analysis. A total of 34 units will thus be available for analysis with the number of patients per unit ranging from 2 to 15.

Table 4.3 contains some summary statistics for this trial. There are no strong differences when comparing both arms, which is to be expected as we are dealing with an equivalence trial. Because the response is in terms of change versus baseline, negative mean and median values for the PANSS score are in line with expectation. There are no strong differences between both groups, which is not surprising given the equivalence-trial status of the study. The CGI score exhibits a larger difference between mean and median values, pointing to the likely skew nature of the outcome.

4.2.8 A Clinical Trial in Cardiovascular Disease

These data come from the Lipid Research Clinics Coronary Primary Prevention Trial (Lipid Research Clinics Program 1984, Freedman, Graubard, and Schatzkin 1992). The trial investigated the effect of the drug cholestyramine (Z) on serum cholesterol levels at one year (S) and on cardiovascular events defined as either death from coronary heart disease or occurrence of a myocardial infarction (T). Here, the true endpoint is binary (cardiovascular event or not), while the surrogate endpoint has been categorized into 5 ordered levels ($<$180, [180;230), [230;280), [280;330), $\geq$330 mg/dl). Hence the surrogate can be considered as an ordinal variable or as a continuous variable (due to the non-availability of individual-patient data, the surrogate will be treated as grouped continuous data). The data are presented in Table 4.4.

4.2.9 Acute Migraine: A Meta-analysis of 10 Clinical Trials

This is a meta-analysis of 10 early phase (dose-escalating and dose- ranging) trials assessing the efficacy of several therapies for the treatment of acute migraine crises. Each trial was placebo-controlled and aimed at evaluating one of three experimental treatments. Two trials also had an active control (Sumatriptan) as comparator. Overall, 801 patients were available in this meta-analysis. These were recruited by 38 different centers, with between 1 and 86 patients enrolled per center.

Severity of headache and migraine-related symptoms was measured prior to and at several occasions after dose administration. Severity was rated on a four-grade intensity scale (0 = no, 1 = mild, 2 = moderate, 3 = severe). Clinically relevant endpoints for efficacy include pain-free (pain score = 0) and pain relief (pain score $\leq$1) two hours post-dose. A question one might ask is to which extent symptoms typically associated with migraine episodes, including nausea, vomiting, increased sensitivity to light (photophobia) and sound (phonophobia), are related to the severity of the migraine. Clearly, this question is not peculiar to surrogate endpoint evaluation, but we will see in Chapter 10 that the tools provided in this book may be helpful to better assess the relationship between migraine-related symptoms and migraine severity.

5

The History of Surrogate Endpoint Validation

Geert Molenberghs, Marc Buyse, and Tomasz Burzykowski

5.1 Introduction

Several authors have argued that if a biomarker is to serve as a surrogate for a clinical endpoint, there should be a causal relationship between them (Lagakos and Hoth 1992, Fleming and DeMets 1996). If there were a causal pathway from the surrogate marker to the clinical endpoint, then any change in the marker (e.g., as a result of treatment) would translate into a corresponding change in the clinical endpoint. Causality, unfortunately, is generally extremely difficult to test for, and it ought to be understood that the statistical criteria, developed to validate a surrogate marker, provide indirect evidence only about the causality of the relationship between the marker and the endpoint.

A first source of evidence is provided by the association, at the level of the individual patient, between the marker and the clinical endpoint. One would expect a good surrogate marker to have a strong association with the clinical endpoint at the individual level, reflecting some biological pathway from the biomarker to the clinical endpoint. In that case, the biomarker could be a plausible surrogate on biological grounds, as the clinical endpoint would be largely determined by the biomarker regardless of any treatment effect. This reasoning, although intuitively appealing, has however been shown to be potentially misleading, for a good correlate is not automatically a good surrogate (Fleming and DeMets 1996). Another source of evidence is needed to quantify the association, at the level of a trial, between the effects of a treatment on the marker and on the clinical endpoint. The distinction between these two levels of evidence has become essential, but has sometimes been missed in attempts to validate surrogate markers in the past (Jacobson *et al.* 1991).

Thus, before a surrogate can replace a true endpoint, it should be *validated* or, more modestly or more realistically, *evaluated.* Several formal methods for this purpose have been proposed (Prentice 1989, Freedman, Graubard, and Schatzkin 1992, Daniels and Hughes 1997, Buyse and Molenberghs 1998, Begg and Leung 2000, Buyse *et al.* 2000a, Gail *et al.* 2000). With the statistical methods available, it ought to be possible to conduct a formal investigation on the quality of various endpoints used as surrogates in clinical practice. Such an investigation can shed light on the feasibility of the use of these endpoints and guide the regulatory agencies, e.g., in the choice of the endpoints that can be used for accelerated approval of investigational drugs. It should be kept in mind that a quantitative evaluation is important but is by no means the only component in the decision process leading to the replacement of the true endpoint by the surrogate one. Several parties are involved, including the regulatory agencies (Chapter 2, Section 2.2) and the industry developing a medicinal product.

5.2 Prentice's Definition and Criteria

In his landmark paper, Prentice (1989) formulated a definition of surrogate endpoints, as well as a set of operational criteria for validating a surrogate endpoint.

5.2.1 Definition

Prentice proposed to define a surrogate endpoint as "a response variable for which a test of the null hypothesis of no relationship to the treatment groups under comparison is also a valid test of the corresponding null hypothesis based on the true endpoint" (Prentice 1989). Symbolically, Prentice's definition can be written

$$f(S|Z) = f(S) \Leftrightarrow f(T|Z) = f(T) \qquad (5.1)$$

where $f(X)$ denotes the probability distribution of random variable X and $f(X|Z)$ denotes the probability distribution of X conditional on the value of Z. Note that this definition involves the triplet (T, S, Z), hence the endpoint S is a surrogate for T only with respect to the effect of some specific treatment Z, except if S were a *perfect* surrogate for T, i.e., if S and T were the same endpoint up to a deterministic transformation ($S \equiv T$). The endpoints T and S can be discrete or continuous, possibly censored, random variables. Prentice (1989) focuses on the case in which T is a time-to-failure endpoint.

As such, this definition is of limited value because a direct verification of a triplet (T, S, Z) poses a number of questions regarding availability of data on the triplet, repetition of experiments, etc. Even if many experiments were available, the equivalence of the statistical tests implied in (5.1) might not be true in all of them because of chance fluctuations and/or lack of statistical power. Operational criteria are therefore needed to check if definition (5.1) is fulfilled.

5.2.2 *Prentice's Criteria*

Prentice (1989) proposed four operational criteria to check if a triplet (T, S, Z) fulfills the definition. Symbolically, they can be written as follows:

$$f(S|Z) \neq f(S), \tag{5.2}$$

$$f(T|Z) \neq f(T), \tag{5.3}$$

$$f(T|S) \neq f(T), \tag{5.4}$$

$$f(T|S, Z) = f(T|S). \tag{5.5}$$

In essence, these criteria require that

- treatment has a significant impact on the surrogate endpoint,
- treatment has a significant impact on the true endpoint,
- the surrogate endpoint has a significant impact on the true endpoint,
- the full effect of treatment upon the true endpoint is captured by the surrogate.

Note that (5.2)–(5.4) are formulated in terms of inequality (rejection a null hypothesis), while (5.5) is in terms of an equality (equivalence setting). We will return to this point later in this chapter.

5.2.3 *Example*

The use of Prentice's criteria for the validation of a surrogate endpoint will be illustrated using the data from the age-related macular degeneration trial described in Chapter 4, Section 4.2.1. Recall that in this example, the binary indicator for treatment for patient j (Z_j) is set to 0 for placebo and to 1 for interferon-α. The surrogate endpoint S_j is the change in visual acuity (which we assume to be normally distributed) at 6 months after starting treatment, while the final endpoint T_j is the change in visual acuity at one year. The first two Prentice's criteria (5.2) and (5.3) can be verified by way of tests of significance of parameters α and β in the following model:

$$S_j = \mu_S + \alpha Z_j + \varepsilon_{Sj}, \tag{5.6}$$
$$T_j = \mu_T + \beta Z_j + \varepsilon_{Tj}, \tag{5.7}$$

where the error terms have a joint zero-mean normal distribution with variance-covariance matrix

$$\Sigma = \begin{pmatrix} \sigma_{SS} & \sigma_{ST} \\ & \sigma_{TT} \end{pmatrix}. \tag{5.8}$$

The third criterion (5.4) can be verified using the test for the parameter γ in the model describing the relationship between S and T:

$$T_j = \mu + \gamma S_j + \varepsilon_j. \tag{5.9}$$

Finally, the fourth criterion (5.5), sometimes called "the" Prentice's criterion, is verified through the conditional distribution of the true endpoint, given treatment *and* surrogate endpoint, derived from (5.6)–(5.7):

$$T_j = \tilde{\mu}_T + \beta_S Z_j + \gamma_Z S_j + \tilde{\varepsilon}_{Tj}, \tag{5.10}$$

where

$$\beta_S = \beta - \sigma_{TS}\sigma_{SS}^{-1}\alpha, \tag{5.11}$$
$$\gamma_Z = \sigma_{TS}\sigma_{SS}^{-1}, \tag{5.12}$$

and the variance of $\tilde{\varepsilon}_T$ is given by

$$\sigma_{TT} - \sigma_{TS}^2\sigma_{SS}^{-1}. \tag{5.13}$$

The criterion, at face value, requires that all treatment effect on T is captured by S. In terms of model (5.10) it means that $\beta_S \equiv 0$.

For the age-related macular degeneration data we get $\alpha = -1.90$ (s.e. 1.87, $p = 0.312$), $\beta = -2.88$ (s.e. 2.32, $p = 0.216$), $\gamma = 0.92$ (s.e. 0.06, $p < 0.001$), and $\beta_S = -1.13$ (s.e. 1.57, $p = 0.529$). Of the three first coefficients, only γ is statistically significant (here and in what follows we assume the conventional 0.05 level of significance), and therefore the validation procedure has to stop inconclusively. Note, however, that the lack of statistical significance of α and β could merely be due to the insufficient number of observations available in this trial. Also note that α and β are negative, indicating a negative effect of interferon-α upon visual acuity.

5.2.4 Theoretical Foundations of Prentice's Criteria

The first two criteria (5.2) and (5.3) verify departures from the null hypotheses implicit in (5.1). Strictly speaking, they are not criteria because having both $f(T|Z) = f(T)$ and $f(S|Z) = f(S)$ is consistent with the definition (5.1). However, in such a case, the validation would practically be impossible because one may fail to detect differences due to lack of power. Thus, in practice, the validation requires Z to have an effect on both T and S. Several authors have pointed out that requiring Z to have a statistically significant effect on T may be excessively stringent, for in that case from the limited perspective of significance testing there would no longer be a need to establish the surrogacy of S (Fleming *et al.* 1994).

Buyse and Molenberghs (1998) reproduce the arguments that establish the sufficiency of conditions (5.5) and (5.4) for binary responses. Consider first the condition required for ($\Rightarrow$) to hold in (5.1). By definition, we have

$$f(T|Z) = \int f(T, S|Z)\, dS = \int f(T|S, Z) f(S|Z)\, dS. \tag{5.14}$$

From (5.1) we have $f(S|Z) = f(S)$, and consequently

$$f(T|Z) = \int f(T|S, Z) f(S)\, dS. \tag{5.15}$$

If (5.5) holds, then (5.15) can be written

$$f(T|Z) = \int f(T|S) f(S)\, dS = \int f(T, S)\, dS = f(T)$$

and ($\Rightarrow$) holds in (5.1).

Consider now the condition required for ($\Leftarrow$) to hold in equation (5.1). If condition (5.5) holds, then (5.14) can be rewritten as follows:

$$\begin{aligned} f(T|Z) &= \int f(T|S, Z) f(S|Z)\, dS \\ &= \int f(T|S) f(S|Z)\, dS. \end{aligned} \tag{5.16}$$

Similarly,

$$f(T) = \int f(T|S) f(S)\, dS. \tag{5.17}$$

Because $f(T|Z) = f(T)$, by subtraction of (5.17) from (5.16),

$$\int f(T|S)[f(S|Z) - f(S)]\, dS = 0. \tag{5.18}$$

For a binary surrogate endpoint $S(0,1)$, expression (5.18) reduces to

$$[f(T|S=0) - f(T|S=1)][f(S=1|Z) - f(S=1)] = 0.$$

Hence, a sufficient condition for ($\Leftarrow$) to hold in (5.1) is that $f(T|S=0) \neq f(T|S=1)$, or (5.4).

It is also easy to show that condition (5.4) is always necessary for (5.1), and that condition (5.5) is necessary for binary endpoints but not in general (Buyse *et al.* 2000a). Indeed, assuming that $f(S|Z) = f(S)$, we have (5.15) and (5.17). But if (5.5) does not hold, then (5.15) and (5.17) are in general not equal to one another, in which case the definition (5.1) is violated. It is possible to construct examples where $f(T|Z) = f(T)$, in which case the definition still holds despite the fact that (5.5) does not hold. Hence, (5.5) is not a necessary condition, except for binary endpoints.

Next, assume (5.5) holds but (5.4) does not. Then,

$$f(T|Z) = \int f(T|S)f(S|Z)\,dS = \int f(T)f(S|Z)\,dS = f(T),$$

and hence $f(T|Z) = f(T)$ regardless of the relationship between S and Z. The simplest example is the situation where T is independent of the pair (S,Z). Thus, (5.4) is necessary to avoid situations where one null hypothesis is true while the other one is not. However, criteria (5.2) and (5.3) already imply that both null hypotheses must be rejected, and therefore criterion (5.4) is of no additional value. In fact, criterion (5.4) indicates that the surrogate endpoint has prognostic relevance for the final endpoint, a condition which will obviously be fulfilled by any sensible surrogate endpoint.

Conditions (5.2)–(5.5) are informative and will tend to be fulfilled for valid surrogate endpoints, but they should not be regarded as strict criteria. They are necessary and sufficient to establish the validity of binary surrogate endpoints, but not of more complex surrogate endpoints. The simplest counterexample is found by considering a multi-categorical surrogate endpoint, as illustrated in Table 5.1.

A reflection on Prentice's criteria can be found in Berger (2004). Despite the reservations mentioned above, criterion (5.5) offers an interesting concept of surrogacy by requiring that the treatment is irrelevant for predicting the true outcome, given the surrogate. In the next section, we discuss how Freedman, Graubard, and Schatzkin (1992) used this concept in estimation rather than in testing.

TABLE 5.1. *Relationship between T, S, and Z in an artificial set of data for which $f(T|S) \neq f(T)$, $f(S|Z) \neq f(S)$, and $f(T|S,Z) = f(T|S)$, yet $f(T|Z) = f(T)$. Cell counts represent numbers of patients.*

S, surrogate endpoint	T, true endpoint	Z, treatment	
		$Z=0$	$Z=1$
$S=0$	$T=0$	40	120
	$T=1$	10	30
$S=1$	$T=0$	150	50
	$T=1$	150	50
$S=2$	$T=0$	30	50
	$T=1$	120	200

5.3 Proportion of Treatment Effect Explained by a Surrogate

Freedman, Graubard, and Schatzkin (1992) argued that criterion (5.5) raises a conceptual difficulty in that it requires the statistical test for treatment effect on the true endpoint to be *non*-significant after adjustment for the surrogate. Hence, criterion (5.5) might be useful to *reject* a poor surrogate endpoint (when the statistical test for treatment effect upon the true endpoint remains statistically significant after adjustment for the surrogate), but it is inadequate to *validate* a good surrogate endpoint, for failing to reject the null hypothesis may be due merely to insufficient power. Note that this observation justifies the use of large numbers of observations for the validation of surrogate endpoints. Even if lack of power were not an issue, the statistical significance of the adjusted and unadjusted tests do not adequately quantify the impact of the surrogate on the analysis of the true endpoint. Because it cannot be *proven* that the effect of treatment upon the true endpoint is *fully* captured by the surrogate, Freedman, Graubard, and Schatzkin (1992) proposed to focus attention on the proportion of the treatment effect explained by the surrogate. A good surrogate is one which explains a large proportion of that effect. Schatzkin *et al.* (1990), in their discussion of the validation of intermediate endpoints in cancer, observe that a valid surrogate endpoint for screening purposes is one for which the "attributable proportion" (the proportion of cases with the disease that can be attributed to the intermediate endpoint) is close to one. Freedman's criterion is similar in spirit, but concentrates on the proportion of the treatment effect that can be explained by the surrogate. Let $PE(T,S,Z)$ stand for the proportion of the effect of Z on T which can be explained by S, or simply *proportion explained*. An estimate of $PE(T,S,Z)$ is as follows:

$$PE(T,S,Z) = \frac{\beta - \beta_S}{\beta} = 1 - \frac{\beta_S}{\beta}, \tag{5.19}$$

where β and β_S are the estimates of the effect of Z on T, respectively, without and with adjustment for S. For example, for normally distributed endpoints, β can be obtained from model (5.9), while β_S can be derived from model (5.10).

PE being the ratio of two parameters, its confidence limits can be calculated using Fieller's theorem or the delta method. Using Fieller's theorem, which is generally preferable (Herson 1975), the $(1-\alpha)\%$ confidence limits of $PE(T,S,Z)$ are given by

$$1 - \frac{A \pm \sqrt{A^2 - BC}}{B}, \tag{5.20}$$

where

$$\begin{aligned} A &= \beta\beta_S - Z_\alpha^2 \mathrm{Cov}(\beta, \beta_S), \\ B &= \beta^2 - Z_\alpha^2 \mathrm{Var}(\beta), \\ C &= \beta_S^2 - Z_\alpha^2 \mathrm{Var}(\beta_S), \end{aligned}$$

and Z_α is the $100(1-\alpha/2)$ percentile of the normal distribution (or, if n were not large enough, of the Student's t distribution with $n-1$ degrees of freedom). The variances of the parameter estimates, $\mathrm{Var}(\beta)$ and $\mathrm{Var}(\beta_S)$ are easily obtained by fitting the unadjusted and adjusted models (5.9) and (5.10), respectively. To determine the covariance between β and β_s, the suggestion of Freedman, Graubard, and Schatzkin (1992) can be followed.

5.3.1 Example

For the age-related macular degeneration data we get $\beta = -2.88$ (s.e. 2.32) and $\beta_s = -1.13$ (s.e. 1.57). Freedman's proportion explained is calculated as $PE = 0.61$ (95% delta-method-based confidence limits $[-0.19, 1.41]$). As we can see, the confidence limits are wide and cover the entire $[0,1]$ interval to which, in principle, a proportion should be limited. This illustrates the remarks about the precision of estimating PE made earlier.

5.3.2 *Properties of the Proportion of Treatment Effect Explained by a Surrogate*

Freedman, Graubard, and Schatzkin (1992) observe that if the treatment effect upon the true endpoint is small, and if in addition the number of observations is not large (as is the case in most randomized clinical trials), the confidence interval of PE will be wide, so there will be substantial uncertainty about the proportion of the effect that is truly mediated by the surrogate. This observation justifies the use of large randomized trials, or a meta-analysis of many related trials, to validate surrogate endpoints. Even when large numbers of observations are available, however, the denominator of the proportion explained (the effect of treatment upon the true endpoint) will be estimated with little precision, for otherwise the need for a surrogate endpoint would no longer exist. Therefore, the proportion explained will generally be too poorly estimated to be of much practical value. This conclusion has been recently supported by the results obtained by Freedman (2001). He reported that, to achieve 80% power for a test of the hypothesis that the surrogate explains more than 50% of treatment effect, the ratio $\beta/\text{SE}(\hat{\beta})$ should equal 5 or more. As noted by Freedman (2001), this requirement makes the use of PE practically infeasible.

Another complication arises when (5.10) is not the correct conditional model, and an interaction term between Z and S needs to be included, as in the following model:

$$T = \breve{\mu}_T + \breve{\beta}_S Z + \breve{\rho}_Z S + \delta ZS + \breve{\varepsilon}_T. \qquad (5.21)$$

With this model, PE ceases to have a single interpretation and the validation process would have to stop (Freedman, Graubard, and Schatzkin 1992).

The poor properties of PE result from a fundamental problem with its definition. In the next section, the problem is explored in more detail by investigating the relationship between PE and other quantities of interest. We will return to issues, common to all single-trial validation efforts, in Section 5.5.

5.4 Relative Effect and Adjusted Association

For a surrogate endpoint to be useful in practice, the investigators must be able to *predict* the effect of treatment upon the true endpoint based on the observed effect of treatment upon the surrogate. Thus, we need to relate the magnitude of the treatment effects upon the true and surrogate endpoints

(Boissel *et al.* 1992). A new treatment could then be tested through its effect on the surrogate endpoint and declared efficacious if its predicted effect on the true endpoint were sufficiently large to be of clinical interest (Ellenberg 1991).

Following this reasoning, Buyse and Molenberghs (1998) suggested to calculate another quantity for the validation of a surrogate endpoint: the *relative effect* (RE), which is the ratio of the effects of treatment upon the final and the surrogate endpoint. Using (5.6)–(5.8), RE is formally defined as follows:

$$RE(T, S, Z) = \frac{\beta}{\alpha}. \tag{5.22}$$

Intuitively, RE is the slope of a regression line between β and α, which has been suggested by other authors (A'Hern *et al.* 1988). If the multiplicative relation (5.22) could be assumed, and if RE were known exactly, it could be used to predict the effect of Z on T based on an observed effect of Z on S. In practice, RE will have to be estimated, and the precision of the estimation will be relevant for the precision of the prediction.

RE associates the effects of Z on T and on S averaged over all subjects. RE will be equal to 1 if the effects of Z on T and on S are of identical magnitude. In such a case, Buyse and Molenberghs (1998) proposed to call a surrogate *"perfect at the population level."* In practice, RE will tend be less than 1 if the true endpoint is more difficult to affect than the surrogate endpoint.

Similarly to PE, RE is a ratio of two parameters. Its confidence limits can thus be calculated using Fieller's theorem or the delta method (Buyse and Molenberghs 1998).

Buyse and Molenberghs (1998) argued further that it might be of interest to also derive the association between S and T after adjustment for the treatment Z, which they termed the *adjusted association* and denoted by ρ_Z. For normally distributed endpoints, the adjusted association is defined as follows:

$$\rho_Z = \frac{\sigma_{ST}}{\sqrt{\sigma_{SS}\sigma_{TT}}}, \tag{5.23}$$

where σ_{ST}, σ_{SS} and σ_{TT} are the elements of matrix Σ given in (5.8). It follows that, if $\rho_Z = 1$, there is a deterministic relationship between S and Z. In such a case, one could call the surrogate *"perfect at the individual level,"* as the knowledge of S and Z would allow for an exact prediction of the value of T for an individual subject. In practice, however, perfection is beyond reach and it is then important to judge, for a given situation, whether the correlation is considered high enough for the surrogate to be trustworthy.

5.4.1 Example

For the age-related macular degeneration trial, the relative effect is $RE = 1.51$ (the delta-method-based 95% C.I.: $[-0.46, 3.49]$), while the adjusted association $\rho_Z = 0.74$ (95% C.I.: $[0.68, 0.81]$). The adjusted association is determined rather precisely, but the confidence limits of RE are too wide to convey any useful information.

5.4.2 Properties of Relative Effect and Adjusted Association and Further Problems

For normally distributed endpoints, a very interesting, simple relationship can be derived between PE, RE, and ρ_Z. Following Molenberghs *et al.* (2002), define $\lambda^2 = \sigma_{TT}\sigma_{SS}^{-1}$. It follows that $\lambda\rho_Z = \sigma_{ST}\sigma_{SS}^{-1}$ and, from (5.11), $\beta_S = \beta - \rho_Z\lambda\alpha$. As a result, using definition (5.19) of PE, we obtain

$$PE = \lambda\rho_Z\frac{\alpha}{\beta} = \lambda\rho_Z\frac{1}{RE}. \tag{5.24}$$

Essentially the same result was developed by Buyse and Molenberghs (1998) and Begg and Leung (2000) for standardized normally distributed endpoints S and T.

The relationship (5.24) indicates that PE amalgamates three sources of information:

- the adjusted association ρ_Z, which is a measure of association between the surrogate and the true endpoints *at the individual level*;
- the RE, which expresses the relationship between the treatment effects on the surrogate and the true endpoint *at the trial level*;
- the variance ratio λ^2, which is a nuisance parameter, not to be viewed as a useful validation measure.

In particular, it is clear that, depending on a particular combination of values of ρ_Z, RE, and λ^2, any value of PE on the real line can be obtained (Molenberghs *et al.* 2002; see also Section 5.5). Hence, as it has been already mentioned and in spite of its relative popularity (Li, Meredith, and Hoseyni 2001, Wang and Taylor 2002, and Chen, Wang, and Snapinn 2003), PE cannot be treated as a proportion, which complicates its interpretation. On the other hand, interpretation of RE is not restricted to any particular range of values.

Based on the decomposition (5.24), Buyse and Molenberghs (1998) suggested to replace PE by the pair (RE, ρ_Z). The two measures allow to get more insight into the properties of a surrogate than PE. The relative effect RE is a useful quantity to predict the effect of treatment upon the true endpoint, having observed the effect of treatment upon the surrogate endpoint. If RE is estimated precisely, then the predicted effect upon the true endpoint will in turn be precise enough to be useful.

Additionally, one would expect a good surrogate to have strong association with the true endpoint *within* individuals, hopefully reflecting some biological pathway from the surrogate endpoint to the true endpoint (Buyse and Molenberghs 1998). Such an association could be captured by ρ_Z. A large value would provide indirect evidence that the surrogate is plausible on biological grounds, as the true endpoint would then be largely determined by the surrogate endpoint regardless of any treatment effect. Of course, such evidence should ideally be supplemented with genuine biological evidence and further work in this area is needed (Albert *et al.* 1997).

In practice, the use of RE and ρ_Z to validate surrogate endpoints is also complicated by a few problems. As noted by Buyse and Molenberghs (1998), the confidence intervals for RE can be wide. This difficulty can be overcome by sufficiently large sample sizes, though. More importantly, however, in order to use the estimate of RE for predicting the treatment effect on T for a new trial (given the effect on S), it is necessary to assume that the relationship between the treatment effects on the surrogate and the true endpoints is multiplicative (Buyse and Molenberghs 1998, Buyse *et al.* 2000a, Molenberghs *et al.* 2002). This assumption may be untenable in practice, and it cannot be checked using data from a single trial. To verify the assumption Buyse and Molenberghs (1998) suggested the use of data from multiple randomized trials.

The use of meta-analytic data in the validation of surrogate endpoints to increase the accuracy of the validation process (for example, to reduce Type II error in testing the Prentice's criteria, or to increase the precision of the estimation of PE or RE) was also postulated by other authors (Freedman, Graubard, and Schatzkin 1992, Lin, Fleming, and DeGruttola 1997, Albert *et al.* 1997). Moreover, it was suggested by Albert *et al.* (1997) and Daniels and Hughes (1997) from the point of view of getting more insight through the modeling of the relationship between the surrogate and the true endpoints. It appears that, while the concept of PE is difficult to generalize to a meta-analytic setting (Molenberghs *et al.* 2002), such a generalization can easily be formulated for RE and ρ_Z and it was proposed by Buyse *et al.* (2000a). This is the basis of the meta-analytic approach to the validation of surrogate endpoints, which will be discussed in Chapter 7 and subsequent chapters.

5.5 Further Problems with Single-trial Validation Measures

Let us discuss some further problems with the single-trial validation measures PE, RE, and adjusted association.

Expression (5.24) allows us to make several useful observations. It is clear from (5.24) that the PE is *not* a proportion. Indeed, each of λ and RE can take values over the entire real line.

The fact that the PE is ill defined, except in trivial cases, and the relationship between the three measures introduced above, will be studied by means of three thought experiments. The first two experiments concentrate on "perfect" conditions, while the last one focuses on general conditions.

Thought Experiment 1. The PE is obviously equal to one in simple situations of perfect surrogacy, for instance if T is linearly related to S ($T = aS + b$), for then (5.6) and (5.7) can be rewritten as

$$S_j = \mu_S + \alpha Z_j + \varepsilon_{Sj}, \quad (5.25)$$
$$T_j = b + a\mu_S + a\alpha Z_j + a\varepsilon_{Sj}, \quad (5.26)$$

and obviously $\rho_Z = 1$, $\lambda = a$ and $RE = a$. Other simple situations are discussed by Day and Duffy (1996).

However, it is possible to construct examples where PE can be chosen to take any arbitrary (positive) value, depending on the values of ρ_Z, λ, and RE. To this end we conduct two further thought experiments.

Thought Experiment 2. Assume $\rho_Z = 1$ and $RE = 1$, and suppose further that we could reduce (increase) the variance of the surrogate endpoint while keeping all other quantities unaffected, say by improving (deteriorating) the precision of its measurement. Then, (5.6)–(5.7) would become

$$S_j = \mu_S + \alpha Z_j + \varepsilon_{Sj}, \quad (5.27)$$
$$T_j = \mu_S + \alpha Z_j + \lambda\varepsilon_{Sj}. \quad (5.28)$$

λ is arbitrary and hence so is PE, despite the fact that (5.27)–(5.28) describe a very desirable situation. The key behind this somewhat artificial and counterintuitive thought experiment is that the systematic components are kept constant, the random error terms are in *perfect* correlation. Then, knowledge about the surrogate endpoint enables exact prediction of the true endpoint: $E[T_j|Z_j, S_j] = T_j$.

Now, we would like to call the situation described by (5.27)–(5.28) "perfect," even though PE may not be equal to one, nor β_S equal to zero.

This casts doubts on the fourth Prentice criterion, which states that the full effect of treatment should be captured by the surrogate, even though this criterion has much intuitive appeal. In the above example, the true endpoint, conditionally on treatment and surrogate endpoint, is

$$T_j = \tilde{\mu}_T + \alpha(1-\lambda)Z_j + \lambda S_j, \tag{5.29}$$

which shows that the true endpoint does depend on treatment, although the residual, unexplained, variability in the true endpoint has been eliminated. In other words, in this perfect situation (at the individual level), (5.13) vanishes, which is equivalent to stating that $\rho_Z = 1$. This suggests to focus on the adjusted association, rather than on the adjusted treatment effect upon the true endpoint. Note that perfection in this context has no implication for the surrogate *across trials*. To study the latter very important quality it is necessary to turn to RE or even to a multi-trial setting (Chapter 7, Section 7.2).

Thought Experiment 3. We will now switch to general conditions and consider two transformations of the surrogate endpoint:

$$S_j^{(1)} = \phi S_j + \psi = (\phi\mu_S + \psi) + \phi\alpha Z_j + \phi\varepsilon_{Sj}, \tag{5.30}$$

$$S_j^{(2)} = \mu_S + \alpha Z_j + \phi\varepsilon_{Sj}. \tag{5.31}$$

It is important to realize that the second transformation is counterfactual. It cannot be conducted through a simple transformation of a dataset variable, but should rather be viewed as an experiment conducted in a parallel world. It might refer to a situation in a sequence of trials where at some point the measurement precision changes due to a change in instrument.

Transformation (5.30) operates on the fixed and random parts of the surrogate endpoint alike, whereas transformation (5.31) operates on the random part only. The second transformation is similar to one in the second thought experiment, except that we now consider the general rather than the perfect situation. It is easy to show that the following relationships hold between the validation measures:

$$RE^{(1)} = RE/\phi, \qquad \rho_Z^{(1)} = \rho_Z, \qquad \lambda^{(1)} = \lambda/\phi, \qquad PE^{(1)} = PE,$$

$$RE^{(2)} = RE, \qquad \rho_Z^{(2)} = \rho_Z, \qquad \lambda^{(2)} = \lambda/\phi, \qquad PE^{(2)} = PE/\phi,$$

with obvious notation. Thus, for transformation (5.30) there is no impact on the PE, but under (5.31), PE is rescaled with an arbitrary amount.

There are also problems with the RE. Indeed, although the adjusted association expresses agreement between both endpoints at the individual level, the trialist will want to know how the *trial-specific* treatment effect on T can be predicted from the treatment effect on S. RE serves this purpose, but it is typically based on information from only one trial. It might not be constant for all trials testing the therapeutic question under consideration. The constancy of RE implies that the relation between α and β is linear through the origin. This assumption may be untenable in practice, and it cannot be verified from a single trial. Therefore, it will prove useful to adopt an alternative definition of surrogacy based on a meta-analysis of several trials.

Another motivation for a multi-trial approach is the issue of measurement error. It can be misleading to assume the surrogate is measured without error, whereas in practice appreciable measurement error occurs in a number of frequently used surrogates (tumor size, CD4 count, ...).

5.6 Discussion

The classical approach to surrogate marker validation, based on Prentice's criteria and measures derived there from, such as the proportion explained and the relative effect, is surrounded with difficulties when applied at face value. Rather, the value of the Prentice-Freedman framework lies in the fact that it started a whole area of research in quantitative evaluation of surrogate endpoints. Freedman, Graubard, and Schatzkin (1992) have brought parameter estimation as an important supplement to the hypothesis testing based proposal of Prentice (1989).

The PE attempts to capture the concept that the treatment effect on the true endpoint is fully explained by the surrogate. In doing so, it focuses on the conditional regression coefficient of the treatment indicator (β_S) and requires that $\beta_S = 0$, or equivalently that $PE = 1$. Unfortunately, this approach fails because it does not appropriately distinguish between different sources of variability. PE is in fact an amalgamation of three quantities: the trial-level relative effect, the individual-level adjusted association, and a nuisance factor related to the ratio of variances of the true and surrogate endpoints. This conceptual difficulty is more worrisome than the confidence interval of PE which, as pointed out by many authors, tends to be too wide to be useful, unless trial sizes are very large or the treatment effect on the true endpoint is very strong (Freedman, Graubard, and Schatzkin 1992).

It seems more meaningful to view the problem from a hierarchical (or, multilevel, or, meta-analytic) point of view. At the individual level, one might focus on the residual variability of the conditional regression of T on S and Z, which is captured by the individual-level adjusted association between the surrogate and true endpoints. If that residual variability vanishes, then knowledge of the surrogate endpoint and treatment indicator allows one to predict the true endpoint without error, which we consider to be a perfect situation (at the individual level).

At the trial level, one might focus on the prediction of the effect of treatment on the true endpoint given its effect on the surrogate endpoint. The quantity aiming at the prediction is RE, the effect of treatment on the true endpoint relative to that on the surrogate endpoint. When only one trial is available, however, an estimate of RE is based on the strong assumption that the relationship between the treatment effects on the surrogate and true endpoints is multiplicative, an assumption that may be too strong to hold and is unverifiable. Again, this difficulty is more fundamental than the limited precision of RE that will typically be obtained in trials of small or moderate size (Buyse and Molenberghs 1998).

A meta-analytic framework is developed in Chapter 7 and subsequent chapters.

6

Validation Using Single-trial Data: Mixed Binary and Continuous Outcomes

Helena Geys

6.1 Introduction

Chapter 5 describes the *RE* and adjusted association, two measures introduced by Buyse and Molenberghs (1998) to assess the quality of a surrogate with single-trial data. They considered the case where both endpoints are of the same data type and suggested a bivariate logistic model for binary endpoints and a bivariate normal model for continuous outcomes.

This chapter describes how the proposals of *RE* and adjusted association (Buyse and Molenberghs 1998) can be extended to cases where the surrogate and the true endpoints are of a different data type (Molenberghs, Geys, and Buyse 2001). First, the theory for binary endpoints is extended to the case of ordinal endpoints, using the Dale model (Dale 1986). Next, the case of mixed binary-continuous endpoints is handled, for which two modeling strategies are proposed. Indeed, the joint distribution of a mixed continuous–discrete outcome vector can always be expressed as the product of the marginal distribution of one of the responses and the conditional distribution of the remaining response given the former response. One can choose either the continuous or the discrete outcome for the marginal model (Olkin and Tate 1961, Cox 1972b, Little and Schluchter 1985, Zeger and Liang 1991, Catalano and Ryan 1992, Cox and Wermuth 1992Fitzmaurice and Laird 1995). The main problem with such approaches is that no easy expressions for the association between both endpoints are obtained. Therefore, Molenberghs, Geys, and Buyse (2001) opted for a more symmetric treatment of the two outcome variables. They treated the case where the surrogate is binary and the true endpoint is continuous. The reverse case is entirely similar.

6.2 Ordinal Endpoints

6.2.1 The Dale Model

Dale (1986) considered a model for bivariate ordinal outcomes. Suppose that S_j and T_j are ordinal random variables observed on N subjects, with levels $0, 1, \ldots, r_S$ and $0, 1, \ldots, r_T$, respectively, and assume the following model:

$$\eta_{jk_T1} = \ln\left(\frac{P(T_j > k_T|Z_j)}{P(T_j \leq k_T|Z_j)}\right) = \mu_{ZT}(k_T) + \beta Z_j, \tag{6.1}$$

$$\eta_{jk_S2} = \ln\left(\frac{P(S_j > k_S|Z_j)}{P(S_j \leq k_S|Z_j)}\right) = \mu_{ZS}(k_S) + \alpha Z_j, \tag{6.2}$$

$$\begin{aligned}\eta_{jk_Tk_S3} &= \ln \psi_{jk_Sk_T} \\ &= \ln\left(\frac{P(S_j \leq k_S, T_j \leq k_T|Z_j)P(S_j > k_S, T_j > k_T|Z_j)}{P(S_j \leq k_S, T_j > k_T|Z_j)P(S_j > k_S, T_j \leq k_T|Z_j)}\right) \\ &= \mu_{STZ} + \delta Z_j, \end{aligned} \tag{6.3}$$

($j = 1, \ldots, N; k_S = 0, \ldots, r_S - 1; k_T = 0, \ldots, r_T - 1$). The proportional odds logistic regression models (6.1) and (6.2) generalize ordinary logistic regression. In Section 6.2.2, it will be illustrated that the treatment effects β and α can vary with the levels of (k_T, k_S). The function $\psi_{jk_Tk_S}$ is called the "global odds ratio" at cutpoint (k_S, k_T). It may be interpreted as the ratio of the odds of the conditional events $\{S_j \leq k_S|T_j \leq k_T, Z_j\}$ versus $\{S_j \leq k_S|T_j > k_T, Z_j\}$. One of the interesting features of this model is that the interpretation of the parameters is invariant if one collapses S_j or T_j over adjacent categories. The relative effect, defined by (5.22), is $RE = \beta/\alpha$ (Molenberghs, Geys, and Buyse 2001).

Maximum likelihood estimates for the parameter vector $\boldsymbol{\nu} = (\boldsymbol{\mu}, \beta, \alpha, \rho)^T$ are found by solving the score equations

$$\mathbf{U}(\boldsymbol{\nu}) = \sum_{j=1}^{N} X_j^T D_j^T V_j^{-1} \boldsymbol{E}_j = \mathbf{0}, \tag{6.4}$$

where X_j is a design matrix reflecting the right hand sides of (6.1)–(6.3),

$$D_j = \left(\frac{\partial \boldsymbol{\eta}_j}{\partial \boldsymbol{\pi}_j}\right)^{-1},$$

V_j is the joint covariance matrix of the binary indicators $S_j = k_S$, $T_j = k_T$, ($k_S = 0, \ldots, r_S - 1; k_T = 0, \ldots, r_T - 1$), and $\boldsymbol{\pi}_j$ is a vector of cell probabilities to be defined in the sequel. Finally, $\boldsymbol{E}_j$ is the vector of differences between observed and expected values of these indicators. The expected values follow directly from $\pi_{jk_Tk_S} = P(S_j = k_S, T_j = k_T|Z_j)$. All quantities needed to evaluate $U(\boldsymbol{\nu})$ are determined from $\boldsymbol{\nu}$. Indeed, $\boldsymbol{\nu}$ determines $\boldsymbol{\eta}_j$,

$$\begin{aligned}\pi_{jk_T+} &= \frac{\exp(\eta_{jk_T1})}{1+\exp(\eta_{jk_T1})},\\ \pi_{j+k_S} &= \frac{\exp(\eta_{jk_S2})}{1+\exp(\eta_{jk_S2})},\end{aligned}$$

and

$$\pi_{jk_Tk_S} = \begin{cases} \frac{1+(\pi_{jk_T+}+\pi_{j+k_S})\psi^\star_{jk_Sk_T} - C(\pi_{jk_T+},\pi_{j+k_S},\psi^\star_{jk_Tk_S})}{2\psi^\star_{jk_Tk_S}} & \text{if } \psi^\star_{jk_Tk_S} \neq 0, \\ \pi_{jk_T+}\pi_{j+k_S} & \text{if } \psi^\star_{jk_Tk_S} = 0, \end{cases} \tag{6.5}$$

where $\psi^\star_{jk_Tk_S} = \psi_{jk_Tk_S} - 1$ and

$$C(q_1, q_2, \psi^\star) = \sqrt{[1+(q_1+q_2)\psi^\star]^2 - 4(\psi^\star+1)\psi^\star q_1 q_2}. \tag{6.6}$$

Expression (6.5) was studied by Plackett (1965) and Mardia (1970). To estimate the covariance matrix of $\boldsymbol{\nu}$, one calculates the matrix of second derivatives of the log-likelihood, i.e., the derivative of $\mathbf{U}(\boldsymbol{\nu})$ and replaces $\boldsymbol{\nu}$ by its maximum likelihood estimate $\hat{\boldsymbol{\nu}}$. The standard error of RE, and hence a 95% confidence interval, is calculated by applying the delta method to the covariance matrix. Details can be found in Molenberghs and Lesaffre (1994, 1995).

Should one want to determine PE, as defined in (5.19), we need to supplement logistic regression (6.1) with

$$\ln\left(\frac{P(T_j > k_T|Z_j, S_j)}{P(T_j \leq k_T|Z_j, S_j)}\right) = \mu_{ZT|S}(k_T) + \beta_S Z_j + \tilde{\gamma}_Z S_j, \tag{6.7}$$

$(k_T = 0, \ldots, r_T - 1)$. The method of Freedman, Graubard, and Schatzkin (1992) to determine the confidence interval for PE is also applicable to the ordinal case. Model (6.7) includes only the linear trend of the ordinal variable S. If this is thought inappropriate, S_j can be included as a qualitative variable (then involving r_S nuisance parameters).

The adjusted association is given by (6.3), with $\eta_{jk_Tk_S3} = \ln\psi_{jk_Sk_T}$. In order to be useful, a constant association needs to be assumed, i.e., $\eta_{jk_Tk_S3} = \mu_{STZ}$.

6.2.2 Application: A Cardiovascular Disease Trial

In this section data are analyzed from a cardiovascular disease trial, described in Section 4.2.8.

Using the data in Table 4.4, we find, in accordance with Freedman, Graubard, and Schatzkin (1992), $\beta = 0.26$ (standard error, s.e. 0.12, $p = 0.0318$), $\beta_S = 0.13$ (s.e. 0.13, $p = 0.3283$), and $\alpha = 1.55$ (s.e. 0.067, $p < 0.0001$). The estimate of PE is 0.50 (95% confidence interval, C.I., $[0.07, 5.91]$) and thus, if we wanted to interpret the PE, cholesterol levels would explain half of the effect of cholestyramine on cardiovascular events. However, the confidence limits of PE are very wide. The estimate of RE is 0.17 (95% C.I. $[0.02, 0.33]$). RE can here be interpreted as follows: the reduction in the odds of a cardiovascular event under cholestyramine is about one sixth of the reduction in the odds of a shift to a lower class of cholesterol with that treatment. Should this value sustain over a class of treatments, then confidence could be put in cholesterol as a surrogate marker, and the benefit of a future treatment on cardiovascular events could be predicted based on its effect on cholesterol levels. This observation points, once more, to the need of a meta-analytic validation framework (Chapter 7). The adjusted log odds ratio is 0.41 (95% C.I. $[0.19, 0.63]$). The corresponding odds ratio is 1.50. This implies a weak but significant association between the surrogate and the true endpoint after correcting for treatment.

The Dale model used to calculate the RE shows severe lack of fit, with a Pearson's χ^2 statistic equal to 222.9 on 10 degrees of freedom. The two potential causes for model misspecification are that (1) the association function $\eta_{k_T k_S 3}$ depends on the level of S, i.e., the global odds ratio depends on the point at which the ordinal surrogate endpoint is dichotomized; or (2) the proportional odds assumption for the marginal logistic regression of S on Z is not valid. Changing the constant global odds ratio to an odds ratio function yields a χ^2 value of 212.6 on 6 degrees of freedom, hardly a better fit than with a constant global odds ratio. Most of the lack of fit is therefore due to a departure from the proportional odds assumption. Indeed, a model with 4 treatment indicators for the regression of Z on S, 1 indicator for Z on T (as T is binary), and a single constant odds ratio, yields $\chi^2 = 11.09$ on 7 degrees of freedom, a very acceptable fit. Four relative effects are estimated with this model, as the relationship between S and Z is now expressed by 4 treatment indicators, as shown in Table 6.1.

The increase of RE with cholesterol level implies that a drug that is active at the highest levels of cholesterol can be expected to have a larger impact on cardiovascular events than one that is equally active at lower levels. This implies that RE becomes a cutoff dependent conversion factor, thereby reducing its simplicity (but not its relevance). A direct test for the

TABLE 6.1. *Cardiovascular Trial. Estimates of the treatment effect on the surrogate* (α) *and of the relative effects (RE, with 95% confidence limits) in a model with 4 treatment indicators for the regression of treatment (cholestyramine) on the surrogate endpoint (cholesterol levels) and one indicator for the regression of treatment on the true endpoint (cardiovascular events) (Lipid Research Clinics Program 1984).*

Indicator	α	RE	95% C.I.
$<180/\geq180$	2.79	0.09	$[0.01; 0.19]$
$<230/\geq230$	2.57	0.10	$[0.01; 0.19]$
$<280/\geq280$	0.99	0.26	$[0.02; 0.51]$
$<330/\geq330$	0.65	0.40	$[0.04; 1.01]$

heterogeneity in the RE is provided by $222.9 - 11.09 = 211.8$ on 3 degrees of freedom, overwhelmingly significant evidence.

6.3 Mixed Continuous and Binary Endpoints

We now turn attention to the situation where one of the outcomes, the surrogate say, is of a binary type. It is convenient to assume that $\tilde{S}_j$ be a latent variable of which S_j is the dichotomized version. Section 6.3.1 describes a bivariate normal model for $\tilde{S}_j$ and T_j, resulting in a probit-linear model for S_j and T_j. Section 6.3.2 presents an alternative formulation based on the bivariate Plackett (1965) density and resulting in a Plackett-Dale model.

6.3.1 A Probit Formulation

In this formulation, the following model is assumed (Molenberghs, Geys, and Buyse 2001):

$$T_j = \mu_T + \beta Z_j + \varepsilon_{Tj}, \quad (6.8)$$

$$\tilde{S}_j = \mu_S + \alpha Z_j + \varepsilon_{Sj}, \quad (6.9)$$

where μ_S and μ_T are fixed intercepts and α and β are the fixed effects of the treatment Z on the surrogate and true endpoints, respectively. Further,

ε_{Sj} and ε_{Tj} are correlated error terms, assumed to satisfy:

$$\begin{pmatrix} \varepsilon_{Tj} \\ \varepsilon_{Sj} \end{pmatrix} \sim N \left[\begin{pmatrix} 0 \\ 0 \end{pmatrix}, \begin{pmatrix} \sigma^2 & \frac{\rho\sigma}{\sqrt{1-\rho^2}} \\ \frac{\rho\sigma}{\sqrt{1-\rho^2}} & \frac{1}{1-\rho^2} \end{pmatrix} \right]. \tag{6.10}$$

Model (6.8)–(6.9) specifies a bivariate normal density. The variance of $\tilde{S}_j$ is chosen for reasons that will be made clear in the sequel. From this model, it is easily seen that the density of T_j is univariate normal with regression given in (6.8) and variance σ^2, implying that the parameters μ_T, β, and σ^2 can be determined using linear regression software with response T_j and single covariate Z_j. Similarly, the conditional density of $\tilde{S}_j$, given Z_j and T_j is

$$\tilde{S}_j | T_j, Z_j \sim N \left(\lambda_0 + \lambda_Z Z_j + \lambda_T T_j ; 1 \right), \tag{6.11}$$

where

$$\lambda_0 = \mu_S - \frac{\rho}{\sigma\sqrt{1-\rho^2}} \mu_T, \tag{6.12}$$

$$\lambda_Z = \alpha - \frac{\rho}{\sigma\sqrt{1-\rho^2}} \beta, \tag{6.13}$$

$$\lambda_T = \frac{\rho}{\sigma\sqrt{1-\rho^2}}. \tag{6.14}$$

The density in (6.11) has unit variance, motivating the earlier choice for the covariance matrix of T_j and $\tilde{S}_j$. The corresponding probability

$$P(S_j = 1 | T_j, Z_j) = \Phi_1(\lambda_0 + \lambda_Z Z_j + \lambda_T T_j), \tag{6.15}$$

where Φ_1 is the standard normal cumulative density function. Note that (6.15) implicitly defines the cutoff value for the dichotomized version. The λ parameters can be found by fitting model (6.15) to S_j with covariates Z_j and T_j. This can be done with standard logistic regression software if it allows to specify the probit rather than the logit link. Given the parameters from the linear regression on T_j (μ_T, β, and σ^2) and the probit regression on S_j (λ_0, λ_Z, and λ_T), the parameters from the linear regression on $\tilde{S}_j$ can now be obtained from (6.12)–(6.14):

$$\mu_S = \lambda_0 + \lambda_T \mu_T, \tag{6.16}$$

$$\alpha = \lambda_Z + \lambda_T \beta, \tag{6.17}$$

$$\rho^2 = \frac{\lambda_T^2 \sigma^2}{1 + \lambda_T^2 \sigma^2}. \tag{6.18}$$

An asymptotic covariance matrix for the parameters involved can easily be derived by means of the delta method. More explicitly, the asymptotic covariance matrix of the parameters (μ_T, β) can be found from standard linear regression output. The variance of σ^2 equals $2\sigma^4/N$. The asymptotic covariance of $(\lambda_0, \lambda_Z, \lambda_T)$ follows from (probit) regression output. These three statements yield the covariance matrix of the six parameters upon noting that it is block-diagonal. In order to derive the asymptotic covariance of (μ_S, α, ρ) it suffices to calculate the derivatives of (6.16)–(6.18) with respect to the six original parameters and apply the delta method. They are:

$$\frac{\partial(\mu_S, \alpha, \rho)}{\partial(\mu_T, \beta, \sigma^2, \lambda_0, \lambda_Z, \lambda_T)} = \begin{pmatrix} \lambda_T & 0 & 0 & 1 & 0 & \mu_T \\ 0 & \lambda_T & 0 & 0 & 1 & \beta \\ 0 & 0 & h_1 & 0 & 0 & h_2 \end{pmatrix},$$

where

$$\begin{aligned} h_1 &= \frac{1}{2\rho} \frac{\lambda_T^2}{(1 + \lambda_T^2 \sigma^2)^2}, \\ h_2 &= \frac{1}{2\rho} \frac{2\lambda_T \sigma^2}{(1 + \lambda_T^2 \sigma^2)^2}. \end{aligned}$$

In addition, a program needs to be developed that performs the joint estimation directly by maximizing the likelihood based on contributions (6.8) and (6.15).

The adjusted association is given by ρ. The relative effect, $RE = \beta/\alpha$, can be determined directly from the output. Determining confidence intervals using the parameter estimates and their covariance matrix is completely analogous to the route taken in Buyse and Molenberghs (1998).

6.3.2 A Plackett-Dale Formulation

Assume that the cumulative distributions of S_j and T_j are given by F_{S_j} and F_{T_j}. The joint cumulative distribution of both these quantities has been studied by Plackett (1965) and is given by:

$$F_{T_j,S_j} = \begin{cases} \dfrac{1 + (F_{T_j} + F_{S_j})\psi_j^\star - C(F_{T_j}, F_{S_j}, \psi_j^\star)}{2\psi_j^\star} & \text{if } \psi_j^\star \neq 0, \\ F_{T_j} F_{S_j} & \text{if } \psi_j^\star = 0, \end{cases}$$

where $\psi_j^\star$ and C are defined similarly to (6.3) and (6.6). Based upon this distribution function, a bivariate Plackett "density" function $G_j(t, s)$ can be derived for mixed continuous-binary outcomes (Molenberghs, Geys, and Buyse 2001). Suppose the success probability for S_j is denoted by π_j, then $G_j(t, s)$ can be defined by specifying $G_j(t, 0)$ and $G_j(t, 1)$ such that they sum to $f_{T_j}(t)$. If $G_j(t,0)$ is defined as $\partial F_{T_j,S_j}(t,0)/\partial t$, then this leads to specifying G_j by:

$$G_j(t,0) = \begin{cases} \frac{f_{T_j}(t)}{2}\left(1 - \frac{1+F_{T_j}(t)\psi_j^\star - F_{S_j}(s)\left(\psi_j^\star+1\right)}{C\left(F_{T_j},1-\pi_j,\psi_j^\star\right)}\right) & \text{if } \psi_j^\star \neq 0, \\ f_{T_j}(t)(1-\pi_j) & \text{if } \psi_j^\star = 0, \end{cases}$$

and

$$G_j(t,1) = f_{T_j}(t) - G_j(t,0).$$

In this formulation, it is assumed that $T_j \sim N(\mu_j, \sigma^2)$, with $\mu_j = \mu_T + \beta Z_j$ and $\text{logit}(\pi_j) = \mu_S + \alpha Z_j$ with similar notation as in the probit case. The global odds ratio is assumed to be constant. Let

$$\boldsymbol{\theta}_j = \begin{pmatrix} \mu_j \\ \sigma^2 \\ \pi_j \\ \psi \end{pmatrix} \text{ and } \boldsymbol{\eta}_j = \begin{pmatrix} \mu_j \\ \ln(\sigma^2) \\ \text{logit}(\pi_j) \\ \ln(\psi) \end{pmatrix},$$

then estimates of the regression parameters $\boldsymbol{\nu} = (\boldsymbol{\mu}, \beta, \alpha, \ln\sigma^2, \ln\psi)$ are easily obtained by solving the estimating equations $\boldsymbol{U}(\boldsymbol{\nu}) = 0$, using a Newton-Raphson iteration scheme, where $\boldsymbol{U}(\boldsymbol{\nu})$ is given by:

$$\sum_{j=1}^{N} \left(\frac{\partial \boldsymbol{\eta}_j}{\partial \boldsymbol{\nu}}\right)^T \left(\frac{\partial \boldsymbol{\eta}_j}{\partial \boldsymbol{\theta}_j}\right)^{-T} \left(\frac{\partial}{\partial \boldsymbol{\theta}_j} \ln G_j(T_j, S_j)\right).$$

Note that the adjusted association is given by ψ in this case, and the relative effect $RE = \beta/\alpha$ can be readily determined.

6.3.3 Application: A Cardiovascular Disease Trial

In addition to the analyses presented in Section 6.2.2, cholesterol levels could also be considered as a continuous variable in order to estimate RE and the adjusted correlation ρ. This is achieved taking the mid-points 155(50)355 for each category. Molenberghs, Geys, and Buyse (2001) analyze these data with the probit model of Section 6.3.1, where the surrogate is now continuous and the true endpoint is dichotomous. They find $\beta = 0.13$ (s.e. 0.06, $p = 0.0281$) and $\alpha = 32.05$ (s.e. 1.30, $p < 0.0001$). The adjusted correlation is estimated with great precision, $\rho = 0.10$ (95% C.I. $[0.05, 0.16]$). As in Section 6.2.2, it indicates a significant but very small correlation between both endpoints, thus casting some doubts on the individual-level validity of cholesterol levels as a surogate for cardiovascular events. The relative effect is estimated to be $RE = 0.0041$ (95% C.I.

TABLE 6.2. *Age-related Macular Degeneration Trial. Mean (standard error) of visual acuity at baseline, at 6 months, and at 1 year according to randomized treatment group (Buyse and Molenberghs 1998).*

Time point	Placebo	Treatment	Total
Baseline	55.3 (1.4)	54.6 (1.3)	55.0 (1.0)
6 months	49.3 (1.8)	45.5 (1.8)	47.5 (1.3)
1 year	44.4 (1.8)	39.1 (1.9)	42.0 (1.3)

$[0.0004, 0.0078]$). The precision of RE is satisfactory owing to the large sample size ($N = 3806$). Precision of RE is however a necessary but not a sufficient condition for establishing the validity of a surrogate endpoint; indeed one would still need to verify that RE is relatively constant over a class of similar trials (or treatments).

6.3.4 Application: Age-related Macular Degeneration

In this section, the data from the age-related macular degeneration trial described in Section 4.2.1 of Chapter 4 are used. First, dichotomized visual acuity at 6 months is used as the surrogate and (continuous) visual acuity at 12 months as the true endpoint. Table 6.2 shows the visual acuity (mean and standard error) by treatment group at baseline, at 6 months, and at 1 year. Dichotomization is achieved by setting a binary variable to 1 if visual acuity at 6 months is larger than the value at baseline and to 0 otherwise.

Let us first present the results of the probit model as it was presented in Molenberghs, Geys, and Buyse (2001). The parameter estimates for the true endpoint are $\mu_T = 11.04$ (s.e. 1.57), $\beta = 4.12$ (s.e. 2.32, $p = 0.0758$), and $\sigma = 15.95$ (s.e. 0.82). The parameter estimates for the surrogate endpoint are $\mu_S = 0.64$ (s.e. 0.20) and $\alpha = 0.39$ (s.e. 0.28, $p = 0.1637$), and the correlation is $\rho = 0.74$ (s.e. 0.05). Note that the parameter estimates for the true endpoint coincide with those in Buyse and Molenberghs (1998), who employed a bivariate normal model for the case where both outcomes are continuous. The relative effect is estimated to be $RE = 10.44$ (95% C.I. $[-1.77, 22.65]$) and the adjusted correlation $\rho = 0.74$ (95% C.I. $[0.64, 0.84]$). Although care has to be taken with the RE as both numerator and denominator are non-significant (leading to a Fieller confidence interval equal to the whole real line), the adjusted correlation is estimated very precisely, and there is clearly a strong correlation between both endpoints. Buyse and Molenberghs (1998) found an adjusted correlation of 0.74 (95% C.I. $[0.68, 0.81]$) which agrees remarkably well with our results. The slightly wider standard error results from the loss of information through dichotomizing the surrogate endpoint.

Molenberghs, Geys, and Buyse (2001) next analyzed the same data using the Plackett-Dale model. The parameter estimates for the true endpoint are $\mu_T = 10.89$ (s.e. 1.56), $\beta = 4.02$ (s.e. 2.32, $p = 0.0831$), and $\sigma = 16.04$ (s.e. 0.81). These results are relatively close to the ones obtained with the probit model, as in both cases a linear regression of T on Z is assumed. The binary regression of S on T and Z contains additional information about the true endpoint parameters as well, which is why the results are not exactly equal. The values for the surrogate endpoint are $\mu_S = 0.74$ (s.e. 0.19) and $\alpha = 0.45$ (s.e. 0.30, $p = 0.1336$) and the log odds ratio $\ln \psi = 2.85$ (s.e. 0.37) with corresponding odds ratio 17.29. The relative effect is estimated to be $RE = 8.92$ (95% C.I. $[-0.41, 18.25]$), in close agreement with the above estimate. Although the adjusted association is relatively large, providing good auxiliary support for surrogacy, the RE is estimated with low precision, indicating that the sample size is too small to conclude on the quality of the surrogate.

Finally, Molenberghs, Geys, and Buyse (2001) considered the more interesting situation of (continuous) visual acuity at 6 months as a surrogate for the binary indicator for loss of at least 3 lines of vision lost at one year. With the probit model, the regression coefficients (standard errors) for the true endpoint are $\mu_T = -0.36$ (s.e. 0.21), $\beta = 0.60$ (s.e. 0.30, $p = 0.0475$). The values for the surrogate endpoint are $\mu_S = 5.53$ (s.e. 1.26), $\alpha = 2.83$ (s.e. 1.87, $p = 0.1287$), and $\sigma = 12.80$ (s.e. 0.66). The correlation is $\rho = 0.81$ (s.e. 0.04). The relative effect is estimated to be $RE = 4.75$ (95% C.I. $[-5.11, 14.61]$). With the Plackett-Dale model, the regression coefficients (standard errors) for the true endpoint are $\mu_T = -0.36$ (s.e. 0.19), $\beta = 0.58$ (s.e. 0.28, $p = 0.0365$), and $\sigma = 12.90$ (s.e. 0.65). The values for the surrogate endpoint are $\mu_S = 5.89$ (s.e. 1.24) and $\alpha = 2.72$ (s.e. 1.84, $p = 0.1403$) and the log odds ratio $\ln \psi = 2.83$ (s.e. 0.29) with corresponding odds ratio 16.93. The relative effect is estimated to be $RE = 4.67$ (95% C.I. $[-5.00, 14.35]$). Qualitatively, the same conclusions are reached as to the surrogacy of the continuous measurement at 6 months for a dichotomized true endpoint.

6.4 Discussion

In this chapter, we have presented an extension of the approach proposed in Buyse and Molenberghs (1998) for the evaluation of surrogate endpoints when the surrogate and the true endpoints are either ordinal or of a different data type.

When the endpoints are of a mixed continuous and discrete nature, a latent variable approach is a natural extension of the likelihood-based approach. Such an approach discretizes one latent response variable and assumes the other one is measured directly. In this chapter, two approaches were presented, one based on a probit–linear model, the other on a Plackett–Dale model. Regarding the adjusted association, one uses either the Pearson correlation coefficient or the log odds ratio, depending on whether a probit or a Plackett-Dale formulation is used. The examples show that the two approaches yield very comparable results, so that in practice one approach can be regarded as a sensitivity analysis for the other. It is interesting to note that, in the examples considered, the discretization of a continuous endpoint into either a binary or an ordinal variable does not lead to a great loss of information for the purposes of evaluating surrogate endpoints. Of course, this need not be the case in general. The reliability of the analyses is primarily driven by the number of observations, rather than by the data type of the endpoints considered.

The two examples used in this chapter underscore one of the greatest practical difficulties of surrogate evaluation, i.e., the need for very large datasets from randomized experiments. The confidence limits of the relative effect will be wide unless the number of observations is large. In the macular degeneration example, for instance, with only 190 patients, the confidence limits of RE are too wide to be useful. In contrast, the confidence limits of the adjusted association will generally be narrow enough to be of practical interest even with small numbers of observations. This is because the surrogate endpoint and the true endpoint are generally strongly correlated (at the individual level). For the evaluation to be complete, however, a strong association between the surrogate and the true endpoint is not sufficient. It is very important that (1) the relative effect be estimated with good precision to permit the reliable prediction of a treatment effect on the true endpoint based on the observation of the treatment effect on the surrogate endpoint and (2) that the relative effect RE remains constant across a meaningful class of trials. Thus, both precision and homogeneity in the RE are required for reliable prediction. This naturally points us to the use of several trials or, at least, several units for analysis. A meta-analytic framework to accommodate for this will be presented in the next chapter and studied further in subsequent chapters.

7

A Meta-analytic Validation Framework for Continuous Outcomes

Geert Molenberghs, Marc Buyse, and Tomasz Burzykowski

7.1 Introduction

In this chapter, we discuss the foundations of the meta-analytic approach to the validation of surrogate endpoints. We focus on surrogate and true endpoints that are assumed to be jointly normally distributed. Subsequent chapters are devoted to non-normal settings.

A meta-analytic approach was called for by several authors, e.g., Albert *et al.* (1998). A first formal proposal, using a Bayesian approach, was given by Daniels and Hughes (1997). Buyse *et al.* (2000a) extended these ideas using the theory of linear mixed-effects models. Gail *et al.* (2000) extended it further using generalized estimating equations methodology. In what follows, we describe the approach as proposed by Buyse *et al.* (2000a).

We assume to have data from N trials at our disposition, in the ith of which n_i subjects are enrolled. T_{ij} and S_{ij} are random variables denoting the true and surrogate endpoints, respectively, for the jth subject in the ith trial or ith center, while Z_{ij} is an indicator variable for treatment.

7.2 A Meta-analytic Approach

The approach is based on a hierarchical, two-stage model. Two distinct modeling strategies can be followed, based on a two-stage fixed-effects representation on the one hand and random effects on the other hand. Computational issues will be discussed in Section 7.4.

Let us describe the two-stage model first. The first stage is based upon a fixed-effects model:

$$S_{ij} = \mu_{Si} + \alpha_i Z_{ij} + \varepsilon_{Sij}, \tag{7.1}$$

$$T_{ij} = \mu_{Ti} + \beta_i Z_{ij} + \varepsilon_{Tij}, \tag{7.2}$$

where μ_{Si} and μ_{Ti} are trial-specific intercepts, α_i and β_i are trial-specific effects of treatment Z on the endpoints in trial i, and ε_{Si} and ε_{Ti} are correlated error terms, assumed to be mean-zero normally distributed with covariance matrix

$$\Sigma = \begin{pmatrix} \sigma_{SS} & \sigma_{ST} \\ & \sigma_{TT} \end{pmatrix}. \tag{7.3}$$

At the second stage, we assume

$$\begin{pmatrix} \mu_{Si} \\ \mu_{Ti} \\ \alpha_i \\ \beta_i \end{pmatrix} = \begin{pmatrix} \mu_S \\ \mu_T \\ \alpha \\ \beta \end{pmatrix} + \begin{pmatrix} m_{Si} \\ m_{Ti} \\ a_i \\ b_i \end{pmatrix}, \tag{7.4}$$

where the second term on the right-hand side of (7.4) is assumed to follow a zero-mean normal distribution with dispersion matrix

$$D = \begin{pmatrix} d_{SS} & d_{ST} & d_{Sa} & d_{Sb} \\ & d_{TT} & d_{Ta} & d_{Tb} \\ & & d_{aa} & d_{ab} \\ & & & d_{bb} \end{pmatrix}. \tag{7.5}$$

Next, the random-effects representation is based upon combining both steps:

$$S_{ij} = \mu_S + m_{Si} + \alpha Z_{ij} + a_i Z_{ij} + \varepsilon_{Sij}, \tag{7.6}$$

$$T_{ij} = \mu_T + m_{Ti} + \beta Z_{ij} + b_i Z_{ij} + \varepsilon_{Tij}, \tag{7.7}$$

where now μ_S and μ_T are fixed intercepts, α and β are the fixed effects of treatment Z on the endpoints, m_{Si} and m_{Ti} are random intercepts, and a_i and b_i are the random effects of treatment Z on the endpoints in trial i. The vector of random effects $(m_{Si}, m_{Ti}, a_i, b_i)$ is assumed to be mean-zero normally distributed with covariance matrix (7.5). The error terms ε_{Sij} and ε_{Tij} follow the same assumptions as in fixed-effects model (7.1)–(7.2), with covariance matrix (7.3). Section 7.4 provides SAS code to fit the random-effects model.

A lot of debate has been devoted to the relative merits of fixed versus random effects, especially in the context of meta-analysis (Thompson and

Pocock 1991, Fleiss 1993, Thompson 1993, Senn 1998). Although the underlying models rest on different assumptions about the nature of the experiments being analyzed, the two approaches yield discrepant results only in pathological situations, or in very small samples where a fixed-effects analysis can yield artificially precise results if the experimental units truly constitute a random sample from a larger population. In our setting, both approaches are very similar, and the two-stage procedure can be used to introduce random effects (Laird and Ware 1982, Verbeke and Molenberghs 2000). As the data analysis in Section 7.5 will illustrate, the choice between random and fixed effects can also be guided by pragmatic arguments. This issue will be discussed further in Section 7.4.

7.2.1 Trial-level Surrogacy

The key motivation for validating a surrogate endpoint is to be able to predict the effect of treatment on the true endpoint based on the observed effect of treatment on the surrogate endpoint. It is essential, therefore, to explore the quality of the prediction of the treatment effect on the true endpoint in trial i by (a) information obtained in the validation process based on trials $i = 1, \ldots, N$ and (b) the estimate of the effect of Z on S in a new trial $i = 0$. Fitting either the fixed-effects model (7.1)–(7.2) or the mixed-effects model (7.6)–(7.7) to data from a meta-analysis provides estimates for the parameters and the variance components. Suppose then the new trial $i = 0$ is considered for which data are available on the surrogate endpoint but not on the true endpoint. We then fit the following linear model to the surrogate outcomes S_{0j}:

$$S_{0j} = \mu_{S0} + \alpha_0 Z_{0j} + \varepsilon_{S0j}. \tag{7.8}$$

Estimates for m_{S0} and a_0 are

$$\begin{aligned} \widehat{m}_{S0} &= \widehat{\mu}_{S0} - \widehat{\mu}_S, \\ \widehat{a}_0 &= \widehat{\alpha}_0 - \widehat{\alpha}. \end{aligned}$$

We are interested in the estimated effect of Z on T, given the effect of Z on S. To this end, observe that $(\beta + b_0 | m_{S0}, a_0)$ follows a normal distribution with mean and variance:

$$\begin{aligned} & E(\beta + b_0 | m_{S0}, a_0) \\ &= \beta + \begin{pmatrix} d_{Sb} \\ d_{ab} \end{pmatrix}^T \begin{pmatrix} d_{SS} & d_{Sa} \\ d_{Sa} & d_{aa} \end{pmatrix}^{-1} \begin{pmatrix} \mu_{S0} - \mu_S \\ \alpha_0 - \alpha \end{pmatrix}, \end{aligned} \tag{7.9}$$

$$\text{Var}(\beta + b_0 | m_{S0}, a_0)$$

$$= \quad d_{bb} - \begin{pmatrix} d_{Sb} \\ d_{ab} \end{pmatrix}^T \begin{pmatrix} d_{SS} & d_{Sa} \\ d_{Sa} & d_{aa} \end{pmatrix}^{-1} \begin{pmatrix} d_{Sb} \\ d_{ab} \end{pmatrix}. \qquad (7.10)$$

This suggests to call a surrogate *"perfect at the trial level"* if the conditional variance (7.10) is equal to zero. Of course, in practice, perfection will not be reached, and a pragmatic approach is to select a surrogate for which the coefficient of determination, to be introduced next, is sufficiently high. A measure to assess the quality of the surrogate at the trial level is the coefficient of determination

$$R^2_{\text{trial(f)}} = R^2_{b_i|m_{Si},a_i} = \frac{\begin{pmatrix} d_{Sb} \\ d_{ab} \end{pmatrix}^T \begin{pmatrix} d_{SS} & d_{Sa} \\ d_{Sa} & d_{aa} \end{pmatrix}^{-1} \begin{pmatrix} d_{Sb} \\ d_{ab} \end{pmatrix}}{d_{bb}}. \qquad (7.11)$$

Coefficient (7.11) is unitless and ranges in the unit interval if the corresponding variance-covariance matrix is positive definite, two desirable features for its interpretation.

Intuition can be gained by considering the special case where the prediction of b_0 can be done independently of the random intercept m_{S0}. Expressions (7.9) and (7.10) then reduce to

$$\begin{aligned} E(\beta + b_0|a_0) &= \beta + \frac{d_{ab}}{d_{aa}}(\alpha_0 - \alpha), \\ \text{Var}(\beta + b_0|a_0) &= d_{bb} - \frac{d_{ab}^2}{d_{aa}} \end{aligned}$$

with corresponding

$$R^2_{\text{trial(r)}} = R^2_{b_i|a_i} = \frac{d_{ab}^2}{d_{aa}d_{bb}}. \qquad (7.12)$$

Now, $R^2_{\text{trial(r)}} = 1$ if the trial level treatment effects are simply multiples of each other. We will refer to this simplified version as the reduced random-effects model, whereas the original expression (7.11) will be said to derive from the full random-effects model.

Coefficient (7.12) results, in particular, if the matrix D, given by (7.5), assumes the following structure:

$$D_0 = \begin{pmatrix} d_{SS} & d_{ST} & 0 & 0 \\ & d_{TT} & 0 & 0 \\ & & d_{aa} & d_{ab} \\ & & & d_{bb} \end{pmatrix} \qquad (7.13)$$

or if the linear mixed-effects model (7.6)–(7.7) does not contain the random intercepts m_{Si} and m_{Ti} at all. Note that in the latter case the fitting of the linear mixed-effects model might be somewhat easier. On the other hand, the structure of the model based on the matrix D_0 is slightly more general, as it still allows for a heterogeneity in the intercepts. We will come back to this issue in the next chapters.

In both cases, (7.12) might be computed using a simplified two-stage representation of (7.6)–(7.7), where the second-stage model is reduced to:

$$\begin{pmatrix} \alpha_i \\ \beta_i \end{pmatrix} = \begin{pmatrix} \alpha \\ \beta \end{pmatrix} + \begin{pmatrix} a_i \\ b_i \end{pmatrix}, \tag{7.14}$$

with $(a_i, b_i)^T$ following a zero-mean normal distribution with dispersion matrix

$$D_r = \begin{pmatrix} d_{aa} & d_{ab} \\ & d_{bb} \end{pmatrix}. \tag{7.15}$$

Additionally, if the linear mixed-effects model (7.6)–(7.7) does not contain the random intercepts m_{Si} and m_{Si}, the first-stage model can be simplified to

$$S_{ij} = \mu_S + \alpha_i Z_{ij} + \varepsilon_{Sij}, \tag{7.16}$$
$$T_{ij} = \mu_T + \beta_i Z_{ij} + \varepsilon_{Tij}. \tag{7.17}$$

In what follows we will refer to the mixed-effects model without the random intercepts as the reduced mixed-effects model and assume it implies the use of the simplified coefficient of determination (7.12). The original expression (7.11) will be said to derive from the full mixed-effects model. Similarly, we will refer to model (7.1)–(7.2), with the second-stage model (7.4), as the full fixed-effects model, while model (7.16)–(7.17), with the simplified second-stage model (7.14), will be termed the reduced fixed-effects model.

Similar to the logic in (7.9) and (7.10), the conditional model for β_i given μ_{Si} and α_i can be written:

$$\beta_i = \theta_0 + \theta_a \alpha_i + \theta_m \mu_{Si} + \varepsilon_i, \tag{7.18}$$

where expressions for the coefficient $(\theta_0, \theta_a, \theta_m)$ follow from (7.4) and (7.5). In case the surrogate is perfect at the trial level ($R^2_{\text{trial}} = 1$), the error term in (7.18) vanishes and the linear relationship becomes deterministic, implying that β_i *equals* the systematic component of (7.18).

In more detail, the prediction interval for treatment effect $\beta + b_0$ in the new trial is constructed as follows. Denote $f = E(\beta + b_0 | m_{S0}, a_0) = \beta + D_1 D_2^{-1} D_3$ where D_1, D_2, and D_3 refer to the corresponding matrices in (7.9). Let f_d be the derivate of f w.r.t. the parameter vector

$$(\beta, \mu_S, \alpha, d_{Sb}, d_{ab}, d_{SS}, d_{Sa}, d_{aa}, \mu_{S0}, \alpha_0)^T.$$

The components of f_d are

$$
\begin{aligned}
\frac{\partial f}{\partial \beta} &= 1, \\
\frac{\partial f}{\partial \mu_{s0}} &= -\frac{\partial f}{\partial \mu_s} = D_1 D_2^{-1} \begin{pmatrix} 1 \\ 0 \end{pmatrix}, \\
\frac{\partial f}{\partial \alpha_0} &= -\frac{\partial f}{\partial \alpha} = D_1 D_2^{-1} \begin{pmatrix} 0 \\ 1 \end{pmatrix}, \\
\frac{\partial f}{\partial d_{sb}} &= \begin{pmatrix} 1 \\ 0 \end{pmatrix}^T D_2^{-1} D_3, \\
\frac{\partial f}{\partial d_{ab}} &= \begin{pmatrix} 0 \\ 1 \end{pmatrix}^T D_2^{-1} D_3, \\
\frac{\partial f}{\partial d_{ss}} &= -D_1 D_2^{-1} \begin{pmatrix} 1 & 0 \\ 0 & 0 \end{pmatrix} D_2^{-1} D_3, \\
\frac{\partial f}{\partial d_{sa}} &= -D_1 D_2^{-1} \begin{pmatrix} 0 & 1 \\ 1 & 0 \end{pmatrix} D_2^{-1} D_3, \\
\frac{\partial f}{\partial d_{aa}} &= -D_1 D_2^{-1} \begin{pmatrix} 0 & 0 \\ 0 & 1 \end{pmatrix} D_2^{-1} D_3.
\end{aligned}
$$

Denoting the asymptotic covariance matrix of the estimated parameter vector by V, the asymptotic variance of f is given by $f_d^T V f_d$, producing a confidence interval in the usual way. For a prediction interval, the variance to be used is $f_d^T V f_d + \text{Var}(\beta + b_0 | m_{s0}, a_0)$.

There is a close connection between the prediction approach followed here and empirical Bayes estimation (Verbeke and Molenberghs 2000). To see this, consider a similar but non-identical approach where all data are analyzed together. This means that a meta-analysis is performed of the surrogate data on trials $i = 0, \ldots, N$ and of the true endpoint data on trials $i = 1, \ldots, N$. The estimate of b_0 will be based only on the surrogate data, as the true endpoint is unknown for trial $i = 0$, and on the parameter estimates. The expression for the empirical Bayes estimate of b_0 is identical to (7.9), but the numerical value will be slightly different, as the parameters of the linear mixed model are determined on a larger set of data. For example, with the MIXED procedure in SAS, obtaining the empirical Bayes estimate of b_0 is immediate, but its conditional variance requires some additional computation (Littell *et al.* 1996).

7.2.2 Individual-level Surrogacy

To validate a surrogate endpoint, Buyse and Molenberghs (1998) suggested to consider the association between the surrogate and the final endpoints after adjustment for the treatment effect. To this end, we need to construct the conditional distribution of T, given S and Z. From (7.1)–(7.2) we derive

$$\begin{aligned} T_{ij}|Z_{ij}, S_{ij} \sim & \; N\{\mu_{Ti} - \sigma_{TS}\sigma_{SS}^{-1}\mu_{Si} + (\beta_i - \sigma_{TS}\sigma_{SS}^{-1}\alpha_i)Z_{ij} \\ & + \sigma_{TS}\sigma_{SS}^{-1}S_{ij}; \sigma_{TT} - \sigma_{TS}^2\sigma_{SS}^{-1}\}. \end{aligned} \quad (7.19)$$

Similarly, the random-effects model (7.6)–(7.7) yields

$$\begin{aligned} T_{ij}|Z_{ij}, S_{ij} \sim & \; N\{\mu_T + m_{Ti} - \sigma_{TS}\sigma_{SS}^{-1}(\mu_S + m_{Si}) \\ & + [\beta + b_i - \sigma_{TS}\sigma_{SS}^{-1}(\alpha + a_i)]Z_{ij} \\ & + \sigma_{TS}\sigma_{SS}^{-1}S_{ij} \; ; \; \sigma_{TT} - \sigma_{TS}^2\sigma_{SS}^{-1}\}, \end{aligned} \quad (7.20)$$

where conditioning is also on the random effects. The association between both endpoints after adjustment for the treatment effect is in both (7.19) and (7.20) captured by

$$R_{\text{indiv}}^2 = R_{\varepsilon_{Ti}|\varepsilon_{Si}}^2 = \frac{\sigma_{ST}^2}{\sigma_{SS}\sigma_{TT}}, \quad (7.21)$$

the squared correlation between S and T after adjustment for both the trial effects and the treatment effect. Note that $R_{\varepsilon_{Ti}|\varepsilon_{Si}}$ generalizes the adjusted association ρ_Z, discussed in Chapter 5, Section 5.4, to the case of several trials.

7.2.3 A New Approach to Surrogate Evaluation

The development in Section 7.2.1 and Section 7.2.2 suggests to term a surrogate *"trial-level valid"* if $R_{\text{trial(f)}}^2$ (or $R_{\text{trial(r)}}^2$) is sufficiently close to one, and to call it *"individual-level valid"* if R_{indiv}^2 is sufficiently close to one. Finally, a surrogate is termed *"valid"* if it is both trial-level and individual-level valid. In order to replace the words *"valid"* with *"perfect,"* the corresponding R-squared values are required to equal one.

To be useful in practice, a valid surrogate must be able to predict the effect of treatment upon the true endpoint with sufficient precision to distinguish safely between effects that are clinically worthwhile and effects that are not. This requires both that the estimate of $\beta + b_0$ be sufficiently large and that the prediction interval of this quantity be sufficiently narrow.

It should be noted that the validation criteria proposed here do not require the treatment to have a significant effect on either endpoint. In particular, it is possible to have $\alpha \equiv 0$ and yet have a perfect surrogate. Indeed, even though the treatment may not have any effect on the surrogate endpoint as a whole, the fluctuations around zero in individual trials (or other experimental units) can be very strongly predictive of the effect on the true endpoint. However, such a situation is unlikely to occur since the heterogeneity between the trials is generally small compared to that between individual patients.

7.3 Single-trial Measures versus Multi-trial Measures

If data are available on a single trial (or, more generally, on a single experimental unit), the above developments are only partially possible. Although the individual-level reasoning, producing ρ_Z as in (7.21), carries over by virtue of the within-trial replication, the trial-level reasoning breaks down and one cannot go beyond the relative effect (RE) as suggested in Buyse and Molenberghs (1998). Recall that the RE is defined as the ratio of the effects of Z on S and T, respectively, as expressed in (5.22). The confidence limits of RE can be used to assess the uncertainty about the value of β predicted from that of α, but in contrast to the above developments, no prediction interval can be calculated for β.

It has been argued in Chapter 5 that, although the concept behind the fourth Prentice criterion has intuitive appeal, it is not captured by the PE. It has been also argued that RE is based on too strong assumptions to be useful. Having introduced measures of surrogacy at the trial-level and at the individual-level, it is now possible to explore these issues further.

The proportion explained (5.24), derived for the single-trial case, can now be calculated for each trial within the meta-analysis:

$$PE_i = \lambda \rho_Z \frac{1}{RE_i}, \tag{7.22}$$

where $RE_i = \beta_i/\alpha_i$.

Let us now examine how the PE_i behaves relative to the R^2 measures. To make the point clearly, it is useful to concentrate on a "perfect" surrogate, i.e., one for which $R^2_{\text{trial}} = 1$ and $R^2_{\text{indiv}} = \rho^2_Z = 1$.

Perfect Surrogate at the Trial Level. Let us first assume that the surrogate is perfect at the trial level, i.e., $R^2_{\text{trial}} = 1$. Then the relationship between α_i and β_i, expressed by (7.18), is deterministic, and (7.22) becomes

$$PE_i = \rho_Z \lambda \frac{\alpha_i}{\theta_0 + \theta_a \alpha_i + \theta_m \mu_{Si}}. \tag{7.23}$$

Thus, even if the important condition $R^2_{\text{trial}} = 1$ is satisfied, and one can predict the treatment effect on the true endpoint without error from the treatment effect on the surrogate endpoint, PE_i cannot be constant across trials, and consequently would not be equal to unity in all of them. Note that also RE_i is not constant across trial. The reason is that for RE_i to be constant the relationship between α_i and β_i must be multiplicative.

Perfect Surrogate at the Individual Level. Let us now make the additional assumption that the surrogate is also perfect at the individual level, i.e., $\rho_Z = 1$.

In this case, (7.23) becomes

$$PE_i = \lambda \frac{\alpha_i}{\theta_0 + \theta_a \alpha_i + \theta_m \mu_{Si}} \tag{7.24}$$

and the property of non-constant PE_i and RE_i persists, again due to the linear but non-multiplicative relationship between α_i and β_i.

Constant Relative Effect. Let us make the final assumption that a simple multiplicative relationship holds between α_i and β_i, i.e., $\theta_0 = \theta_m = 0$ and hence $RE_i = \theta_a$. Thus,

$$PE = PE_i = \frac{\lambda}{\theta_a}. \tag{7.25}$$

Now, RE_i is constant and so is PE_i, but the latter is still a function of two quantities:

- the multiplicative factor θ_a linking the treatment effects in each trial and
- the multiplicative factor λ linking the two error terms in each patient.

Clearly, under the three assumptions made above, the surrogate and true endpoints are identical, up to scaling factors that translate the treatment effects within a trial and the subject-specific deviations within each patient. Yet, depending on the values of θ_a and λ, the PE can assume any positive real value.

7.4 Computational Issues

In this section, we investigate convergence properties of the random-effects approach as proposed in Section 7.2. The need for such an investigation arises from the observation that in many practical instances, convergence of the Newton-Raphson algorithm yielding (restricted) maximum likelihood solutions could hardly be achieved. Therefore, it is worth knowing what features of the problem at hand may be of influence in easing convergence of the algorithm, as this may be an additional factor to decide between a two-stage or a random-effects model. These ideas are then taken further in Section 7.4.2, where a number of simplifying model fitting approaches are proposed.

7.4.1 Initial Simulation Study

Buyse *et al.* (2000a) explored the following factors: number of trials, size of the between-trial variability (compared to residual variability), number of patients per trial, normality assumption, and strength of the correlation between random treatment effects. Because only the first two factors were found significantly to affect convergence of the algorithm, only those are discussed in the remainder of this paragraph.

Table 7.1 shows the number of runs for which convergence could be achieved within 20 iterations. In each case, 500 runs were performed, assuming the following model:

$$\begin{aligned} S_{ij} &= 45 + m_{S_i} + (3 + a_i)Z_{ij} + \epsilon_{Sij}, \\ T_{ij} &= 50 + m_{Ti} + (5 + b_i)Z_{ij} + \epsilon_{Tij}, \end{aligned}$$

where $(m_{Si}, m_{Ti}, a_i, b_i) \sim N(0, D)$ with

$$D = \sigma^2 \begin{pmatrix} 1 & 0.8 & 0 & 0 \\ & 1 & 0 & 0 \\ & & 1 & 0.9 \\ & & & 1 \end{pmatrix},$$

and $(\epsilon_{Sij}, \epsilon_{Tij}) \sim N(0, \Sigma)$ with

$$\Sigma = 3 \begin{pmatrix} 1 & 0.8 \\ & 1 \end{pmatrix}.$$

The number of trials was fixed to either 10, 20, or 50, each trial involving 10 subjects randomly assigned to treatment groups. The σ^2 parameter was set to 0.1 or 1.

TABLE 7.1. *Number of runs for which convergence was achieved within 20 iterations.*

	Number of trials		
σ^2	50	20	10
1	500 (100%)	498 (100%)	412 (82%)
0.1	491 (98%)	417 (83%)	218 (44%)

NOTE: Total number of runs: 500; percentages are given in parentheses.

From Table 7.1, we see that when the between-trial variability is large ($\sigma^2 = 1$), no convergence problems occur, except when the number of trials gets very small. When the between-trial variability gets smaller, convergence problems do arise and worsen as the number of trials decreases.

These simulation results indicate that there should be enough variability at the trial level, and a sufficient number of trials, to obtain convergence of the Newton-Raphson algorithm for fitting mixed-effects models. When these requirements are not fulfilled, one must rely on simpler fixed-effects models, or mixed-effects models with random treatment effects but no random intercepts.

We describe now how to use the SAS statistical software package to fit the random-effects model proposed in Section 7.2. Notice that other packages such as MLwiN are also particularly well-suited for fitting this type of multivariate multilevel models and could therefore be utilized instead.

The SAS code to fit model (7.6)–(7.7) may be written as follows:

```
proc mixed data=dataset covtest;
class endpoint subject trial;
model outcome = endpoint endpoint*treat / Solution noint;
random endpoint endpoint*treat / subject=trial type=un;
repeated endpoint / subject=subject(trial) type=un;
run;
```

The above syntax presumes that there are two records per subject in the input data set, one corresponding to the surrogate endpoint and the other to the true endpoint. The variable ENDPOINT is an indicator for the kind of endpoint (coded -1 for surrogate and 1 for true endpoint) and the variable OUTCOME contains measurements obtained from each endpoint. The variable TREAT is also assumed to be $-1/1$ coded. This is better than a 0/1 coding, as otherwise the group with code 0 is assumed to have a smaller total variance than the other one, as the contribution coming from the random-effects variance is multiplied with zero and hence annihilated. The $-1/1$

coding, on the other hand, leads to equal variances in both groups.

The RANDOM statement defines the covariance matrix D in (7.5) of random effects at the trial level, while the REPEATED statement builds up the residual covariance matrix Σ in (7.3). Note that the nesting notation in the 'subject=' option is necessary for SAS to recognize the nested structure of the data (subjects are clustered within trials). Acknowledgment of the hierarchical nature of the data enables SAS to build a block-diagonal covariance matrix, with diagonal blocks corresponding to the different trials, which speeds up computations considerably.

7.4.2 Simplified Modeling Strategies

Fitting random-effects model (7.6)–(7.7) can be a surprisingly difficult task in a number of situations. This is particularly true when the number of trials or the number of patients per trial is small. Also, situations with extreme correlations pose problems. It is therefore imperative to explore approximate strategies with better computational properties. Buyse *et al.* (2000a) studied one alternative approach in the sense that they replaced the random effects by their fixed-effect counterparts. Such a two-stage approach is very similar in spirit to the original proposal of Laird and Ware (1982). Tibaldi *et al.* (2003) embedded this ad-hoc strategy in a more formally developed system of model simplifications. We will describe it here.

In more detail, Tibaldi *et al.* (2003) considered three dimensions along which simplifications can be made:

Trial dimension: whether the trial-specific effects are treated as either random or fixed. A full random-effects is then distinguished from a two-stage approach.

Endpoint dimension: whether the surrogate and true endpoints are modeled as a bivariate outcome or two univariate ones. In the latter case the correlation between both endpoints is not incorporated into the modeling strategy, rendering the study of the individual-level surrogacy more involved. However, usually the trial-level surrogacy is of most interest, in which case the investigation of the individual-level surrogacy may be considered of secondary importance.

Measurement error dimension: whenever the full random-effects model is abandoned, one is confronted with measurement error, as the treatment effects in the various trials are estimated with error. The magnitude of this error is likely to depend on several characteristics, such as trial size, which will vary across trials. Tibaldi *et al.* (2003) considered three ways to account for measurement error: unadjusted (i.e.,

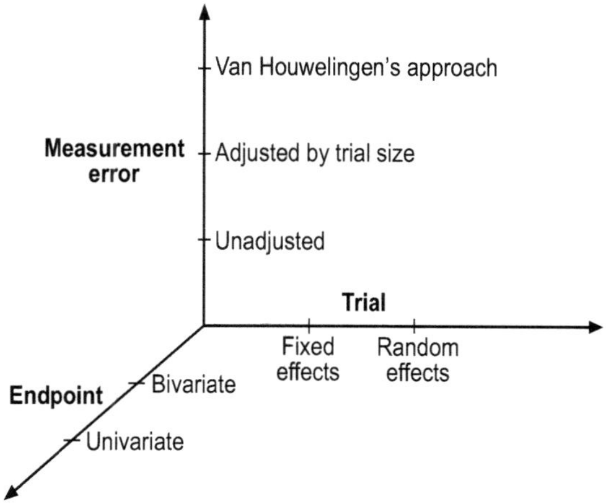

FIGURE 7.1. *Graphical representation of the different modelling approaches.*

no correction at all), adjustment by trial size, and an approach based on the results developed by van Houwelingen, Arends, and Stijnen (2002) and explained in the sequel.

The combination of these three dimensions are graphically represented in Figure 7.1 and gives rise to twelve strategies. However, some do not have to be considered. For example, when one chooses for a bivariate (endpoint dimension) random-effects (trial dimension) approach, measurement error is automatically accounted for, whence explicit corrections are no longer needed. In the special case when sample size is constant across trials, further simplifications arise (see Section 7.4.3).

We will now discuss each of the three simplifying dimensions in turn.

The Trial Dimension

As stated before, the parameters of the full random-effects model (7.6)–(7.7) can be estimated by maximum likelihood or restricted maximum likelihood, using standard linear mixed model software such as the SAS procedure MIXED.

In case the trial-level parameters are treated as fixed, exactly as Buyse *et al.* (2000a), one can rewrite the model as

$$S_{ij} = \mu_{S_i} + \alpha_i Z_{ij} + \varepsilon_{S_{ij}}, \quad (7.26)$$

$$T_{ij} = \mu_{T_i} + \beta_i Z_{ij} + \varepsilon_{T_{ij}}, \quad (7.27)$$

where μ_{S_i}, μ_{T_i}, α_i, and β_i are trial-specific intercepts and treatment effects.

The assumption about the error terms depends on the choice made on the *endpoint dimension*. Indeed, when the univariate approach is opted for, both errors are assumed independent. Otherwise, a bivariate unstructured covariance matrix is considered.

At the second stage, a regression model is fitted to the treatment effects, estimated at the first stage, for example:

$$\widehat{\beta}_i = \lambda_0 + \lambda_1 \widehat{\mu}_{S_i} + \lambda_2 \widehat{\alpha}_i + \varepsilon_i. \tag{7.28}$$

This model can then be employed to assess trial-level surrogacy, using the $R^2_{\text{trial(f)}}$ associated with this regression. This is not calculated as in (7.11), but is merely the classical coefficient of determination found by regressing $\widehat{\beta}_i$ on $\widehat{\mu}_{S_i}$ and $\widehat{\alpha}_i$.

In case the trial-specific intercept from surrogate model (7.26) is not used, λ_1 would be dropped and an $R^2_{\text{trial(r)}}$ is obtained, similar in spirit to (7.12).

The Measurement Error Dimension

Recall that this dimension is irrelevant when the full random-effects model is assumed but is crucial when a fixed-effects approach is selected on the *trial dimension* and/or when a univariate model is chosen on the *endpoint dimension*.

Tibaldi *et al.* (2003) allowed for three possible choices. First, a simple linear model can be assumed to determine the relationship between β_i, α_i, and μ_{S_i}, whereby the errors in (7.28) are assumed to be zero-mean normally distributed with constant variance σ^2.

Clearly, this approach ignores the fact that the estimated treatment effects α_i and β_i will typically come from trials with large variations in size. One way to address this issue is by weighing the contributions according to trial size, resulting in a weighted linear regression. Such an approach may account for some but not all of the heterogeneity in information content between trial-specific contributions. A nice way to overcome this can be obtained using the results developed by van Houwelingen, Arends, and Stijnen (2002).

To this end, one can introduce models for the estimated trial-specific treatment effects $(\widehat{\mu}_{S_i}, \widehat{\alpha}_i, \widehat{\beta}_i)^T$, given the true trial-specific treatment effects $(\mu_{S_i}, \alpha_i, \beta_i)^T$:

$$\begin{pmatrix} \widehat{\mu}_{S_i} \\ \widehat{\alpha}_i \\ \widehat{\beta}_i \end{pmatrix} \sim N\left[\begin{pmatrix} \mu_{S_i} \\ \alpha_i \\ \beta_i \end{pmatrix}, \Omega_i\right]. \tag{7.29}$$

Here, Ω_i is the variance-covariance matrix of the estimated treatment effects. In case both treatment-effect estimates are assumed to be independent (which would result from a univariate choice on the *endpoint dimension*), Ω_i would be taken to be diagonal, even though this may be unrealistic.

Further, a normal model for the true trial-specific treatment effects around the true overall treatment effects is assumed:

$$\begin{pmatrix} \mu_{S_i} \\ \alpha_i \\ \beta_i \end{pmatrix} \sim N\left[\begin{pmatrix} \mu_S \\ \alpha \\ \beta \end{pmatrix}, \Sigma\right]. \tag{7.30}$$

The resulting marginal model, combining (7.29) and (7.30), is:

$$\begin{pmatrix} \widehat{\mu}_{S_i} \\ \hat{\boldsymbol{\alpha}}_i \\ \hat{\boldsymbol{\beta}}_i \end{pmatrix} \sim N\left[\begin{pmatrix} \mu_S \\ \alpha \\ \beta \end{pmatrix}, \Sigma + \Omega_i\right]. \tag{7.31}$$

Maximum likelihood estimation for this model can be quite easily carried out by using mixed model software, provided the values for Ω_i can be input and held fixed, as is the case in the SAS procedure MIXED. An example program is provided by Tibaldi *et al.* (2003).

Endpoint Dimension

It seems natural to assume both endpoints to be correlated. However, this assumption will almost always complicate modelling and corresponding parameter estimation. In addition, the bivariate nature of the outcome is related for the better part with individual-level surrogacy, whereas our main goal is trial-level surrogacy. This suggests an additional simplification, i.e., by considering separate, independent models for each of the endpoints. It then remains to be seen inhowfar such a simplification hampers estimation of trial-level surrogacy.

One needs to make a distinction between two cases, according to the corresponding choice on the *trial dimension*. In the random-effects approach, this simplification would lead to a pair of *univariate* hierarchical models, one for each endpoint. In the fixed-effects approach, one would fit a separate linear regression model per endpoint and per trial. It is easy to show that the parameter estimates as well as the estimated variances are identical to the ones obtained from fitting a fixed-effects *bivariate* model to each trial separately. This follows from standard multivariate normal theory (Johnson and Wichern 1992).

TABLE 7.2. *Means of the estimated trial-level surrogacy and 95% simulation-based confidence intervals for $R^2 = 0.90$. Column numbers refer to the columns of Table 7.6.*

	Variance 10		
No. Sub	1, 2, 7, 8	3	4, 5
50	0.898 (0.894;0.902)	0.895 (0.890;0.900)	0.898 (0.895;0.902)
60	0.900 (0.897;0.904)	0.899 (0.896;0.903)	0.901 (0.897;0.904)
70	0.898 (0.894;0.902)	0.896 (0.892;0.901)	0.898 (0.894;0.902)
80	0.899 (0.895;0.903)	0.898 (0.894;0.902)	0.899 (0.895;0.903)
90	0.900 (0.896;0.903)	0.899 (0.895;0.902)	0.900 (0.896;0.903)
100	0.901 (0.898;0.905)	0.901 (0.897;0.904)	0.901 (0.898;0.905)
No. Sub	6	9	10–12
50	0.894 (0.890;0.898)	0.898 (0.894;0.902)	0.896 (0.892;0.900)
60	0.897 (0.893;0.900)	0.900 (0.896;0.903)	0.897 (0.894;0.901)
70	0.894 (0.890;0.899)	0.897 (0.893;0.902)	0.895 (0.891;0.900)
80	0.895 (0.891;0.899)	0.898 (0.894;0.902)	0.896 (0.892;0.900)
90	0.896 (0.892;0.899)	0.899 (0.896;0.903)	0.897 (0.893;0.901)
100	0.897 (0.894;0.901)	0.901 (0.897;0.904)	0.898 (0.895;0.902)

7.4.3 Additional Simulation Study

Tibaldi *et al.* (2003) studied performance of the various approaches prsented in the previous section, in terms of estimation (point and interval) of $R^2_{\text{trial(f)}}$, and in terms of convergence through a simulation study. To make their results comparable with those from Buyse *et al.* (2000a), the same configuration setting was adopted.

In more detail, model (7.6)–(7.7) is considered with $(m_{S_i}, m_{T_i}, a_i, b_i) \sim N(0, D)$, $\mu_S = 50$, $\mu_T = 45$, $m_{S_i} = 5$, $m_{T_i} = 3$,

$$D = \sigma^2 \begin{pmatrix} 1 & 0.8 & 0 & 0 \\ 0.8 & 1 & 0 & 0 \\ 0 & 0 & 1 & \rho \\ 0 & 0 & \rho & 1 \end{pmatrix}, \tag{7.32}$$

with $\rho^2 = 0.5$ or $\rho^2 = 0.9$, and $(\varepsilon_{S_{ij}}, \varepsilon_{T_{ij}}) \sim N(0, \Sigma)$ with

$$\Sigma = 3 \begin{pmatrix} 1 & 0.8 \\ 0.8 & 1 \end{pmatrix}.$$

The parameter σ^2 was chosen to be either 3 or 10. Five hundred runs were completed for every setting, consisting of 25 trials each. The true R^2,

TABLE 7.3. *Means of the estimated trial-level surrogacy and 95% simulation-based confidence intervals for* $R^2 = 0.90$. *Column numbers refer to the columns of Table 7.6.*

	Variance 3		
No. Sub	1, 2, 7, 8	3	4, 5
50	0.893 (0.889;0.897)	0.889 (0.885;0.894)	0.894 (0.890;0.898)
60	0.896 (0.893;0.900)	0.893 (0.889;0.897)	0.897 (0.893;0.901)
70	0.894 (0.890;0.898)	0.890 (0.886;0.895)	0.894 (0.890;0.898)
80	0.895 (0.891;0.899)	0.892 (0.888;0.896)	0.896 (0.892;0.900)
90	0.897 (0.893;0.900)	0.894 (0.890;0.898)	0.897 (0.894;0.901)
100	0.898 (0.895;0.902)	0.896 (0.892;0.899)	0.899 (0.895;0.902)
No. Sub	6	9	10–12
50	0.892 (0.888;0.896)	0.892 (0.888;0.896)	0.896 (0.891;0.900)
60	0.896 (0.892;0.899)	0.895 (0.892;0.899)	0.897 (0.893;0.901)
70	0.891 (0.887;0.896)	0.893 (0.889;0.897)	0.895 (0.890;0.899)
80	0.894 (0.890;0.898)	0.895 (0.891;0.899)	0.896 (0.892;0.900)
90	0.893 (0.889;0.897)	0.896 (0.893;0.900)	0.897 (0.893;0.901)
100	0.895 (0.891;0.899)	0.898 (0.894;0.901)	0.898 (0.894;0.902)

following from (7.11) and (7.32) is set equal to either 0.5 or 0.9. Results are presented in Tables 7.2–7.5. In all settings, convergence was 100%, which is slightly different from the analysis of the examples.

The approach based on the results by van Houwelingen, Arends, and Stijnen (2002) exhibits a small amount of bias. In case $R^2 = 0.9$ and $\sigma^2 = 3$, there is a hint of underestimation in column 3, 6, and somehow also 9. The situation is more dramatic in the case of $R^2 = 0.5$, where indeed we observe now overestimation in all but one columns, the exception being the full model (columns 10–12).

7.5 Case Studies

We apply the hierarchical methods introduced here to three of the case studies introduced in Chapter 4: the age-related macular degeneration study (Section 4.2.1) and the studies in advanced colorectal (Section 4.2.3) and advanced ovarian (Section 4.2.2) cancer. To all three, the full hierarchical method as well as the simplified methods will be applied. Summary results are provided in Table 7.6.

TABLE 7.4. *Means of the estimated trial-level surrogacy and 95% simulation-based confidence intervals for* $R^2 = 0.50$. *Column numbers refer to the columns of Table 7.6.*

Variance 10			
No. Sub	1, 2, 7, 8	3	4, 5
50	0.527 (0.515;0.539)	0.526 (0.514;0.538)	0.528 (0.516;0.540)
60	0.532 (0.520;0.544)	0.531 (0.519;0.543)	0.533 (0.521;0.544)
70	0.525 (0.513;0.538)	0.524 (0.512;0.537)	0.526 (0.513;0.538)
80	0.522 (0.509;0.536)	0.522 (0.509;0.535)	0.523 (0.510;0.536)
90	0.524 (0.512;0.535)	0.523 (0.511;0.535)	0.524 (0.512;0.536)
100	0.526 (0.514;0.538)	0.525 (0.513;0.538)	0.527 (0.514;0.539)
No. Sub	6	9	10–12
50	0.523 (0.511;0.535)	0.526 (0.514;0.538)	0.498 (0.485;0.510)
60	0.529 (0.517;0.540)	0.531 (0.519;0.543)	0.502 (0.490;0.515)
70	0.522 (0.509;0.535)	0.525 (0.512;0.537)	0.500 (0.487;0.513)
80	0.520 (0.506;0.533)	0.522 (0.509;0.535)	0.498 (0.484;0.511)
90	0.520 (0.509;0.532)	0.523 (0.511;0.535)	0.501 (0.488;0.513)
100	0.523 (0.510;0.535)	0.525 (0.513;0.538)	0.503 (0.490;0.516)

7.5.1 Age-related Macular Degeneration Study (ARMD)

In this section, the data from the age-related macular degeneration trial, described in Section 4.2.1, are used. The data come from a single multicenter trial. Therefore, it is natural to consider the center in which the patients were treated as the unit of analysis. A total of 36 centers were thus available for analysis, with a number of individual patients per center ranging from 2 to 18.

Figure 7.2(a) shows a plot of the raw data (true endpoint versus surrogate endpoint for all individual patients).

Buyse *et al.* (2000a) experienced problems in fitting the full random-effects models, irrespective of whether standard statistical software or user developed alternatives were used. Therefore, they entertained a (unweighted) fixed-effects approach instead. This produced a moderate trial-level surrogacy: $R^2_{\mathrm{trial(f)}} = 0.692$ (standard error, s.e., 0.087). The standard error was calculated by means of a straightforward application of the delta method. Let us now compare their result to the ones obtained by Tibaldi *et al.* (2003) from the approaches described in Section 7.4.2.

As mentioned earlier, for the fixed-effects approaches, univariate and bivari-

TABLE 7.5. *Means of the estimated trial-level surrogacy and 95% simulation-based confidence intervals for $R^2 = 0.50$. Column numbers refer to the columns of Table 7.6.*

	Variance 3		
No. Sub	1, 2, 7, 8	3	4, 5
50	0.539 (0.527;0.551)	0.535 (0.523;0.547)	0.542 (0.530;0.554)
60	0.542 (0.531;0.554)	0.539 (0.527;0.551)	0.545 (0.534;0.557)
70	0.533 (0.521;0.546)	0.530 (0.518;0.543)	0.535 (0.522;0.547)
80	0.531 (0.517;0.544)	0.529 (0.516;0.542)	0.533 (0.519;0.546)
90	0.531 (0.519;0.542)	0.529 (0.517;0.540)	0.532 (0.520;0.544)
100	0.531 (0.519;0.544)	0.530 (0.518;0.542)	0.534 (0.521;0.546)
No. Sub	6	9	10–12
50	0.534 (0.522;0.546)	0.538 (0.526;0.550)	0.496 (0.483;0.510)
60	0.538 (0.526;0.550)	0.542 (0.530;0.553)	0.501 (0.488;0.514)
70	0.528 (0.516;0.541)	0.532 (0.520;0.545)	0.497 (0.484;0.511)
80	0.527 (0.514;0.540)	0.530 (0.517;0.543)	0.497 (0.483;0.511)
90	0.527 (0.515;0.538)	0.530 (0.518;0.542)	0.500 (0.487;0.512)
100	0.528 (0.516;0.541)	0.531 (0.519;0.543)	0.502 (0.489;0.515)

ate results values are equal. Of course, the univariate approach prohibits the assessment of individual-level surrogacy but, as mentioned earlier, in many trials the main interest is on trial-level surrogacy.

For the $R^2_{\text{trial(f)}}$, the approach based on the van Houwelingen, Arends, and Stijnen (2002) results is more difficult to fit in the sense that the random-effects values cannot be obtained.

The reduced-model values are generally higher than the full-model values, suggesting that the trial-specific intercept terms for the surrogate model does convey information and, if possible, full models should be used. Within the reduced-model approach, the van Houwelingen, Arends, and Stijnen univariate random-effects approach yields a low value. This is in line with intuition, as it corrects for measurement error present in the estimated treatment effects. Simulations will have to weigh costs and benefits from this approach. In general computational terms, a choice for univariate models and/or fixed-effects approaches is less expensive.

Figure 7.2(b) shows a plot of the treatment effects on the true endpoint by the treatment effects on the surrogate endpoint. These effects are moderately correlated. Figure 7.2(c) shows that the correlation of the measurements at 6 months and at 1 year is indeed rather poor at the individual level. Therefore, even with the limited data available, it is clear that the

TABLE 7.6. *Results of the trial-level surrogacy analysis for the ARMD, advanced colorectal, and advanced ovarian studies.* R^2_{trial} *(a – symbol indicates non-convergence). Unw'd: Unweighted; W'd: Weighted; vH'n: the van Houwelingen, Arends, and Stijnen method.*

	Full model					
	Univariate approach					
	Fixed effects			Random effects		
	Unw'd	W'd	vH'n	Unw'd	W'd	vH'n
Study	1	2	3	4	5	6
ARMD	0.692	0.693	0.689	0.664	0.801	-
Colorectal	0.473	0.488	0.466	-	-	-
Ovarian	0.939	0.917	0.937	0.911	0.905	-
	Bivariate approach					
	Fixed effects			Random effects		
	Unw'd	W'd	vH'n			
Study	7	8	9	10–12		
ARMD	0.692	0.693	0.698	-		
Colorectal	0.473	0.488	0.472	-		
Ovarian	0.939	0.917	0.938	-		
	Reduced model					
	Univariate approach					
	Fixed effects			Random effects		
Study	Unw'd	W'd	vH'n	Unw'd	W'd	vH'n
ARMD	0.776	0.758	0.775	0.659	0.786	0.623
Colorectal	0.527	0.497	0.596	-	-	-
Ovarian	0.928	0.909	0.925	0.911	0.905	0.900
	Bivariate approach					
	Fixed effects			Random effects		
Study	Unw'd	We'd	vH'n			
ARMD	0.776	0.758	0.719	-		
Colorectal	0.527	0.497	0.471	-		
Ovarian	0.928	0.909	0.938	0.951		

assessment of visual acuity at 6 months is not a good surrogate for the same assessment at 1 year.

7.5.2 Advanced Colorectal Cancer

We consider data from two randomized multicenter trials in colorectal cancer, introduced in Section 4.2.3. In this example, we will use $Z_{ij} = 0$ to

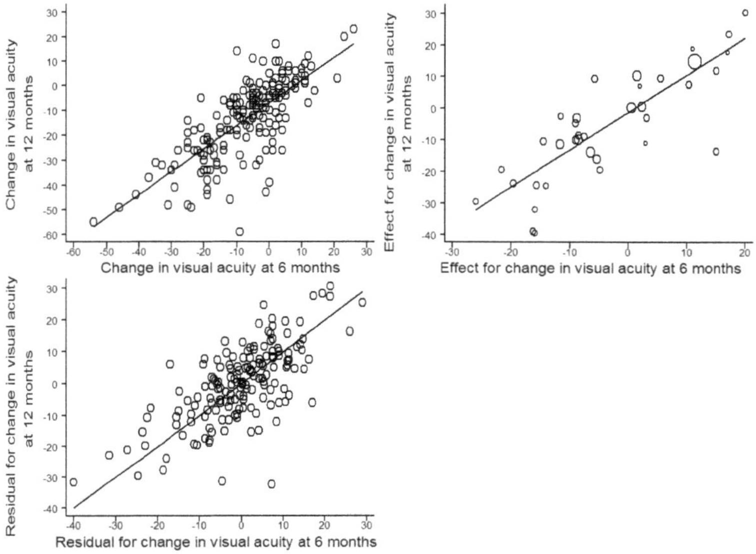

FIGURE 7.2. *Age-related macular degeneration trial. (a) True endpoint (change in visual acuity at 1 year) versus surrogate endpoint (change in visual acuity at 6 months) for all individual patients, raw data (top left). (b) Treatment effects on the true endpoint versus treatment effects on the surrogate endpoint in all centers. The size of each point is proportional to the number of patients in the corresponding center (top right). (c) True endpoint versus surrogate endpoint for all individual patients, after correction for treatment effect (bottom left).*

denote 5FU plus interferon and for 5FU alone. The final endpoint T_{ij} will be survival time in years. The surrogate endpoint S_{ij} will be progression-free survival time, i.e., the years between the randomization to clinical progression of the disease or death. For the purposes of the analysis, censoring is ignored and the logarithms of the two times are considered as continuous, normally distributed endpoints. In agreement with previous analyses, only centers with at least 3 patients on each treatment arm are considered. The data include 48 centers, with a total sample size of 642 patients.

Using the bivariate unweighted fixed-effects approach model proposed by Buyse *et al.* (2000a) we obtain $R^2_{\text{trial(f)}} = 0.473$ (s.e. 0.108), which is, of course, too low to be useful.

Results of fitting the various approaches, obtained by Tibaldi *et al.* (2003) and reported in Table 7.6, largely confirm the results from the ARMD study in terms of ease of convergence for the univariate and/or fixed-effects approaches. All coefficients are relatively close to each other, although the reduced versions tend to be a bit higher than the full versions.

7.5.3 Advanced Ovarian Cancer

In this section, the meta-analytic approach is illustrated using the data from the meta-analysis of four clinical trials in advanced ovarian cancer, described in Section 4.2.2 of Chapter 4. The results were reported by Buyse *et al.* (2000a). Recall that the surrogate endpoint S is progression-free survival time, while the true endpoint T is survival time. For the purposes of the analysis in this chapter, censoring is ignored and the logarithms of the two times are considered as continuous, normally distributed endpoints. All analyses have been performed with and without the two smaller trials. Excluding the two smaller trials has very little impact on the estimates of interest, and therefore the results reported are those obtained with all four trials. Two-stage fixed-effects models (7.1)–(7.2) could be fitted, as well as a reduced version of the mixed-effects model (7.6)–(7.7), with random treatment effects but no random intercepts. Point estimates for the two types of model are in close agreement, although standard errors are smaller by roughly 35% in the random-effects model. Figure 7.3 shows a plot of the treatment effects on the true endpoint (logarithm of survival) by the treatment effects on the surrogate endpoint (logarithm of progression-free survival time). These effects are highly correlated. Similarly to the random-effects situation, we refer to the models with and without the intercept used for determining R^2 as the reduced and full fixed-effects models. The reduced fixed-effects model provides $R^2_{\text{trial(r)}} = 0.939$ (s.e. 0.017). When the sample sizes of the experimental units are used to weigh the pairs (a_i, b_i), then $R^2_{\text{trial(r)}} = 0.916$ (s.e. 0.023). The full fixed-effects model yields $R^2_{\text{trial(f)}} = 0.940$ (s.e. 0.017). In the reduced random-effects model, $R^2_{\text{trial(r)}} = 0.951$ (s.e. 0.098).

Predictions of the effect of treatment on log(survival), based on the observed effect of treatment on log(progression-free survival time) are of interest. Table 7.7 reports prediction intervals for several experimental units: six centers taken at random from the two large trials, and the two small trials in which center is unknown. Note that none of the predictions is significantly different from zero. The predicted values for $\beta + b_0$ agree reasonably well with the effects estimated from the data. The ratio $\widehat{\beta}_0/\widehat{\alpha}_0$ ranges from 0.69 to 0.73.

At the individual level, $R^2_{\text{indiv}} = 0.886$ (s.e. 0.006) in the fixed-effects model, and $R^2_{\text{indiv}} = 0.888$ (s.e. 0.006) in the reduced random-effects model. The square roots of these quantities are respectively 0.941 and 0.942.

Thus, we conclude that progression-free survival time can be used as a surrogate for survival in advanced ovarian cancer. The effect of treatment can be observed earlier if time to progression is used instead of survival, and it is also more pronounced as shown by the overall Kaplan-Meier estimates of

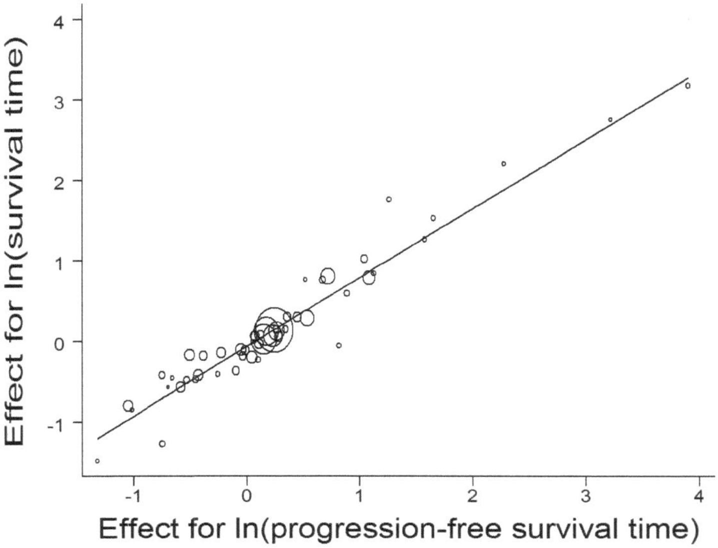

FIGURE 7.3. *Advanced ovarian cancer. Treatment effects on the true endpoint (logarithm of survival time) versus effects on the surrogate endpoint (logarithm of progression-free survival time) for all units of analysis.*

Figure 4.3 (Chapter 4). Hence, a trial that used time to progression would require less follow-up time and less patients to establish the statistical significance of a truly superior treatment than a trial that used survival (Chen *et al.* 1998).

The difference between the various approaches, as fitted by Tibaldi *et al.* (2003) and reported in Table 7.6, is even smaller than in the other two case studies. Further, the relative computational complexity, suggested by the other case studies, is confirmed here as well.

7.6 Discussion

The approach described in this chapter provides a quantitative assessment of the value of a surrogate, as well as predictions of the expected effect of treatment upon the true endpoint (Boissel *et al.* 1992, Chen *et al.* 1998). It evaluates the "validity" of a surrogate in terms of coefficients of determination, which are intuitively appealing quantities in the unit interval. Such an approach is more informative than a mere dichotomization of surrogate endpoints as being "valid" or "invalid." Moreover, the validation procedure no longer requires statistical tests to be statistically significant:

TABLE 7.7. *Predictions for the Advanced Ovarian Cancer data.*

Unit	No. pts.	No. trials	$\widehat{\alpha}_0$(s.e.)	$E(\beta + b_0 \mid a_0)$ (s.e.)	$\widehat{\beta}_0$ (s.e.)
Center 6	17	2	-0.58 (0.33)	-0.45 (0.29)	-0.56 (0.32)
		4		-0.45 (0.29)	
Center 8	10	2	0.67 (0.76)	0.49 (0.57)	0.76 (0.39)
		4		0.47 (0.56)	
Center 37	12	2	1.02 (0.61)	0.76 (0.54)	1.04 (0.70)
		4		0.73 (0.53)	
Center 49	40	2	0.54 (0.34)	0.39 (0.26)	0.28 (0.28)
		4		0.37 (0.25)	
Center 55	31	2	1.08 (0.56)	0.80 (0.44)	0.79 (0.45)
		4		0.77 (0.44)	
Center BB	21	2	-1.05 (0.55)	-0.80 (0.46)	-0.79 (0.51)
		4		-0.79 (0.46)	
DACOVA	274	2	0.25 (0.15)	0.17 (0.13)	0.14 (0.14)
GONO	125	2	0.15 (0.25)	0.10 (0.20)	0.03 (0.22)

NOTE: The number of patients is reported for each unit, as well as which sample is used for the estimation (only 2 trials or all 4). $\widehat{\alpha}_0$ and $\widehat{\beta}_0$ are values estimated from the data; $E(\beta + b_0 \mid a_0)$ is the predicted effect of treatment on survival (β_0), given its effect upon time to progression($\widehat{\alpha}_0$). The DACOVA and GONO trials are the two smaller studies, for which predictions are based on parameter estimates from the centers in the two larger studies.

for instance, an endpoint with a low individual-level coefficient of determination ($R^2_{\text{indiv}} \ll 1$) is unlikely to be a good surrogate (even if $R^2_{\text{trial(f)}} = 1$), a conclusion that may be reached with a limited number of observations.

The need for validated surrogate endpoints is as acute as ever, particularly in diseases where an accelerated approval process is deemed necessary (Cocchetto and Jones 1998, Weihrauch and Demol 1998). Some surrogate endpoints or combinations of endpoints, such as viral load measures combined with CD4+ lymphocyte counts, have in fact already replaced assessment of clinical outcomes in AIDS clinical trials (O'Brien *et al.* 1996, Mellors *et al.* 1997). The approach presented in this chapter offers a better understanding of the worth of a surrogate endpoint, provided that large enough sets of data from multiple randomized experiments are available to estimate the required parameters (Daniels and Hughes 1997). Large numbers of observations are needed for the estimates to be sufficiently precise, while multiple studies are needed to distinguish individual-level from trial-level associations between the endpoints and effects of interest. However, it has to be emphasized that, even if the results of a surrogate evaluation seem encouraging based on several trials, applying these results to a new trial requires a certain amount of extrapolation that may or may not be deemed acceptable. In particular, when a new treatment is under investigation, is it reasonable to assume that the quantitative relationship between its effects on the surrogate and true endpoints will be the same as with other treatments? The leap of faith involved in making that assumption rests primarily on biological considerations, although the type of statistical information presented above may provide essential supporting evidence. This and similar reservations lead to the following perspective.

However, while we like to underscore the integrity of such a meta-analytic framework, important questions remain open. First, the hierarchical framework is computationally more involved, and requires the number of trials and the number of patients per trials to be sufficiently large. In Section 7.4, we have considered a number of simplified approaches, where a fully hierarchical analysis is replaced by a two-stage approach and/or the two endpoints are analyzed separately. The latter is convenient when only the trial-level is of interest. Second, in several of the analyzed examples, by way of poor man's choice, "center" or "investigator" was used as sub-unit, rather than trial. Cortiñas *et al.* (2004) have investigated the impact of either ignoring or shifting between hierarchical levels. They have found that, the choice of the unit can be important if there are large differences in the magnitude of the variability in treatment effects at different levels. These results are reported in Chapter 8. Thus, it is of great interest, both to the public and to the scientific community, that data be shared to undertake the widest possible meta-analytic evaluations, rather than being considered the sole propriety of pharmaceutical companies. Third, the use of complex hierarchical models implies that different surrogacy measures are proposed for different types of outcomes, especially at the individual level. Indeed, while R^2 measures are used throughout at the trial level, individual-level measures include R^2, the odds ratio, Kendall's τ, etc. Alonso *et al.* (2004a) initiated the investigation to unify the various approaches (see Section 14.5.3). Fourth, the models considered so far reflect practice within later phase clinical trials, in the sense that, apart from treatment assignment, no other explanatory information is used. It is conceivable, especially in earlier phase trials and in preclinical research, that more elaborate models be used, incorporating explanatory (baseline) covariates, (molecular) biological, pharmacokinetic, or pharmacodynamic information. Fifth, Gail *et al.* (2000) have indicated that not properly accounting for measurement error may paint too optimistic a picture about surrogacy. It remains to be explored, theoretically and empirically, how useful surrogate markers are when all sources of measurement error are taken into account. Sixth, and linked to the previous issue, is the question how a properly evaluated surrogate endpoint could be used when designing a new trial. For example, one may want to determine the sample size to allow prediction of a significant effect on the true endpoint, without actually measuring it. Seventh, a properly evaluated surrogate endpoints will rarely be universally valid. The difficult question remains as to how broad the class of drugs is within which it can be used.

7.7 Extensions

In Section 7.2 we focused on the methodologically appealing case of normally distributed endpoints. In practice, situations abound where are the surrogate endpoint, or the true endpoint, or both, are of a non-Gaussian type. Indeed, binary, time-to-event, and longitudinal endpoints abound. Whereas the linear mixed model (Verbeke and Molenberghs 2000) provides a unified and flexible framework to analyze Gaussian multivariate and/or repeated measurements, similar tools for non-normal outcomes are unfortunately less well developed. In all non-Gaussian settings, one typically has to make a choice between marginal models on the one hand, where each outcome is modeled directly, without conditioning on other outcomes or on unobserved latent variables, and random-effects models on the other hand, where a vector of repeated measures is modeled, conditional upon one or a few unobserved random effects. For example, with binary outcomes, there are both marginal models such as generalized estimating equations (Liang and Zeger 1986) or full likelihood approaches (Fitzmaurice and Laird 1993, Lang and Agresti 1994, Molenberghs and Lesaffre 1994, Glonek and McCullagh 1995) and random-effects models (Stiratelli, Laird, and Ware 1984, Zeger, Liang, and Albert 1988, Breslow and Clayton 1993, Wolfinger and O'Connell 1993, Lee and Nelder 1996). Reviews are given in Diggle *et al.* (2002), Fahrmeir and Tutz (2002), and Molenberghs and Verbeke (2004). Similar choices need to be made with time-to-event outcomes, where marginal models are often based on the use of copulas, and random-effects models are based on so-called *frailties* (Genest and McKay 1986, Shih and Louis 1995a, Joe 1997, Nelsen 1999). Of course, specific attention needs to be given to those situations where the surrogate and the true endpoints are of a different type of outcome. Subsequent chapters will consider main situations in turn. In particular, two binary endpoints are treated in Chapter 10, while two time-to-event endpoints are discussed in Chapter 11. The combination of categorical surrogates with time-to-event endpoints is treated in Chapter 12. A longitudinal surrogate, combined with a survival true endpoint is the subject of Chapter 13, and the situation where both are longitudinal is the topic of Chapter 14.

8

The Choice of Units

José Cortiñas Abrahantes, Tomasz Burzykowski, and Geert Molenberghs

8.1 Introduction

In the previous chapter, we have introduced a hierarchical modeling framework to evaluate surrogate markers. As a general paradigm, trial was taken as the level of replication. However, in several of the examples, the unit of choice was center. This effectively implies extension of the framework to a three-level model, with patients nested within centers, and then centers within trials. Thus, it is important to assess the impact of omitting one of the levels in such a three-way hierarchy. An extended meta-analytic setting, to be used in this chapter, is introduced in Section 8.2. The different analytic approaches are presented in Section 8.3. A simulation study is reported in Section 8.4. With the results of the simulation study in mind, the data from a clinical study in schizophrenia, introduced in Section 4.2.6, are analyzed in Section 8.5. Note that the case study is based on a meta-analysis containing only five trials. This is insufficient to apply the meta-analytic methods. In all of the trials, information is also available on the investigators that treated the patients. Thus, we can also use investigator as the unit of analysis. For this case a total of 138 units are available for analysis, with the number of patients per unit ranging from 2 to 30. The true endpoint is Clinician's Global Impression (CGI), and as a surrogate measure, we consider the Positive and Negative Syndrome Scale (PANSS). Clearly, the majority of units consists of less than 5 patients. Alternatively, one could also consider the main investigator as unit of analysis. For 4 out of the 5 trials, only one main investigator was used, leading to extremely large investigator sites. This leads to a total number of 29 units with the number of patients per unit ranging from 4 to 450, 4 of which represent trials. Another possibility is to consider the countries where patients were treated, which fortunately is also available. Hence, we can also use country within trial as the unit of analysis. In this case a total of 19 units are available, with the number of patients per unit ranging from 9 to 128. The comparison of the three different choices will be used as an empirical assessment as to the importance the choice of unit can have on the results. In addition, data from the international equivalence trial on schizophrenic patients, introduced in Section 4.2.7, are analyzed. The trial included 206 schizophrenic patients. All patients received an equal daily amount of risperidone during 8 weeks, but 103 patients were randomized to a one-time daily intake (O.D.), while the remaining 103 patients were randomized to receive risperidone twice a day (B.I.D.). The surrogate and true endpoints are again PANSS and CGI, respectively. We will consider the investigator as the unit of analysis. This leads to a total of 34 units available for analysis with the number of patients per unit ranging from 2 to 15.

8.2 Model Description and Setting

In this section, we will introduce a three-level model for normally distributed endpoints. This model will allow us to consider the fully general case of a three-way hierarchy (e.g., patients within centers and centers within trials), as well as sub-cases that are of a two-level type. The emphasis will be on the surrogate marker situation, where such a model is needed for both the surrogate as well as the true endpoint. At the same time, the impact of misspecification by modeling the data as if they arose from a two-way structure, even though they were generated under a three-way model, can be assessed. In addition, the impact of considering the sub-unit effects as fixed, even though they are generated using a random-effects model, is studied.

Let T_{ijk} and S_{ijk} be random variables denoting the true and the surrogate endpoints for subject $k = 1, \ldots n_{ij}$ in center $j = 1, \ldots N_i$ within trial $i = 1, \ldots M$. Further, let Z_{ijk} denote a binary treatment indicator. The full three-way random-effects model can then be written as

$$\begin{cases} S_{ijk} = \mu_S + m_{S_i} + m_{S_{ij}} + (\alpha + a_i + a_{ij})Z_{ijk} + \varepsilon_{S_{ijk}}, \\ T_{ijk} = \mu_T + m_{T_i} + m_{T_{ij}} + (\beta + b_i + b_{ij})Z_{ijk} + \varepsilon_{T_{ijk}}, \end{cases} \quad (8.1)$$

where μ_S and μ_T are fixed intercepts, m_{S_i} and m_{T_i} are random intercepts for trial i, and $m_{S_{ij}}$ and $m_{T_{ij}}$ are random intercepts for center j in trial i. The parameters α and β are fixed treatment effects, a_i and b_i are random treatment effects associated with trial, and a_{ij} and b_{ij} are random treatment effects related to center. The individual-specific error terms are $\varepsilon_{S_{ijk}}$ and $\varepsilon_{T_{ijk}}$. The vector of random effects associated with trial, $(m_{S_i}, m_{T_i}, a_i, b_i)^T$, is assumed to be zero-mean normally distributed with covariance matrix

$$D = \begin{pmatrix} d_{SS} & d_{ST} & d_{Sa} & d_{Sb} \\ d_{ST} & d_{TT} & d_{Ta} & d_{Tb} \\ d_{Sa} & d_{Ta} & d_{aa} & d_{ab} \\ d_{Sb} & d_{Sa} & d_{ab} & d_{bb} \end{pmatrix}. \tag{8.2}$$

The vector of random effects associated with center, $(m_{S_{ij}}, m_{T_{ij}}, a_{ij}, b_{ij})^T$, is also assumed to be zero-mean normally distributed with covariance matrix

$$D' = \begin{pmatrix} d'_{SS} & d'_{ST} & d'_{Sa} & d'_{Sb} \\ d'_{ST} & d'_{TT} & d'_{Ta} & d'_{Tb} \\ d'_{Sa} & d'_{Ta} & d'_{aa} & d'_{ab} \\ d'_{Sb} & d'_{Sa} & d'_{ab} & d'_{bb} \end{pmatrix}. \tag{8.3}$$

Finally, the individual-level error terms $(\varepsilon_{S_{ijk}}, \varepsilon_{T_{ijk}})^T$ are also zero-mean normally distributed with variance-covariance matrix

$$\Sigma = \begin{pmatrix} \sigma_{SS} & \sigma_{ST} \\ \sigma_{ST} & \sigma_{TT} \end{pmatrix}. \tag{8.4}$$

Parameter estimation can be based on, for example, maximum likelihood or restricted maximum likelihood (Verbeke and Molenberghs 2000).

Clearly, (8.1) is not free from modeling assumptions. For example, one might want to entertain fixed effects rather than random effects. This will be considered in Section 8.3, where the second strategy would then be very appropriate. Indeed, fitting a random-effects model in such a case might lead to incorrectly attributing components of variability. Further, the joint normality of (8.1) implies that the regression of T_{ijk} on S_{ijk} is linear, whereas in reality a nonlinear association might apply. In practice, therefore, one may want to carefully assess the fit of the model. For the purpose of this chapter, model (8.1) is considered a versatile paradigm.

We will now shortly describe the use of these models in surrogate endpoint validation, expanding the methodology presented in Chapter 7. The next step considered in the methodology proposed by Buyse *et al.* (2000a) focused on prediction. Precisely, assuming one considers a new trial, for which data are available on the surrogate endpoint but not on the true endpoint, the goal is to predict the outcome on the true endpoint. Using two-level model (7.6)–(7.7) with trial- and individual-level random effects, and considering the implied conditional distribution of the treatment effect on the true endpoint given the treatment effect on the surrogate, Buyse *et al.* (2000a) proposed to assess the quality of the surrogate at the trial level by the coefficient of determination (see also equation (7.11))

$$R^2_{\text{trial(f)}} = R^2_{b_i|m_{Si},a_i} = \frac{\begin{pmatrix} d_{sb} \\ d_{ab} \end{pmatrix}^T \begin{pmatrix} d_{SS} & d_{Sa} \\ d_{Sa} & d_{aa} \end{pmatrix}^{-1} \begin{pmatrix} d_{Sb} \\ d_{ab} \end{pmatrix}}{d_{bb}} \tag{8.5}$$

or by its "reduced" variant (see equation (7.12))

$$R^2_{\text{trial(r)}} = R^2_{b_i|a_i} = \frac{d^2_{ab}}{d_{aa}d_{bb}}. \tag{8.6}$$

Similarly, to measure individual-level surrogacy, Buyse *et al.* (2000a) proposed to use the coefficient of determination given by (see also equation (7.21))

$$R^2_{\text{indiv}} = \frac{\sigma^2_{ST}}{\sigma_{SS}\sigma_{TT}}, \tag{8.7}$$

where σ_{ST}, σ_{SS} and σ_{TT} are components of variance-covariance matrix (8.4).

In our *three-level* context, the same procedure can be followed for the center level and $R^2_{\text{center(f)}}$ and $R^2_{\text{center(r)}}$ can be computed a way similar to (8.5) and (8.6) using matrix (8.3), providing us with an assessment of the *center-level* surrogacy.

8.3 Modeling Strategies

Tibaldi *et al.* (2003) showed that, in the two-level hierarchy, fitting random-effects model (8.1) can be replaced by simplified computational methods. In the remainder of this chapter, simplified methods will be used to face the computational challenges. In particular, we consider three strategies:

Strategy I: Two-level Only. This pertains to the case where, in spite of the three-level data generating mechanism, we consider either the trial level or center level for analysis and for validation, but not both. The trial and center-specific effects are treated as fixed.

Strategy II: Three Levels, Fixed Effects. A model in which the full three-level structure of the data is included. Both the trial-specific and the center-specific effects are treated as fixed.

Strategy III: Three Levels, Random Effects. A model in which the full three-level structure of the data is included. Both the trial-specific and center-specific effects are treated as random.

We will now discuss each of these three strategies in turn.

8.3.1 Strategy I: Two-level Only

As stated before, the parameters of the full random-effects model (8.1) can be estimated by maximum likelihood or restricted maximum likelihood, using standard linear mixed model software such as the SAS procedure MIXED (Verbeke and Molenberghs 2000).

Trial Level Only

In case we only consider the trial level for the validation process, exactly as Tibaldi *et al.* (2003), we can rewrite and simplify the model as

$$\begin{cases} S_{ijk} = \mu_{S_i} + \alpha_i Z_{ijk} + \varepsilon_{S_{ijk}}, \\ T_{ijk} = \mu_{T_i} + \beta_i Z_{ijk} + \varepsilon_{T_{ijk}}, \end{cases} \tag{8.8}$$

where μ_{S_i}, μ_{T_i}, α_i, and β_i are trial-specific intercepts and treatment effects. In addition, the univariate approach is opted for and hence errors $(\varepsilon_{S_{ijk}}, \varepsilon_{T_{ijk}})$ in (8.8) are assumed independent, rather than correlated. Tibaldi *et al.* (2003) showed that this approach is computationally advantageous, while resulting in little or no loss of efficiency when emphasis is on the trial-level surrogacy. Of course, if one is interested in individual-level surrogacy as well, the correlation between the outcomes needs to be accounted for. At the second stage, a regression model is fitted to the treatment effects, estimated at the first stage. For example,

$$\widehat{\beta}_i = \lambda_0 + \lambda_1 \widehat{\mu}_{S_i} + \lambda_2 \widehat{\alpha}_i + \varepsilon_i. \tag{8.9}$$

As Tibaldi *et al.* (2003) stated, this model can then be employed to assess the trial-level surrogacy, using the $R^2_{\text{trial(f)}}$ associated with the model. The coefficient is not calculated as in (8.5), but it merely is the classical coefficient of determination found by regressing $\widehat{\beta}_i$ on $\widehat{\mu}_{S_i}$ and $\widehat{\alpha}_i$.

If trial-specific intercept from the surrogate model (8.8) is not used, λ_1 is dropped from (8.9) and an $R^2_{\text{trial(r)}}$ is obtained, similar in spirit to (8.6).

Center Level Only

In case we only consider the center level for the validation process, and analogous to the previous case, the model can be rewritten as:

$$\begin{cases} S_{ijk} = \mu_{S_{ij}} + \alpha_{ij} Z_{ijk} + \varepsilon_{S_{ijk}}, \\ T_{ijk} = \mu_{T_{ij}} + \beta_{ij} Z_{ijk} + \varepsilon_{T_{ijk}}, \end{cases} \tag{8.10}$$

where now $\mu_{S_{ij}}$, $\mu_{T_{ij}}$, α_{ij}, and β_{ij} are center-specific intercepts and treatment effects. As in the previous case, the models are fitted separately and the errors are assumed to be independent. At the second stage, a regression model similar to (8.9) is fitted to the treatment effects, obtained from the estimation at the first stage:

$$\widehat{\beta}_{ij} = \lambda_0' + \lambda_1'\widehat{\mu}_{S_{ij}} + \lambda_2'\widehat{\alpha}_{ij} + \varepsilon_{ij}. \tag{8.11}$$

The model can be used to assess the center-level surrogacy, using the $R^2_{\text{center(f)}}$ associated with this regression. In case that center-specific intercept from surrogate model is not used, a reduced $R^2_{\text{center(r)}}$ is obtained.

8.3.2 Strategy II: Three Levels, Fixed Effects

We now include both trial as well as center effects in the first-stage model, but they are considered to be fixed rather than random. The model then reads:

$$\begin{cases} S_{ijk} = \mu_{S_i} + \mu_{S_{ij}} + (\alpha_i + \alpha_{ij})Z_{ijk} + \varepsilon_{S_{ijk}}, \\ T_{ijk} = \mu_{T_i} + \mu_{T_{ij}} + (\beta_i + \beta_{ij})Z_{ijk} + \varepsilon_{T_{ijk}}, \end{cases} \tag{8.12}$$

where both errors ($\varepsilon_{S_{ijk}}$,$\varepsilon_{T_{ijk}}$) are to be dependent.

At the second stage, an appropriate set of regressions is fitted to the treatment effects, estimated at the first stage:

$$\widehat{\beta}_i = \lambda_0 + \lambda_1\widehat{\mu}_{S_i} + \lambda_2\widehat{\alpha}_i + \varepsilon_i, \tag{8.13}$$

$$\widehat{\beta}_{ij} = \lambda_0' + \lambda_1'\widehat{\mu}_{S_{ij}} + \lambda_2'\widehat{\alpha}_{ij} + \varepsilon_{ij}. \tag{8.14}$$

Model (8.13) is used, when the trial-level association is of interest. Model (8.14) is used, when the focus is on the association at the center level. Both regressions produce an R^2 measure of surrogacy.

8.3.3 Strategy III: Three Levels, Random Effects

Buyse *et al.* (2000a) assumed the availability of individual-patient data and formulated a two-stage model, with the joint distribution $[T, S|Z]$ specified at the first stage and the joint distribution of the treatment effects $[\beta, \alpha]$ specified at the second stage. Shkedy *et al.* (2003) employed this methodology and developed a Bayesian approach under the assumption that individual data are available (Browne *et al.* 2002, Liao 2002). We will extend their methodology for model (8.1).

Generally, consider linear predictors for T and S:

$$\begin{cases} E(S_{ijk}|m_{S_i}, m_{S_{ij}}, a_i, a_{ij}) \\ \qquad = \mu_S + m_{S_i} + m_{S_{ij}} + (\alpha + a_i + a_{ij})Z_{ijk}, \\ E(T_{ijk}|m_{T_i}, m_{T_{ij}}, b_i, b_{ij}) \\ \qquad = \mu_T + m_{T_i} + m_{T_{ij}} + (\beta + b_i + b_{ij})Z_{ijk}. \end{cases} \tag{8.15}$$

The coefficients m_{S_i}, m_{T_i}, a_i, b_i, $m_{S_{ij}}$, $m_{T_{ij}}$, a_{ij}, b_{ij} have a similar meaning as those in model (8.1). Further, the vector of random effects associated to trial, $(m_{S_i}, m_{T_i}, a_i, b_i)^T$, is assumed to be zero-mean normally distributed with covariance matrix (8.2), while the vector of random effects associated to center, $(m_{S_{ij}}, m_{T_{ij}}, a_{ij}, b_{ij})^T$, is assumed to be zero-mean normally distributed with covariance matrix (8.3).

Shkedy *et al.* (2003) proposed to combine (8.15) and (8.2)–(8.3), defining a hierarchical Bayesian model (see also Chapter 15). Thus, at the first stage of the hierarchical model, we specify the following joint distribution of T_{ijk} and S_{ijk}:

$$\begin{pmatrix} S_{ijk} \\ T_{ijk} \end{pmatrix} \sim \mathrm{N}\left\{\begin{bmatrix} \mu_S + m_{S_i} + m_{S_{ij}} + (\alpha + a_i + a_{ij})Z_{ijk} \\ \mu_T + m_{T_i} + m_{T_{ij}} + (\beta + b_i + b_{ij})Z_{ijk} \end{bmatrix}, \Sigma\right\}, \tag{8.16}$$

where Σ is given by (8.4).

At the second stage of the model the priors for the "fixed" effects are specified:

$$\begin{aligned} \mu_S &\sim \mathrm{N}(0, \theta^2_{\mu_S}), \\ \mu_T &\sim \mathrm{N}(0, \theta^2_{\mu_T}), \\ \alpha &\sim \mathrm{N}(0, \tau^2_\alpha), \\ \beta &\sim \mathrm{N}(0, \tau^2_\alpha). \end{aligned} \tag{8.17}$$

For the precision parameters in (8.17) (flat) hyperprior models can be specified using Gamma distributions, e.g., $\theta^{-2}_{\mu_S} \sim \mathrm{gamma}(0.001, 0.001)$, etc. As the hyperprior distribution for the covariance matrices D, D' and Σ, a Wishart distribution is assumed:

$$\begin{aligned} D^{-1} &\sim \mathrm{Wishart}(R_D), \\ D'^{-1} &\sim \mathrm{Wishart}(R_{D'}), \\ \Sigma^{-1} &\sim \mathrm{Wishart}(R_\Sigma). \end{aligned} \tag{8.18}$$

To assess the trial-level surrogacy, the coefficient of determination defined by (8.5) will be used. The center-level surrogacy can be assessed using the coefficient of determination computed from (8.5) with matrix D', given in (8.3), in place of matrix D. Finally, to measure individual-level surrogacy, the coefficient of determination given in (8.7) can be used.

To avoid computational problems, Buyse *et al.* (2000a) proposed a reduced model in which the linear predictors of S and T do not include trial and center specific intercepts. In the hierarchical model, the likelihood at the first stage of the model can be specified by omitting the trial-specific random intercepts from (8.16). This leads to the specification:

$$\begin{pmatrix} S_{ij} \\ T_{ij} \end{pmatrix} \sim \mathrm{N}\left\{ \begin{bmatrix} \mu_S + (\alpha + a_i + a_{ij}) Z_{ijk} \\ \mu_T + (\beta + b_i + b_{ij}) Z_{ijk} \end{bmatrix}, \Sigma \right\}. \tag{8.19}$$

At the second stage of the model, the prior distribution of the random effects, $(a_i, b_i)^T$, is assumed to be bivariate normal with mean 0 and covariance matrix D_r. Note that the covariance matrix D_r is the 2×2 lower right submatrix in (8.2) and is assumed to follow a Wishart distribution, $D_r^{-1} \sim \text{Wishart}(R_{D_r})$. Other prior and hyperprior models remain the same as in the full model. For the reduced model, the coefficient of determination, measuring the trial-level surrogacy, reduces to (8.6). Similar considerations can be made for $(a_{ij}, b_{ij})^T$, which is assumed normal with zero mean and covariance matrix D_r', which is the 2×2 right bottom sub matrix of D' defined in (8.3).

8.4 A Simulation Study

We assess the performance of the various strategies in terms of both point estimation, as well as precision, of $R^2_{\text{trial(r)}}$ and of $R^2_{\text{center(r)}}$, by means of a simulation study. A setting, similar to the one used in Chapter 7 is adopted.

8.4.1 Simulation Settings

Generating Mechanism I

Under Mechanism I, data are generated using model (8.1) with

$$(m_{S_i}, m_{T_i}, a_i, b_i) \sim N(0, D)$$

and

$$(m_{S_{ij}}, m_{T_{ij}}, a_{ij}, b_{ij}) \sim N(0, D'),$$

where

$$D = \sigma_T^2 \begin{pmatrix} 1 & 0.8 & 0 & 0 \\ 0.8 & 1 & 0 & 0 \\ 0 & 0 & 1 & \rho_T \\ 0 & 0 & \rho_T & 1 \end{pmatrix},$$

$$D' = \sigma_C^2 \begin{pmatrix} 1 & 0.8 & 0 & 0 \\ 0.8 & 1 & 0 & 0 \\ 0 & 0 & 1 & \rho_C \\ 0 & 0 & \rho_C & 1 \end{pmatrix}, \tag{8.20}$$

and $\mu_S = 50$, $\mu_T = 45$, $\alpha = 5$, $\beta = 3$.

Further, the true R^2, following from (8.5) and (8.20), is set equal to either 0.5 or 0.9 at the trial or at the center level. Thus, for both ρ_T^2 and ρ_C^2, the values of 0.5 or 0.9 are considered. Parameters σ_T^2 and σ_C^2 are assigned values of 0.1 or 10. Regarding the individual-level variability, $(\varepsilon_{S_{ij}}, \varepsilon_{T_{ij}}) \sim N(0, \Sigma)$ with

$$\Sigma = \sigma^2 \begin{pmatrix} 1 & 0.8 \\ 0.8 & 1 \end{pmatrix}.$$

The parameter σ^2 equals either 0.1 or 3.

For every choice of values for ρ_T, ρ_C, σ_T^2, σ_C^2 and σ^2, simulated datasets were obtained assuming 5, 10, 20, or 100 trials, with 10 or 100 centers per trial and with 10 or 100 subjects per center. In total, 250 datasets were simulated for each setting.

Generating Mechanisms II and III

Further, a simulation was performed in which, instead of considering model (8.1) to generate the data, we used a model in which we have random effects associated to either trial or to center, but not to both of them.

The first of these, termed Mechanism II and where only trial-level random effects are considered, is given by:

$$\begin{cases} S_{ijk} = \mu_S + m_{S_i} + (\alpha + a_i) Z_{ijk} + \varepsilon_{S_{ijk}}, \\ T_{ijk} = \mu_T + m_{T_i} + (\beta + b_i) Z_{ijk} + \varepsilon_{T_{ijk}}. \end{cases} \tag{8.21}$$

Alternatively, when only random-effects at the center level are present (Mechanism III), (8.1) simplifies to:

$$\begin{cases} S_{ijk} = \mu_S + m_{S_{ij}} + (\alpha + a_{ij}) Z_{ijk} + \varepsilon_{S_{ijk}}, \\ T_{ijk} = \mu_T + m_{T_{ij}} + (\beta + b_{ij}) Z_{ijk} + \varepsilon_{T_{ijk}}. \end{cases} \tag{8.22}$$

The random vectors associated to trial and center were considered, as in Mechanism I, to follow mean-zero normal distributions: $(m_{S_i}, m_{T_i}, a_i, b_i) \sim N(0, D)$, $(m_{S_{ij}}, m_{T_{ij}}, a_{ij}, b_{ij}) \sim N(0, D')$.

A setting of simulation parameters similar to the one used for Mechanism I was considered, i.e., 5, 10, 20, or 100 trials, with 10 or 100 centers and 10 or 100 subjects per center; σ_T^2 and σ_C^2 equal to 10 or 0.1; $\sigma^2 = 3$ or 0.1; $\rho_T^2 = 0.5$ or 0.9 and $\rho_C^2 = 0.5$ or 0.9.

8.4.2 Simulation Results, Equal Trial- and Center-level Association

Generating Mechanism I

The results of the simulations for Mechanism I, assuming $\rho_T^2 = \rho_C^2 = 0.5$ or 0.9, $\sigma_T^2 = \sigma_C^2 = 10$, and $\sigma^2 = 3$ for 5, 10 or 20 trials with 10 centers per trial and 10 subjects per center are shown in Figure 8.1. Results for other settings of the parameters are similar.

Figure 8.1 shows the results obtained when Strategies I and II were used. In particular, the use of Strategy I means that the association at the trial level was evaluated using a model without the center level (see (8.8) in Section 8.3.1), whereas the association at the center level was assessed using a model without the trial level (see (8.10) in Section 8.3.1).

Figure 8.1 indicates that both strategies give comparable results. One can observe that Strategy II has larger bias in the estimation than Strategy I. It is important to point out that when $\rho_T^2 = \rho_C^2 = 0.5$, both methods tend to overestimate the strength of the association, whereas if $\rho_T^2 = \rho_C^2 = 0.9$, the strategies underestimate it.

Generating Mechanisms II and III

When only one level of association is present in the data generating mechanism, we can try to estimate the effects at this particular level using Strategy I, with either the correct or the incorrect level included in the model. That is, if Mechanism II was used, which involved only the trial-level association, we could try to capture this association using center as the unit of analysis. A similar approach could be used for Mechanism III, but in this case the center-level association could be evaluated using trial as the unit of analysis. This would correspond to realistic situations where our interest lies at another level than at which data are available from. For example, the first scenario (Mechanism II with center as the unit of analy-

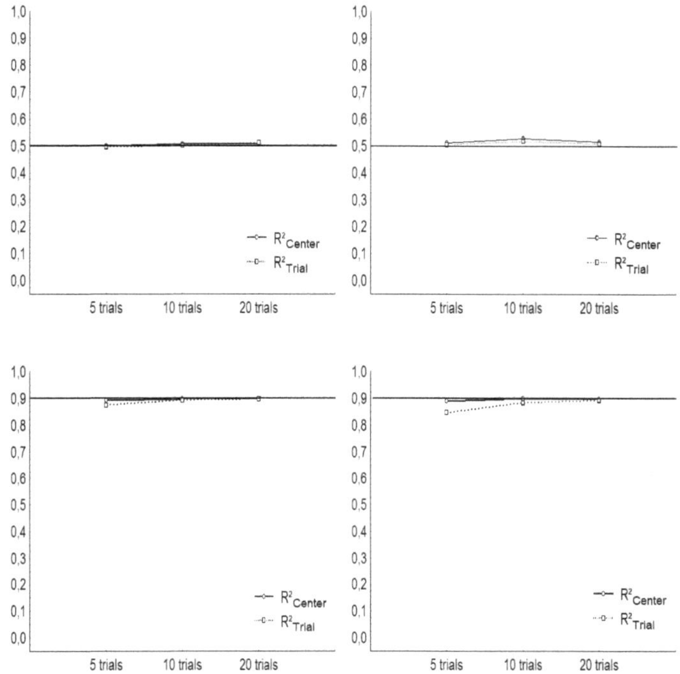

FIGURE 8.1. *Simulation study. The estimation of* R^2 *and its precision for* $R^2_{trial(r)} = R^2_{center(r)}$ *and* $\sigma_T^2 = \sigma_C^2 = 10$. *Data were generated using Mechanism I. Left column: Strategy I (two-level only); right column: Strategy II (three-levels, fixed effects). Top row: estimation of* $R^2 = 0.5$; *bottom row: estimation of* $R^2 = 0.9$.

sis) is of practical interest when there are too few trials available and, to assess the trial-level surrogacy, data for centers is used instead. The results for 5, 10 or 20 trials with 10 centers per trial and 10 subjects per center and $\rho_T^2 = \rho_C^2 = 0.5$ or 0.9, $\sigma_T^2 = \sigma_C^2 = 10$, $\sigma^2 = 3$ are shown in Figure 8.2. Results for other settings of the parameters are similar.

From Figure 8.2, it can be seen that when the data were generated using Mechanism II (graphs on the left-hand side of Figure 8.2), the strategies proposed in Section 8.3.1 using either equation (8.9) and (8.11) led to very similar results. That is, the estimated strength of the (trial-level) association was similar irrespectively of whether trial (correctly) or center (incorrectly) was used as the unit of analysis. On the other hand, when Mechanism III was used to generate the data (graphs on the right-hand side of Figure 8.2), the method based on equation (8.11), in which center was (correctly) used as the unit of analysis, performed much better than

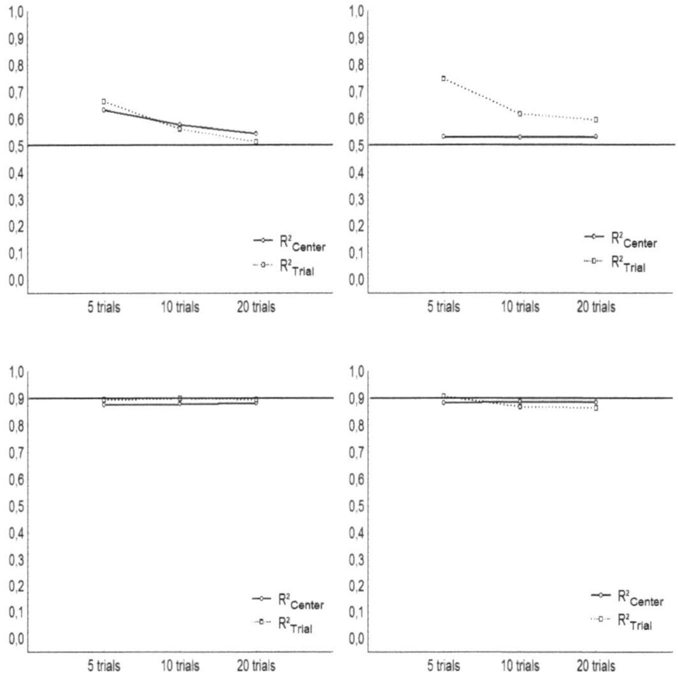

FIGURE 8.2. *Simulation study. The estimation of* R^2 *and its precision for Strategy I (two-level only) when* $R^2_{trial(r)} = R^2_{center(r)}$ *and* $\sigma_T^2 = \sigma_C^2 = 10$. *Left column: Generating Mechanism II; Right column: Generation Mechanism III. Top row: estimation of* $R^2 = 0.5$*; bottom row: estimation of* $R^2 = 0.9$.

the method based on equation (8.9), in which trial was (incorrectly) used as the unit of analysis. To be precise, for the analysis based on centers the estimates were closer to the true parameter. It can be also noted that, as it has been observed in the case of Mechanism I (see Figure 8.1), when ρ_T^2 and ρ_C^2 were equal to 0.5, Strategy I tended to overestimate the strength of the association, whereas when ρ_T^2 and ρ_C^2 were equal to 0.9, it was generally underestimated.

In addition, Strategy II was also applied to the simulated datasets. In this case, first three-level fixed-effects model (8.12) was fitted to the data, and then models (8.13) and (8.14) were used to compute the determination coefficients assessing the strength of association at the trial and center level, respectively. The results for 5, 10 or 20 trials with 10 centers per trial and 10 subjects per center and $\rho_T^2 = \rho_C^2 = 0.5$ or $\rho_T^2 = \rho_C^2 = 0.9$, $\sigma_T^2 = \sigma_C^2 = 10$, $\sigma^2 = 3$ are shown in Figure 8.3. Results for other settings of the parameters are similar.

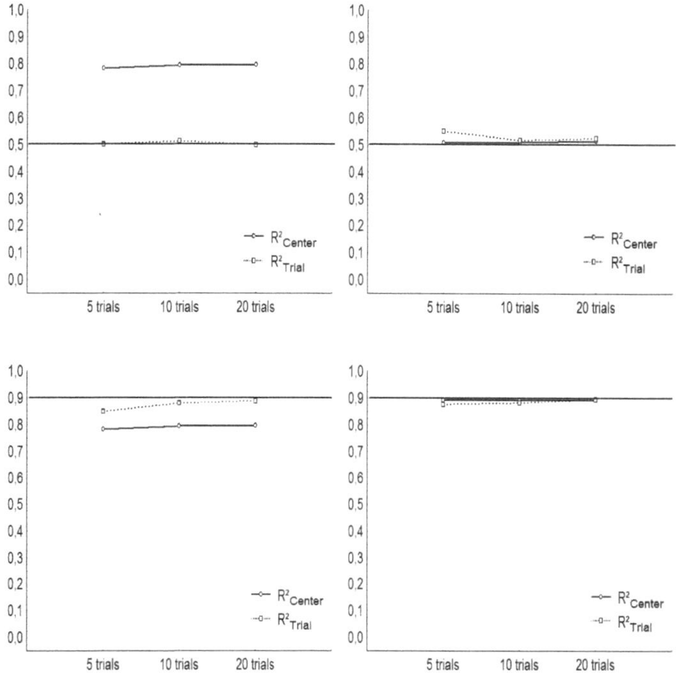

FIGURE 8.3. *Simulation study. The estimation of R^2 and its precision for Strategy II (three-levels, fixed effects) when $R^2_{trial(r)} = R^2_{center(r)}$ and $\sigma^2_T = \sigma^2_C = 10$. Left column: Generating Mechanism II; Right column: Generating Mechanism III. Top row: estimation of $R^2 = 0.5$; bottom row: estimation of $R^2 = 0.9$.*

From Figure 8.3 it is clear that, when Mechanism II was used, Strategy II with model (8.13) at the second stage (based on trial-specific estimates) was giving satisfactory results in terms of the bias of the estimation. On the other hand, for model (8.14), based on center-specific estimates, the results were poor. Figure 8.3 also shows that when Mechanism III was used to generate the data, Strategy II gave similar results in terms of bias irrespectively of the model used at the second stage.

8.4.3 Simulation Results, Unequal Trial- and Center-level Association

The results of simulations presented in Section 8.4.2 allow to conclude that both Strategy I and Strategy II performed reasonably well when the association at the trial and at the center levels were equal. In this section,

TABLE 8.1. *Simulation study. Results for Strategies I and II for $\sigma_T^2 = \sigma_C^2 = 10$, with 10 patients per center and 10 centers per trial. Mean estimates of ρ_T^2 and ρ_C^2 with model-based and empirical standard errors (in parentheses).*

ρ_T^2	ρ_C^2	No. trials	Trial as unit*	Center as unit**
			Strategy I	
0.5	0.9	5	0.521(0.309,0.317)	0.706(0.158,0.169)
0.5	0.9	10	0.528(0.220,0.226)	0.700(0.116,0.121)
0.5	0.9	20	0.540(0.147,0.151)	0.698(0.077,0.079)
0.9	0.5	5	0.830(0.179,0.186)	0.655(0.113,0.118)
0.9	0.5	10	0.851(0.098,0.099)	0.676(0.085,0.088)
0.9	0.5	20	0.856(0.064,0.065)	0.681(0.059,0.058)
			Strategy II	
0.5	0.9	5	0.623(0.296,0.301)	0.891(0.050,0.054)
0.5	0.9	10	0.676(0.182,0.183)	0.900(0.034,0.040)
0.5	0.9	20	0.681(0.122,0.121)	0.898(0.025,0.027)
0.9	0.5	5	0.663(0.268,0.273)	0.511(0.139,0.145)
0.9	0.5	10	0.685(0.190,0.196)	0.527(0.119,0.122)
0.9	0.5	20	0.686(0.123,0.124)	0.518(0.092,0.093)

* Gives estimates of ρ_T^2.

** Gives estimates of ρ_C^2.

we present the case in which the associations at both levels differ.

Performance of Strategies I and II

To study further the performance of Strategies I and II, we simulated data using Mechanism I, with $\rho_T^2 \neq \rho_C^2$. In particular, we considered $\rho_T^2 = 0.5$ with $\rho_C^2 = 0.9$ and $\rho_T^2 = 0.9$ with $\rho_C^2 = 0.5$. The values for the other parameters were similar to those used for the simulations presented in Section 8.4.2. The results for 5, 10 or 20 trials with 10 centers per trial and 10 subjects per center and $\sigma_T^2 = \sigma_C^2 = 10$ and $\sigma^2 = 3$ are shown in Table 8.1. In terms of bias, the results from Table 8.1 are reasonable for the estimation of the trial-level association when Strategy I was applied (i.e., using trial as the unit of analysis at both stages) and of the center-level association when Strategy II was applied (i.e., a three-level fixed-effects model at the first stage with center-specific effects analyzed at the second stage).

The above conclusions were drawn for the case when $\sigma_T^2 = \sigma_C^2 = 10$. It is also of interest to study what would happen if σ_C^2 were much smaller

TABLE 8.2. *Simulation study. Results for Strategies I and II for $\sigma_T^2 = 10$ and $\sigma_C^2 = 0.1$ and 10 patients per center and 10 centers per trial. Mean estimates of ρ_T^2 and ρ_C^2 with model-based and empirical standard errors (in parentheses).*

ρ_T^2	ρ_C^2	No. trials	Trial as unit*	Center as unit**
			Strategy I	
0.5	0.9	5	0.535(0.305,0.315)	0.537(0.294,0.312)
0.5	0.9	10	0.504(0.228,0.235)	0.516(0.220,0.231)
0.5	0.9	20	0.507(0.151,0.157)	0.519(0.145,0.153)
0.9	0.5	5	0.894(0.122,0.131)	0.880(0.123,0.134)
0.9	0.5	10	0.891(0.094,0.102)	0.884(0.087,0.092)
0.9	0.5	20	0.897(0.043,0.047)	0.890(0.042,0.046)
			Strategy II	
0.5	0.9	5	0.526(0.312,0.320)	0.819(0.075,0.079)
0.5	0.9	10	0.508(0.231,0.238)	0.822(0.060,0.062)
0.5	0.9	20	0.513(0.156,0.161)	0.822(0.044,0.045)
0.9	0.5	5	0.870(0.151,0.154)	0.722(0.109,0.111)
0.9	0.5	10	0.882(0.088,0.090)	0.730(0.087,0.089)
0.9	0.5	20	0.888(0.048,0.047)	0.731(0.068,0.070)

* Gives estimates of ρ_T^2.

** Gives estimates of ρ_C^2.

than σ_T^2. From a practical point of view this situation is desirable, since a large variance for the center level means existence of a strong center-specific treatment effect, what makes difficult to draw general conclusions. Table 8.2 presents results for Strategies I and II for the case of $\sigma_T^2 = 10$ and $\sigma_C^2 = 0.1$.

Table 8.2 indicates that, when the variability at the center level was much smaller than at the trial level, the estimates obtained using either Strategy I or Strategy II for the trial-level association were close to the true value of the parameter of interest. On the other hand, for the center-level association, reasonable results were obtained only for Strategy II when $\rho_C^2 = 0.9$. For other cases using center as the unit of the analysis, either at both stages (Strategy I) or only at the second one (Strategy II), produced results that, on average, were close to the value of the coefficient of determination related to the trial-level association.

Insights in the Performance of Strategy I

The bad performance of Strategy I, especially for the center level, can be explained by the fact that ignoring a level can lead to overestimation of the variability at the levels surrounding the level being ignored. To this aim, we will use the results obtained by Hutchison and Healy (2001). For example, consider the following model:

$$S_{ijk} = \mu_S + m_{S_i} + m_{S_{ij}} + (\alpha + \alpha_i + \alpha_{ij})Z_{ijk} + \varepsilon_{S_{ijk}}.$$

This model is similar to model (8.1), but contains only three random effects: random intercepts m_{S_i} and $m_{S_{ij}}$ associated to trial and center, respectively, and the random error $\varepsilon_{S_{ijk}}$. Assume that the data are balanced ($N_i \equiv N$, $n_{ij} \equiv n$) and the variances of the random effects corresponding to the trial, center and individual level are equal to σ_T^2, σ_C^2 and σ^2, respectively. It can be then shown that the two variance components of the model in which the center level is ignored are:

$$\tilde{\sigma}_T^2 = \sigma_T^2 + \frac{n-1}{N \cdot n - 1} \cdot \sigma_C^2 \approx \sigma_T^2 + \frac{1}{N} \cdot \sigma_C^2, \quad (8.23)$$

$$\tilde{\sigma}^2 = \sigma^2 + \frac{n \cdot (N-1)}{N \cdot n - 1} \cdot \sigma_C^2 \approx \sigma^2 + \frac{N-1}{N} \cdot \sigma_C^2. \quad (8.24)$$

Thus, they can be seen as the true variance, plus a certain fraction of the variance of the random effect associated to the level that has been ignored. For this particular case not much variability is added to the variance corresponding to the level above the one ignored (trial), as most of the information is sent to the level below. This is the reason why in Tables 8.1 and 8.2 the trial-level association is generally well estimated when Strategy I is used. On the other hand, if the trial level is ignored, the center-level variance becomes

$$\tilde{\sigma}_C^2 = \sigma_C^2 + \frac{N \cdot (M-1)}{M \cdot N - 1} \cdot \sigma_T^2 \approx \sigma_C^2 + \frac{M-1}{M} \cdot \sigma_T^2. \quad (8.25)$$

The individual-level variability remains unchanged. Thus, most of the variability contained in the trial level is sent to the center level, which affects the estimation of the association at the center level. This is the reason why in Tables 8.1 and 8.2 the center-level association is poorly estimated when Strategy I is used.

Performance of Strategy II in a Large Dataset

To explore further the behavior of Strategy II observed in Tables 8.1 and 8.2, an additional simulation study was conducted. Table 8.3 shows results

TABLE 8.3. *Simulation study. Results for* Strategy II *for different values of variance components associated to trial and center random effects, with 100 subjects per center, 100 centers per trial, and 100 trials. Mean estimates of* ρ_T^2 *and* ρ_C^2 *with model-based and empirical standard errors (in parentheses).*

σ_T^2	σ_C^2	σ^2	ρ_T^2	ρ_C^2	Trial as unit*	Center as unit**
10	10	3	0.5	0.9	0.685(0.030,0.033)	0.900(0.004,0.009)
10	10	3	0.9	0.5	0.684(0.031,0.035)	0.501(0.014,0.021)
10	10	0.1	0.5	0.9	0.685(0.030,0.033)	0.900(0.004,0.009)
10	10	0.1	0.9	0.5	0.683(0.031,0.035)	0.499(0.014,0.020)
10	0.1	3	0.5	0.9	0.508(0.028,0.030)	0.877(0.010,0.012)
10	0.1	3	0.9	0.5	0.896(0.010,0.013)	0.565(0.024,0.027)
10	0.1	0.1	0.5	0.9	0.506(0.028,0.031)	0.899(0.005,0.007)
10	0.1	0.1	0.9	0.5	0.896(0.010,0.013)	0.503(0.015,0.017)
0.1	0.1	0.1	0.5	0.9	0.686(0.030,0.032)	0.899(0.005,0.008)
0.1	0.1	0.1	0.9	0.5	0.684(0.031,0.033)	0.503(0.015,0.0017)

* Gives estimates of ρ_T^2.
** Gives estimates of ρ_C^2.

for several different combinations of the values of parameters σ_T^2, σ_C^2, σ^2, ρ_T^2, and ρ_C^2, for 100 trials with 100 centers per trial and 100 subjects per center. The idea is to investigate the behavior of the strategy in a large dataset.

Results presented in Table 8.3 indicate that, the center-level association was in general estimated reasonably well. It is worth noting that the bias, observed in Table 8.2 for the combination of $\rho_T^2 = 0.9$ and $\rho_C^2 = 0.5$, was greatly reduced when $\sigma^2 = 3$, and essentially disappeared when $\sigma^2 = 0.1$. This suggests that, for Strategy II, the bias in the estimation of the center-level surrogacy may be negligible as long as the variability at the level of center is at least as large as the variability at the lower (individual) level.

On the other hand, from Table 8.3, one can see that, when the variability at the trial and center level was of the same magnitude, the trial-level association was poorly estimated, even though the sizes of the units were large. The bias generally disappeared when the variability at the center level became much smaller than that at the level of trial. This suggest that, as for the center-level association, bias in the assessment of the trial-level association for Strategy II may be negligible as long as the variability at the lower (center) level is smaller.

Comparison of Strategies II and III

Finally, we attempted to compare Strategy II with Strategy III. Because using a maximum-likelihood approach to implement Strategy III was numerically too complex, we considered the use of a Bayesian approach. Unfortunately, performing an extensive simulation using the latter approach turned out to be too time-consuming. Therefore, the simulation study was limited to the random generation of only one dataset for different parameter settings, and the comparison of the results obtained for Strategy II and Strategy III to the true values of the parameters used for simulations. The results are shown in Table 8.4. By comparing the estimates of the coefficients of determination to their actual values (i.e., the values computed from the actual, simulated random effects) in Table 8.4 we can observe that, when the variability at the center and trial level was of the same magnitude, Strategy II did not estimate the trial-level association well, in contrary to Strategy III. Even when the variability at the center level was smaller than that at the level of trial, estimates obtained for Strategy III were closer to the actual values than the estimates produced by Strategy II. One can conclude, admittedly based on the anecdotal evidence obtained by generating a single dataset under each setting, that Strategy III gives better results, which is reasonable if we take into account that the other two strategies are ignoring levels and are using fixed effects as representation of random effects.

8.5 Analysis of Schizophrenia Trials

In the first psychiatric study, several options were studied considering the units available. The first row in Table 8.5 shows the results obtained when Strategy I was applied. That is, the coefficient of determination associated to a particular level (indicated in the header of the column) was estimated using a (two-stage) model including only this level and individual variability. We observe that, in general, there is relatively little difference between the estimates obtained.

Strategy II, using a fixed-effects model with all three levels included at the first stage, was fitted as well. In this model the estimate of the magnitude of the association at the highest level (country) is close to that obtained using Strategy I. For the other two levels more substantial differences can be observed.

Finally, a random-effects (Strategy III) analysis, based on the Bayesian approach, was performed. The results are shown in the last row of Table 8.5.

TABLE 8.4. *Simulation study. Results for* Strategy II *and* Strategy III *for a simulated sets of data with 10 subjects per center and 10 centers per trial and* $\sigma_T = 10$ *(Mean = posterior mean; StDev = posterior standard deviation; Median = posterior median).*

σ_C	No. trials	ρ_T^2	ρ_C^2	R^2	Actual value	Strategy II	Strategy III Mean	StDev	Median
10	5	0.5	0.9	Trial	0.750	0.840	0.653	0.2420	0.7127
10	5	0.5	0.9	Center	0.927	0.914	0.934	0.0210	0.9381
10	5	0.9	0.5	Trial	0.916	0.822	0.917	0.0856	0.9430
10	5	0.9	0.5	Center	0.443	0.539	0.497	0.1079	0.5012
10	10	0.5	0.9	Trial	0.263	0.501	0.260	0.2128	0.2234
10	10	0.5	0.9	Center	0.930	0.951	0.929	0.0154	0.9311
10	10	0.9	0.5	Trial	0.872	0.725	0.826	0.1207	0.8572
10	10	0.9	0.5	Center	0.431	0.454	0.399	0.0837	0.3999
10	20	0.5	0.9	Trial	0.358	0.719	0.425	0.1697	0.4329
10	20	0.5	0.9	Center	0.912	0.938	0.901	0.0153	0.9018
10	20	0.9	0.5	Trial	0.915	0.747	0.894	0.0667	0.9109
10	20	0.9	0.5	Center	0.502	0.557	0.524	0.0532	0.5250
0.1	5	0.5	0.9	Trial	0.777	0.760	0.777	0.1871	0.8355
0.1	5	0.5	0.9	Center	0.914	0.810	0.907	0.1112	0.9482
0.1	5	0.9	0.5	Trial	0.941	0.948	0.960	0.0504	0.9751
0.1	5	0.9	0.5	Center	0.533	0.635	0.534	0.1889	0.5572
0.1	10	0.5	0.9	Trial	0.444	0.421	0.447	0.2169	0.4628
0.1	10	0.5	0.9	Center	0.932	0.760	0.892	0.1082	0.9265
0.1	10	0.9	0.5	Trial	0.795	0.776	0.792	0.1276	0.8217
0.1	10	0.9	0.5	Center	0.488	0.551	0.494	0.1513	0.5054
0.1	20	0.5	0.9	Trial	0.292	0.288	0.311	0.1652	0.3063
0.1	20	0.5	0.9	Center	0.915	0.819	0.951	0.0468	0.9668
0.1	20	0.9	0.5	Trial	0.950	0.933	0.952	0.0250	0.9574
0.1	20	0.9	0.5	Center	0.466	0.691	0.465	0.1325	0.4698

One can see that the estimates of the magnitude of the association for the two highest levels (main investigator and country) are lower than those obtained for the two other strategies. As for Strategy I, there is relatively little difference in the estimates obtained for different levels.

Let us turn attention to the second psychiatric case study, where data from an equivalence trial are used. The result for the investigator level ($R^2 = 0.70$, bootstrap-based 95% confidence interval [0.44, 0.96]), obtained using Strategy I, is within the range of the estimates observed for the first study (see Table 8.5). This observation supports the claim that might have

TABLE 8.5. *R^2 values (with 95 % confidence/credible intervals) at different levels for the first psychiatric study, using different modeling strategies.*

	Unit of analysis		
	Investigator (138 units)	Main investigator (29 units)	Country (19 units)
Strategy I	0.56 [0.43, 0.68]†	0.69 [0.41, 0.86]†	0.62 [0.25, 0.88]†
Strategy II	0.42 [0.30, 0.55]†	0.77 [0.49, 0.89]†	0.56 [0.15, 0.86]†
Strategy III	0.52 [0.24, 0.74]††	0.66 [0.31, 0.88]††	0.51 [0.11, 0.83]††

† Bootstrap confidence interval.

†† Credible set.

been able to quantify reasonably accurately the surrogacy of PANSS for CGI in the context of certain compounds for schizophrenia. Of course, the R^2 values are not terribly high, so that a mere replacement of CGI by PANSS may be questionable.

8.6 Concluding Remarks

In this chapter, we have investigated several strategies to deal with hierarchical linear models. We have been interested primarily in the estimation of the strength of the association between random effects at different levels. This interest has been motivated in the context of validating surrogate markers.

Three different strategies have been considered: (1) applying fixed-effects models with only the trial level or the center level used in the validation process (Strategy I); (2) including both levels in a fixed-effects model at the first stage (Strategy II); and (3) including both levels in a random-effects model at the first stage (Strategy III). The strategies differ in the complexity of the models. Consequently, they also differ in the ease of their practical implementation.

In general terms, the results indicate that the performance of the strategies depends on the sample sizes, as well as on the magnitude of variability present at different levels. The latter dependency, especially for Strategy I, can be explained using theoretical results on the effect of ignoring levels when fitting multi-level models presented in a recent article by Hutchison and Healy (2001).

In particular, from the simulations conducted we could conclude that, when data were generated according to a model with random effects present at both levels, and when the strength of association between the random effects was the same at both levels, all the strategies produced reasonable results. When the association was different, Strategy I, with trials as the units of analysis, produced satisfactory estimates of the trial-level association. On the other hand, using centers as the units of analysis resulted in biased estimates of the center-level association. The estimates were, in fact, close to the true value of the measure of the strength of the trial-level association, when the variability of center-specific random effects was smaller than the variability of trial-specific effects. This observation gives some justification to the use of, e.g., centers instead of trials as the units of analysis in practical applications of the meta-analytic approach to the validation of surrogate endpoints.

On the other hand, to obtain plausible estimates of the strength of the association at a particular level for Strategy II, the variability at the level below the one of interest had to be smaller.

A limited investigation of the performance of Strategy III suggested that it was able to identify correctly different sources of variability and association. The estimates obtained under Strategy III were closer to the actual values than, e.g., those for Strategy II. In view of the structure of the model used in Strategy III, these conclusions were not surprising. However, an important problem associated with the practical use of this strategy is its numerical complexity. From this point of view, a possibility to use, e.g., Strategy I might be very advantageous.

9

Extensions of the Meta-analytic Approach to Surrogate Endpoints

Mitch Gail

9.1 Introduction

Whether an endpoint S is a good surrogate for a true clinical endpoint T depends on the intended use of the surrogate. Our primary goal is to use a surrogate in a clinical trial to estimate the trial-level effect of a new treatment on T without having to measure T. Another possible use of a surrogate is to predict the outcome T on an individual patient.

For clinical management of an individual patient, it would be valuable if S could be used to predict that individual's outcome T reliably, regardless of what treatment, Z, or other covariates, X, might be present. This assumption that T be conditionally independent of Z (and X) given S is the essential component in Prentice's (1989) criteria that define a good surrogate for hypothesis testing. This assumption holds if S is on the sole causal pathway leading to T, and all factors that influence T do so only through their effects on S. Although this strong assumption and ancillary conditions guarantee the validity of hypothesis tests for no treatment effect, they do not insure that S can predict T well at the individual level. Instead, Buyse, Molenberghs, Burzykowski, Renard, and Geys (2000a), which we abbreviate BMBRG, propose the within individual squared correlation, R^2_{indiv}, of T on S as a measure of the adequacy of S for predicting an individual's outcome (see also Chapter 7).

If S could be shown to satisfy the conditional independence assumption and to have a high R^2_{indiv}, one would have powerful evidence for a causal biological role for S and its close biological connection to T. Moreover, one could hope not only to test for treatment effects on T based on those on S, but also to estimate treatment effects on T from those on S. For example, suppose one wishes to estimate $\delta = E(T|Z = 1) - E(T|Z = 2)$ where

$Z = 1$ corresponds to an experimental treatment and $Z = 2$ to a control or standard treatment, possibly a placebo. We assume $Z = 1$ or 2 is assigned at random with equal probability. Suppose a previous study on control subjects has been done that yields an estimate of the density $f(T|S, Z = 1, X)$ that equals $f(T|S)$ by the conditional independence assumption. In the new study population

$$\delta = \int tf(t|s)h(s|Z = 1, x)dG(x)dt - \int tf(t|s)h(s|Z = 2, x)dG(x)dt,$$

where $h(s|z, x)$ is the conditional density of S given Z and X, and $G(x)$ is the distribution function of X. Because $f(t|s)$ is assumed known from previous studies on (T, S) and because $h(s|Z = 2, x)$ and $h(s|Z = 1, x)$ are estimable from the current study using the surrogate endpoint only, one can calculate the effect of the treatment Z on T in this new study without measuring the true clinical endpoint T.

All this depends on the strong conditional independence assumption $T \amalg Z$, X given S, however. It is impossible to verify this assumption empirically, because one would need to examine an infinite number of treatments and covariates. Even for a single study and treatment comparison, there is limited ability to rule out a dependence of T on Z given S with regression methods, leading Freedman, Graubard, and Schatzkin (1992) and Lin *et al.* (1997) to explore the related criterion of percentage of the treatment effect explained (see Chapter 5 for a discussion of this criterion and allied concepts). But without conditional independence, some other basis is needed to attain the central goal of estimating the magnitude of the treatment effect on T in a new trial from data on S only.

The meta-analytic approach to evaluating surrogate markers, introduced by Daniels and Hughes (1997) and BMBRG, leads to an empirical assessment of how well a surrogate can be used to estimate trial-level treatment effects on T. The basic idea is that one can use information from previous similar studies in which both T and S are measured in treated $(Z = 1)$ and control $(Z = 2)$ groups to learn how well the treatment effect on T is predicted by outcomes S in the treated and control groups. In a trial of a new treatment similar to those in the previous studies, one measures only the effects of Z on S and uses data from the previous studies and from the results on S in the new study to estimate the effects of Z on T.

In order to carry out this program, one needs to posit a superpopulation of similar trials from which the new trial and the previous trials are drawn. For example, Daniels and Hughes (1999) studied various retroviral therapies against HIV/AIDS. In some applications it may be unclear whether the new trial with its new experimental treatment is similar enough to previous studies and their treatments to regard it as a sample from the same superpopulation of trials. Even if there is agreement on the class of similar trials, a serious practical limitation may be the small number of previous trials with data on T and S. One relies on superpopulation parameters, which reflect trial to trial variation, in order to infer trial-level treatment effects on T from those on S. Having too few previous trials limits the precision with which superpopulation parameters can be estimated and hence the precision of meta-analytic inference (Gail, Pfeiffer, van Houwelingen, and Carroll 2000, which we abbreviate GPHC).

A second meta-analytic issue concerns the degree to which models describe the joint distribution of T and S at the individual level. Chapters 7 and 10–14 in this book present such detailed models. GPHC describe a marginal approach in which the distributions of S given Z, and T given Z, are modeled separately. They argue that this approach allows great flexibility for describing trial-level treatment effects and avoids having to specify the joint distribution of T and S given Z, which may be poorly understood. The marginal approach also captures most of the available information about trial-level treatment effects. Tibaldi *et al.* (2003) show that estimates of the proportion of variability in the estimated trial-level treatment effect that is explained by the surrogate, R^2_{trial}, is almost identical for marginal ("univariate") and bivariate linear models, as discussed further in Section 9.3.

In Section 9.2 we illustrate these concepts for normal models for S and T, in Section 9.3 we discuss the flexibility of the marginal model approach, and in Section 9.4 we recount some potential practical and theoretical limitations of the meta-analytic approach.

9.2 The Normal Model

Many of the previous ideas are illustrated by the normal model. Let T_{zij} denote the true clinical response of patient j ($j = 1, 2, \ldots$) in trial i on treatment $Z = z$ ($z = 1$ or 2) and define S_{zij} similarly for the surrogate. Here j ranges from 1 to n_i for $Z = 1$ and from 1 to m_i for $Z = 2$. Given $\theta_i = (\theta_{1T_j}, \theta_{1S_j}, \theta_{2T_j}, \theta_{2S_j})^T$, the vector $(T_{1ij}, S_{1ij}, T_{2ij}, S_{2ij})^T$, is normally distributed with mean θ_i and variance-covariance matrix Σ_i, which is block diagonal with non-zero components Σ_{11i} and Σ_{22i}, corresponding respectively to $(T_{1ij}, S_{1ij})^T$ and $(T_{2ij}, S_{2ij})^T$, which are independent. The θ_i come from a normal superpopulation with mean μ and variance ϕ. This model is very similar to that of BMBRG except that it allows for $\Sigma_{11i} \neq \Sigma_{22i}$, whereas BMBRG require $\Sigma_{11i} = \Sigma_{22i}$.

A series of N "previous" trials permits one to estimate the parameters of the superpopulation, μ and ϕ. Within the ith such trial, the mean is estimated as $\widehat{\theta}_i = (T_{1i}, S_{1i}, T_{2i}, S_{2i})^T$, where, for example, $T_{1i} = n_i^{-1} \sum_j T_{1ij}$.

The quantities Σ_{11i} and Σ_{22i} are estimated from the within-trial empirical variance-covariance matrices of $(T_{1ij}, S_{1ij})^T$ and $(T_{2ij}, S_{2ij})^T$, respectively. Because θ_i is normally distributed with mean μ and variance-covariance matrix $\phi + \Sigma_i$, various methods such a maximum likelihood, REML or empirical Bayes can be used to estimate μ and ϕ.

Now suppose we consider a new trial ($i = 0$) drawn from the superpopulation and only get to observe (S_{10j}, S_{20j}), which have within trial components of variance σ_{220} from Σ_{11i} and σ_{440} from Σ_{22i}. We seek to estimate θ_0 and especially the components that correspond to the unmeasured clinical outcomes T. Let $\theta_{T0} = (\theta_{1T0}, \theta_{2T0})^T$ be the means of T_{10j} and T_{20j}, respectively, and let $\theta_{S0} = (\theta_{1S0}, \theta_{2S0})^T$ be the means of S_{10j} and S_{20j}, respectively. Because $(\theta_{T0}^T, \widehat{\theta}_{S0}^T)^T$ is multivariate normal, the conditional mean and variance of θ_{T0} can be expressed in terms of $\widehat{\theta}_{S0}$ and parameters $\psi = (\mu, \phi, \sigma_{220}, \sigma_{440})$. Indeed, letting D and W be known matrices defined so that $\theta_{T0} = D\theta_0$ and $\theta_{S0} = W\theta_0$ (see Section 2 of GPHC for details),

$$E(\theta_{T0} \mid \widehat{\theta}_{S0}) = D\mu + D\phi W^T[W(\phi + \Sigma_0)W^T]^{-1}(\widehat{\theta}_{S0} - W\mu) \tag{9.1}$$

and

$$\mathrm{Cov}(\theta_{T0} \mid \widehat{\theta}_{S0}) = D\phi D^T - D\phi D^T[W(\phi + \Sigma_0)W^T]^{-1}W\phi D^T, \tag{9.2}$$

where (9.1) and (9.2) only depend on the elements σ_{220} and σ_{440} of Σ_0. The variances σ_{220} and σ_{440} can be estimated from the empirical variances of S_{10j} and S_{20j}, respectively, and μ and ϕ can be estimated from the previous trials. Assuming the elements of ψ are known, one knows the distribution of the means of the unmeasured true clinical outcomes θ_{T0} from the conditional normal distribution defined by (9.1) and (9.2). In particular, for $R = (1, -1)$, one can calculate the distribution of the treatment effect $\delta_0 \equiv R\theta_0 \equiv \theta_{1T0} - \theta_{2T0}$, which is normal with mean $M(\psi) \equiv RE(\theta_{T0} \mid \widehat{\theta}_{S0})$ and variance $V(\psi) \equiv R\,\mathrm{cov}(\theta_{T0} \mid \widehat{\theta}_{S0})R^T$, which can be calculated easily from (9.1) and (9.2).

If no measurements on the surrogate were available in the new study, but if the parameters of the superpopulation were known without error from many similar previous studies, one could still estimate the new treatment effect as $\mu_{1T} - \mu_{2T}$, with variance $RD\phi D^T R^T$. The proportion by which this variance is reduced by measuring the surrogate in the new study is, from equation (9.2),

$$R^2_{\mathrm{trial}} = \frac{RD\phi W^T[W(\phi + \Sigma_0)W^T]^{-1}W\phi D^T R^T}{RD\phi D^T R^T}. \tag{9.3}$$

If σ_{220} and σ_{440} are negligible, so that Σ_0 is omitted from (9.3), this definition of R^2_{trial} reduces to that given by BMBRG. BMBRG propounded the version of R^2_{trial} (with $\Sigma_0 = 0$) as a measure of the adequacy of the surrogate S at the trial level.

The difference $\delta_0 = \theta_{1T0} - \theta_{2T0}$ is a natural measure of treatment effect, but the distribution of an arbitrary treatment effect function $\delta_0 = \delta(\theta_{1T0}, \theta_{2T0})$ can be obtained analytically or by simulating from the conditional normal distribution of θ_{T0} given ψ and $\widehat{\theta}_{S0}$. An estimate of δ_0 might be $\widehat{\delta}_0 = \delta[E(\theta_{1T0}|\psi, \widehat{\theta}_{S0}), E(\theta_{2T0}|\psi, \widehat{\theta}_{S0})]$, and confidence intervals could be based on the quantiles of the distribution of δ_0 given ψ and $\widehat{\theta}_{S0}$.

9.2.1 *Precision of Estimates of* $\boldsymbol{\delta_0}$ *Based on the Meta-analytic Approach*

Using the surrogate to estimate the true treatment effect δ_0 can lead to severe loss of precision compared to measuring T directly. Even if a large number of previous trials have been conducted so that μ and ϕ are known without error, and even if the sample size in the new trial on the surrogate tends to infinity, so that $\sigma_{220} = \sigma_{440} = 0$, there is irreducible variability in $\widehat{\theta}_0$ that reflects trial-to-trial variation in θ_i in the superpopulation, as quantified by ϕ. For example, with $\delta_0 = R\theta_{T0}$ defined as above, the variance of $\widehat{\theta}_0$ is

$$RD\phi D^T R^T - RD\phi W^T (W\phi W^T)^{-1} W\phi D^T R^T,$$

which is strictly positive unless θ_{1Ti} and θ_{2Ti} are linearly dependent on θ_{1Si} and θ_{2Si}. In contrast, measuring true endpoints T will yield an estimate of δ_0 with variance tending to zero.

A realistic assessment of the variability of $\widehat{\theta}_0$ also needs to acknowledge uncertainty in $\widehat{\mu}$ and $\widehat{\phi}$, the estimates of superpopulation parameters. GPHC considered a 95% confidence interval on $\delta_0 = \theta_{1T0} - \theta_{2T0}$. A naïve 95% confidence interval that assumes known $\psi = (\mu, \phi, \sigma_{220}, \sigma_{440})$ is $M(\psi) \pm 1.96V^{1/2}(\psi)$ with M and V as defined previously. For $N = 5, 10, 25, 50$ and 100 previous trials, this naïve confidence interval had coverage 0.64, 0.61, 0.82, 0.90 and 0.92 respectively. Thus, with a small number of previous trials, confidence intervals that assume ψ is known without error have subnominal size and can be seriously misleading. GPHC provide bootstrap procedures that give confidence intervals with nominal coverage. These intervals ranged from 4% to 293% longer than the naïve confidence interval, however, as the number of previous trials decreased from $N = 100$ to $N = 5$.

To illustrate further the loss in precision from the meta-analytic approach, GPHC discussed a comparison of pravastatin ($Z = 1$) with placebo ($Z = 2$) on a true clinical outcome (T), namely change in coronary artery diameter over a two-year period, and on a surrogate (S), change in total cholesterol. The example was favorable to the meta-analytic approach because, rather than take different trials of similar agents ("statins") from the literature, GPHC chose 10 centers from a single trial, the REGRESS Trial (Jukema *et al.* 1995) as the "previous" studies, and one remaining center as the "new" study. Because all centers were using the same protocol and studying the exact same agent, there was probably less "between-trial" variability, captured in ϕ, than would be expected in a real meta-analysis based on different trials with different agents. Using the clinical endpoint T, the "new study" indicated a favorable treatment effect on decreases in coronary diameter of $\widehat{\theta}_{1T0} - \widehat{\theta}_{2T0} = 0.0381\,\text{mm}$ with 95% confidence interval $[-0.0138, 0.0900]$. Based on the surrogate data only in the "new study", GPHC estimated the true treatment effect as 0.0402 with naïve confidence interval $[-0.0552, 0.1355]$ and with bootstrap confidence interval that takes variation of ψ into account: $[-0.1346, 0.2149]$. Thus, there is a huge loss in precision from relying on S to estimate treatment effects on T.

9.3 Flexibility of the Marginal Approach

In Section 9.2, we made no mention of the ability of the surrogate to predict individual outcomes, which can be assessed in each trial by examining correlations between T and S in Σ_{11i} and Σ_{22i}. The quantities Σ_{11i} and Σ_{22i}, however, only influence estimates of trial-level treatment effects through their impact on estimating μ and ϕ in the superpopulation model and through σ_{220} and σ_{440}. Especially if all the component trials are large, Σ_{11i}, Σ_{22i}, σ_{220}, and σ_{440} have little influence on superpopulation parameters, and inference on trial-level effects is unrelated to how well S predicts T at the individual level. Because the main interest is in estimating effects on T at the trial level, and in order to avoid specification of the joint distribution of T and S, GPHC adopted a marginal approach to modeling.

Suppose θ_{zTi} represents some feature(s) of the marginal distribution of T in treatment group z in trial i, such as the mean, and define θ_{zSi} similarly for features of the marginal distribution of S. Assume that the components of $\theta_i = (\theta_{1T_j}, \theta_{1Sj}, \theta_{2Tj}, \theta_{2Sj})^T$ satisfy separate estimating equations

$$\sum_{j=1}^{n_i} U_{1Tij}(\theta_{1Ti}) = 0, \qquad \sum_{j=1}^{n_i} U_{1Sij}(\theta_{1si}) = 0,$$

$$\sum_{j=1}^{m_i} U_{2Tij}(\theta_{2Ti}) = 0, \qquad \sum_{j=1}^{m_i} U_{2Sij}(\theta_{2Si}) = 0.$$

We assume that U_{1Tij} is functionally independent of θ_{1Si}, θ_{2Ti}, and θ_{2si}, and that other estimating equations likewise depend only on the parameters shown in their arguments. As in GPHC, it is possible to estimate within experiment variance-covariance matrices Σ_i, namely the conditional covariance of $\widehat{\theta}_i$ given θ_i, from the empirical covariances of terms like U_{1Tij} and U_{1Sij}. Moreover, if θ_i is drawn from a normal $N(\mu, \phi)$ superpopulation, the methods in Section 9.2 can be applied to obtain inference on $\delta_0 = \delta(\theta_{1T0}, \theta_{2T0})$.

The marginal approach is very flexible. For example, if T and S are dichotomous with values 1 or 0, we might choose θ_{zSi} to be the logarithms of the marginal odds that $T = 1$ on treatment z in trial i and θ_{zSi} to be marginal odds that $S = 1$. Inference on the log odds ratio, $\delta_0 = \theta_{1T0} - \theta_{2T0}$ follows directly from (9.1) and (9.2) with allowance for uncertainty in ψ. The risk difference

$$\delta_0 = \exp(\delta_{1T0})/[1 + \exp(\delta_{1T0})] - \exp(\theta_{2T0})/[1 + \exp(\theta_{2T0})]$$

is non-linear in θ_{1T0} and θ_{2T0}, and inference can be based on simulations from the conditional distribution of θ_{T0} given $\widehat{\theta}_{S0}$, with allowance for uncertainty in ψ, as in GPHC.

Marginal models can also be used for survival data. For example, T_{zij} might have a Weibull distribution, $P(T_{zij} \leq y) = 1 - \exp(-\lambda_{2Ti} y^{\alpha_{zTi}})$. Likewise, S_{zij} might have a Weibull distribution with parameters λ_{zSi} and α_{zSi}. The alternative parameters $\theta_{zTi} = (\ln(\lambda_{zTi}), \alpha_{zTi})^T$ and $\theta_{zSi} = (\ln(\lambda_{zSi}), \alpha_{zSi})^T$ might plausibly conform to the multivariate normal distribution. The distribution of the difference in median survival in groups with $Z = 1$ and $Z = 2$, $\delta_0 = [\ln(2)/\lambda_{1T0}]^{\alpha_{1T0}} - [\ln(2)/\lambda_{2T0}]^{\alpha^{2T0}}$, can be estimated by simulations from the conditional distribution of θ_{T0} given $\widehat{\theta}_{S0}$ and $\widehat{\psi}$, with bootstrap methods used to account for variability in $\widehat{\psi}$, as in GPHC. Similar methods can be used for piecewise exponential models, as in GPHC. A subtlety arises if S can censor T or T can censor S and the censoring is informative. Then it may be necessary to posit a joint distribution for (T, S), rather than work simply with the marginal distributions, in order to account for informative censoring.

The marginal-level approach can be used for many other types of endpoints (GPHC).

The trial-level correlation R^2_{trial} in equation (9.3) does not depend on within individual correlations, namely correlations between T and S calculable from Σ_{11i} and Σ_{22i}. It is not surprising, therefore, that marginal models yield almost identical estimates of R^2_{trial} as do corresponding bivariate models for T and S (Tibaldi *et al.* 2003, who use the term "univariate" model, instead of marginal model). This is also an indication that marginal models capture most if not all of the surrogate information for predicting treatment effects on T at the trial level. The quantity R^2_{trial} does not account for uncertainty in $\widehat{\psi}$. As pointed out by GPHC, a more realistic measure would be 1 minus the ratio of the variance of $\widehat{\delta}_0$ based on $\widehat{\theta}_{S0}$ and $\widehat{\psi}$, with bootstrap calculations to account for uncertainty in $\widehat{\psi}$, to the variance of $\widehat{\delta}_0$ based only on $\widehat{\mu}_{1T}$ and $\widehat{\mu}_{2T}$, again with bootstrap calculations to account for variability in $\widehat{\mu}_{1T}$ and $\widehat{\mu}_{2T}$. Typically, this assessment of the value of the surrogate will be less optimistic than that provided by R^2_{trial}.

9.4 Discussion

The meta-analytic approach provides an empirical alternative to having to make the strong assumption that T is independent of Z and X given S in order to estimate effects of a new intervention on T from its effects on S. Marginal models that allow one to estimate features of the marginal distributions of T and S in treated and control groups capture most of the available surrogate information on trial-level effects on T, without the need for elaborate bivariate models. Bivariate models may be needed in the presence of informative censoring, however. The ability of the surrogate to predict intervention effects in a new study depends primarily on how tightly summary parameters of the marginal distribution of T are related to such summary parameters for S in a series of studies of interventions similar to the new intervention.

There is a serious price to be paid in loss of precision from the meta-analytic approach. Even with a large number of previous trials to estimate super-population parameters and with a large new experiment on the surrogate, the precision of the estimated treatment effect on T in the new study will typically be much less than from a new study with measurements on T itself. This loss of precision is inherent in the irreducible between-study variation, characterized by ϕ. The loss of precision is compounded when there are 10 or fewer previous studies, because an imprecise estimate of the parameters degrades the precision of estimated treatment effects on T considerably.

Apart from precision, several other limitations of the meta-analytic approach should be mentioned (see GPHC):

1. there may be disagreement as to which studies are similar enough to be used in the meta-analysis;
2. published data may not include estimates of Σ_{11i} and Σ_{22i}, requiring the use of unverified assumptions to estimate ϕ;
3. the normal superpopulation model may not be applicable, even after

transformation of the parameters θ, and more complex methods may be required for non-normal superpopulations models;

4. stopping the new study early on the basis of surrogate information may restrict the ability of the study to detect unanticipated toxicities of the new treatment; and
5. comprehensive evaluation of a new treatment may require examining several clinical endpoints, so that T becomes a vector. In this case, the use of surrogates becomes more complex and less appealing.

Further methodological research and experience with the method will be needed to determine the extent to which meta-analysis can assist in the evaluation and use of surrogate endpoints.

10

Meta-analytic Validation with Binary Outcomes

Didier Renard and Helena Geys

10.1 Introduction

In this chapter, a meta-analytic formulation for binary outcomes is presented. Unlike for continuous outcomes, where the multivariate normal distribution and the linear mixed model provide natural paradigms for model development, there is no such unambiguous model choice for binary outcomes. One typically distinguishes between marginal, conditional, and random-effects models. Which family is to be preferred principally depends on the research question(s) to be answered. In conditionally specified models, the probability of a positive response for one outcome is modeled conditionally on other outcomes for the same unit, whereas marginal models relate the covariates directly to the marginal probabilities. Models for non-normal repeated measures pose non-trivial computational challenges. In this chapter, a particular choice will be made based on a random-effects formulation, to cope with the hierarchical structure of the meta-analytic data, combined with a probit formulation for the pair of surrogate and true endpoints.

10.2 Model Formulation

In order to extend the methodology described in Chapter 7, we adopt a latent variable perspective. That is, we posit the existence of a pair of latent variables $(\tilde{S}_{ij}, \tilde{T}_{ij})$ that are continuously distributed and related to the actual response through a certain threshold. In the context of i.i.d. binary data, this approach motivates a wide class of models, of which the standard logistic and probit regression models are special cases (Cox and Snell 1989). Precisely, we assume that an observed binary response is obtained by dichotomizing an unobserved continuous variable based on the chosen threshold, which can be taken to be 0 without loss of generality. In other words, it is assumed that a success $S_{ij} = 1$ and $T_{ij} = 1$, respectively, is recorded if $\tilde{S}_{ij} > 0$ and $\tilde{T}_{ij} > 0$, respectively, and a failure $S_{ij} = 0$ and $T_{ij} = 0$, respectively, otherwise.

With the additional assumption that $(\tilde{S}_{ij}, \tilde{T}_{ij})$ is normally distributed with mean 0 and covariance matrix Σ, we can consider the following random-effects model for the latent variables:

$$\tilde{S}_{ij} = \mu_S + m_{Si} + (\alpha + a_i)Z_{ij} + \tilde{\varepsilon}_{Sij}, \quad (10.1)$$

$$\tilde{T}_{ij} = \mu_T + m_{Ti} + (\beta + b_i)Z_{ij} + \tilde{\varepsilon}_{Tij}. \quad (10.2)$$

The above model is similar to (7.6)–(7.7) and the resulting model for the observed binary outcomes is

$$\Phi^{-1}[P(S_{ij} = 1|m_{Si}, a_i, m_{Ti}, b_i)] = \mu_S + m_{Si} + (\alpha + a_i)Z_{ij}, \quad (10.3)$$

$$\Phi^{-1}[P(T_{ij} = 1|m_{Si}, a_i, m_{Ti}, b_i)] = \mu_T + m_{Ti} + (\beta + b_i)Z_{ij}, \quad (10.4)$$

where $\Phi(.)$ denotes the standard normal cumulative distribution function.

It is well-known that not all parameters are identifiable in model (10.1)–(10.2). Thus, variance parameters σ_{SS} and σ_{TT} can be fixed, arbitrarily and without loss of generality, to 1 and we can write

$$\Sigma = \begin{pmatrix} 1 & \rho_{ST} \\ \rho_{ST} & 1 \end{pmatrix}. \quad (10.5)$$

Using the above identifiability constraints, model (10.3)–(10.4) takes the form of a multilevel probit model and can be regarded either as a bivariate two-level model or a three-level model for binary response data (Goldstein 1995). It also belongs to the class of so-called generalized linear mixed models (Breslow and Clayton 1993).

The above model formulation allows us to consider coefficients of determination defined in Chapter 7 without any further modification although, formally, their interpretation is bound by the postulated latent variables generating the observed binary responses. The coefficient $R^2_{\text{trial(f)}}$ is calculated using expression (7.11) and R^2_{indiv} is equal to ρ^2_{ST}.

10.3 Parameter Estimation

Two estimation methods are widely used within the family of generalized linear mixed models (GLMMs): maximum (marginal) likelihood (ML) and penalized quasi-likelihood (PQL). Likelihood estimation proceeds by maximizing the marginal likelihood obtained after integrating out random effects. If $\boldsymbol{\theta}$ denotes the vector of all parameters, the contribution of the ith trial to the likelihood, conditionally on $\boldsymbol{b}_i = (m_{S_i}, a_i, m_{T_i}, b_i)^T$, is

$$L_i(\boldsymbol{\theta} \mid \boldsymbol{b}_i) = \prod_{j=1}^{n_i} P(S_{ij}, T_{ij} \mid \boldsymbol{b}_i). \tag{10.6}$$

ML estimators are obtained by maximizing the integrated likelihood, with ith contribution given by

$$L_i(\boldsymbol{\theta}) = \int L_i(\boldsymbol{\theta} \mid \boldsymbol{b}_i)\phi(\boldsymbol{b}_i; D)d\boldsymbol{b}_i, \tag{10.7}$$

where $\phi(\boldsymbol{b}_i; D)$ denotes the joint density function of the normal distribution with mean $\mathbf{0}$ and covariance matrix D.

Unfortunately, (10.7) is intractable and necessitates the use of numerical integration techniques, such as Gauss-Hermite quadrature or Monte Carlo methods. In our context of (meta-analytic) surrogate endpoint validation, this approach will likely demand a great deal of computational resources.

A number of researchers have attempted to circumvent the computational burden caused by the need for numerical integration in the likelihood and have suggested to use approximations. Breslow and Clayton (1993), for instance, exploit the penalized quasi-likelihood (PQL) method by applying Laplace's integral approximation. They also consider marginal quasi-likelihood (MQL), a name they give to a procedure previously proposed by Goldstein (1991). PQL and MQL can be viewed as iterative procedures that entail fitting of linear multilevel models based on a first-order Taylor expansion of the mean function about the current estimated fixed part predictor (MQL) or the current predicted value (PQL).

As shown by Rodríguez and Goldman (1995), the PQL and MQL procedures can be seriously biased. These authors' simulations reveal that both fixed effects and variance components may suffer from substantial, if not severe, attenuation bias with binary response data. Goldstein and Rasbash (1996) showed that including second-order terms in the PQL expansion (PQL2) considerably reduces biases described by Rodríguez and Goldman.

Although PQL is computationally efficient, our personal experience led us to believe that attenuation bias may be more severe in models more complex than those evaluated by Goldstein and Rasbash (1996), and that the algorithm tends to be numerically unstable, the problem being aggravated with the use of PQL2 and/or with more complex models such as (10.3)–(10.4). Because we have direct interest in variance-covariance parameters, another approach to parameter estimation would be preferable, while bearing in mind that computational burden should be kept as low as possible.

A procedure that may fulfill such requirements is maximum pairwise likelihood (MPL). Pairwise likelihood (PL) is a special example of what is called pseudo-likelihood, first proposed by Besag (1975) and also termed composite likelihood by Lindsay (1988). The motivation behind pseudo-likelihood estimation is to replace the likelihood by a function that is easier to evaluate, and hence to maximize. Such a function is a product of conditional or marginal densities. Thus, the main feature of a pseudo-likelihood function is that it is composed of (pieces of) likelihoods and this can be exploited to prove general results about the consistency and asymptotic normality of pseudo-likelihood estimators.

As the name suggests, with PL we aim to replace the likelihood contribution L_i by the product of all possible pairwise probabilities. More formally, if we let $\boldsymbol{Y}_i$ denote the vector $(S_{i1},\ldots,S_{in_i},T_{i1},\ldots,T_{in_i})$, then the contribution of the ith trial to the PL can be written

$$PL_i = \prod_{j=1}^{2n_i} \prod_{k>j} P(Y_{ij}, Y_{ik}). \tag{10.8}$$

The terms in (10.8) reflect different types of association, as illustrated in Figure 10.1:

(i) the association between the surrogate and true endpoints measured on the same individual;

(ii) the association between the surrogate endpoints measured on two distinct individuals;

(iii) the association between the true endpoints measured on two distinct individuals;

(iv) the association between the surrogate and true endpoints measured on two distinct individuals.

We emphasize that the bivariate probabilities in (10.8) are marginal, not conditional. These probabilities can easily be expressed in terms of univariate and bivariate probits. For example, the probability that both S and T yield a positive outcome for subject j in trial i can be written as:

$$\begin{aligned} P[S_{ij}=1, T_{ij}=1] &= P[\tilde{S}_{ij}>0, \tilde{T}_{ij}>0] \\ &= \Phi_2\left(\frac{\mu_S+\alpha Z_{ij}}{\sqrt{\text{var}(\tilde{S}_{ij})}}, \frac{\mu_T+\beta Z_{ij}}{\sqrt{\text{var}(\tilde{T}_{ij})}}; \rho_{ij}\right). \end{aligned}$$

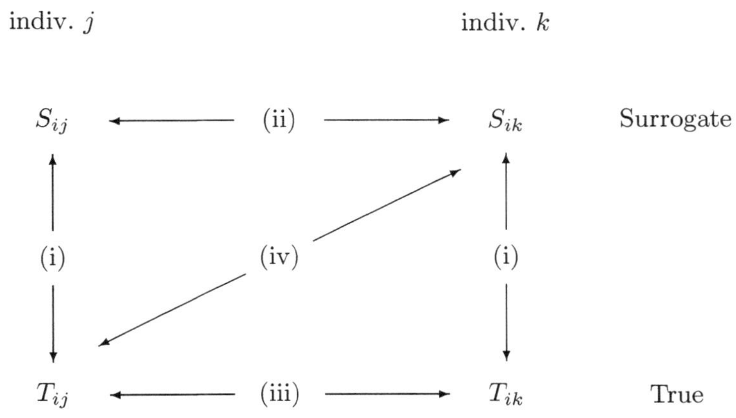

FIGURE 10.1. *Association structure between the surrogate and true endpoints for two distinct individuals j and k in trial i.*

In this expression, $\text{var}(\tilde{S}_{ij})$, $\text{var}(\tilde{T}_{ij})$ and ρ_{ij} are obtained by selecting the appropriate 2×2 submatrix of the (marginal) covariance matrix $V_i = Z_i \boldsymbol{D} Z_i^T + R_i$, where Z_i is a suitable design matrix and R_i is a block-diagonal matrix with blocks equal to $\boldsymbol{\Sigma}$.

Estimates of the parameters $\boldsymbol{\theta}$ can be obtained by maximizing the log PL function

$$p\ell = \sum_{i=1}^{N} p\ell_i = \sum_{i=1}^{N} \log PL_i. \tag{10.9}$$

Under standard regularity conditions, PL estimators are consistent and asymptotically normally distributed. The asymptotic covariance matrix of the PL estimator $\tilde{\boldsymbol{\theta}}$ can be approximated by the "sandwich estimator" $J^{-1}KJ^{-1}$, where

$$J = \sum_{i=1}^{N} \frac{\partial^2 p\ell_i(\tilde{\boldsymbol{\theta}})}{\partial \boldsymbol{\theta} \partial \boldsymbol{\theta}^T} \tag{10.10}$$

and

$$K = \sum_{i=1}^{N} \frac{\partial p\ell_i(\tilde{\boldsymbol{\theta}})}{\partial \boldsymbol{\theta}} \frac{\partial p\ell_i(\tilde{\boldsymbol{\theta}})}{\partial \boldsymbol{\theta}^T}. \tag{10.11}$$

Alternatively, an estimator of

$$E\left[\frac{\partial^2 \log PL}{\partial \boldsymbol{\theta} \partial \boldsymbol{\theta}^T}\right],$$

which does not require evaluation of second-order derivatives is given by

$$J = \sum_{i=1}^{N} \sum_{j=1}^{2n_i} \sum_{k>j} \frac{\partial \ell_{ijk}(\tilde{\boldsymbol{\theta}})}{\partial \boldsymbol{\theta}} \frac{\partial \ell_{ijk}(\tilde{\boldsymbol{\theta}})}{\partial \boldsymbol{\theta}^T}. \tag{10.12}$$

Instead of maximizing (10.9), it might be preferable to maximize the function

$$p\ell^* = \sum_{i=1}^{N} p\ell_i^* = \sum_{i=1}^{N} \frac{1}{2n_i - 1} p\ell_i. \tag{10.13}$$

Weighting corrects for the fact that each response occurs $(2n_i - 1)$ times in PL_i. Renard, Molenberghs, and Geys (2003) compared the weighted and unweighted estimators in a simple random-intercept model and found that the weighted estimator seems to perform slightly better under moderate and strong dependence.

Renard *et al.* (2002) conducted a simulation study to investigate the performance of the MPL estimator with model (10.3)–(10.4). The goal was to evaluate the impact of such factors as number of trials and trial size on $R^2_{\text{trial(f)}}$ and R^2_{indiv} and to examine convergence issues. The results of these simulations showed that both quantities tend to be biased in small samples but, as expected, bias in R^2_{indiv} can be eliminated by increasing overall sample size (i.e., trial size and/or number of trials), whereas bias in $R^2_{\text{trial(f)}}$ can be reduced by increasing replication at the trial level. Convergence problems were observed more frequently when the sample size is small and the magnitude of ρ_{ST} increases. For comparison purposes, the PQL procedure, as implemented in the SAS macro GLIMMIX (Wolfinger and O'Connell 1993), was also utilized to analyze some simulated data sets. The proportion of cases where the algorithm failed to converge was dramatically high (>50%).

To conclude, we briefly comment on the implementation of the algorithm. To remove constraints on the matrix D, which should be positive-definite, and thereby improve convergence properties of the algorithm, a Cholesky decomposition $D^{\star T} D^{\star} = D$ was used and the log PL function maximized with respect to the elements of the Cholesky factor. To constrain the residual correlation parameter ρ_{ST} to lie in the interval $[-1, 1]$, Fisher's z-transformation

$$\eta_{ST} = \log\left(\frac{1 + \rho_{ST}}{1 - \rho_{ST}}\right).$$

was employed. The algorithm was implemented in SAS IML (SAS Institute Inc. 1995) and maximization of the log PL function performed using the NLPDD (Double-Dogleg) optimization routine. This optimization procedure requires only function and gradient calls, which are much faster to

TABLE 10.1. *Acute migraine data. S = photophobia, T = absence of pain relief.*

		T	
Z	S	0	1
Active treatment	0	304 (78)†	87 (22)
	1	7 (3)	203 (97)
Placebo	0	81 (68)	38 (32)
	1	1 (1)	80 (99)

† Frequency (row percentage).

compute than the Hessian. Upon convergence of the algorithm, estimates of the standard errors of $\tilde{\boldsymbol{\theta}}$ can be obtained as indicated above, with J estimated using (10.10) or (10.12). In the former case, the final Hessian matrix was computed using numerical second-order derivatives by forward difference approximations.

10.4 Acute Migraine: A Meta-analysis of Ten Clinical Trials

To illustrate the methodology, we use the data described in Section 4.2.9. Recall that the data come from ten early phase clinical trials evaluating the efficacy of several migraine-abortive therapies. Grouping units considered in this analysis are centers.

Our motivation here is to investigate the relationship between migraine-associated symptoms and migraine severity assessed at 2 hours. Our "true" endpoint is taken to be absence of pain relief (= 1 if score $\geq$2) while our surrogate endpoint is either photophobia, phonophobia, or nausea (= 1 if score $\geq$2). Pooled data from the ten trials are presented in Table 10.1 for photophobia. As can be seen, there is a strong relationship between S and T. Table 10.2 shows MPL parameter estimates and their standard errors obtained after fitting model (10.3)–(10.4) to these data.

Table 10.3 shows R^2 measures for each of the three migraine-associated symptoms versus absence of pain relief. For photophobia, there is a very strong association, both at the individual and at the trial (center) level. Figure 10.2 depicts (naively) the relationship between treatment effects

TABLE 10.2. *Acute migraine data. MPL estimates: S = photophobia, T = absence of pain relief.*

Mean structure			Covariance structure		
Parameter	Estimate	s.e.	Parameter	Estimate	s.e.
μ_S	-0.335	0.101	d_{SS}	0.095	0.087
α	-0.085	0.053	d_{ST}	0.091	0.077
μ_T	0.091	0.115	d_{TT}	0.097	0.077
β	-0.145	0.060	d_{Sa}	0.018	0.012
			d_{Ta}	0.026	0.017
			d_{aa}	0.041	0.015
			d_{Sb}	0.034	0.018
			d_{Tb}	0.047	0.028
			d_{ab}	0.048	0.021
			d_{bb}	0.060	0.036
			ρ_{ST}	0.931	0.102

TABLE 10.3. *Acute migraine data. R^2 measures.*

	Photophobia	Phonophobia	Nausea
R^2_{indiv}	0.87 (0.19)	0.72 (0.20)	0.56 (0.19)
R^2_{trial}	0.96 (0.13)	0.95 (0.08)	0.79 (0.03)

on S (photophobia) and T (absence of pain relief). Circles represented on this plot were obtained by fitting a probit regression model for each center separately, with size of the circle being proportional to size of the center. Table 10.3 shows that photophobia also exhibits a rather strong association at the trial level with reduced association at the individual level. Finally, the association at both levels is lower for nausea symptoms, especially at the individual level. From this analysis it seems that photophobia symptoms are most closely related to severity of the migraine.

10.5 Concluding Remarks

Extension of the methodology discussed in Chapter 7 to the case of two binary endpoints was based on a latent variable approach that allows us to

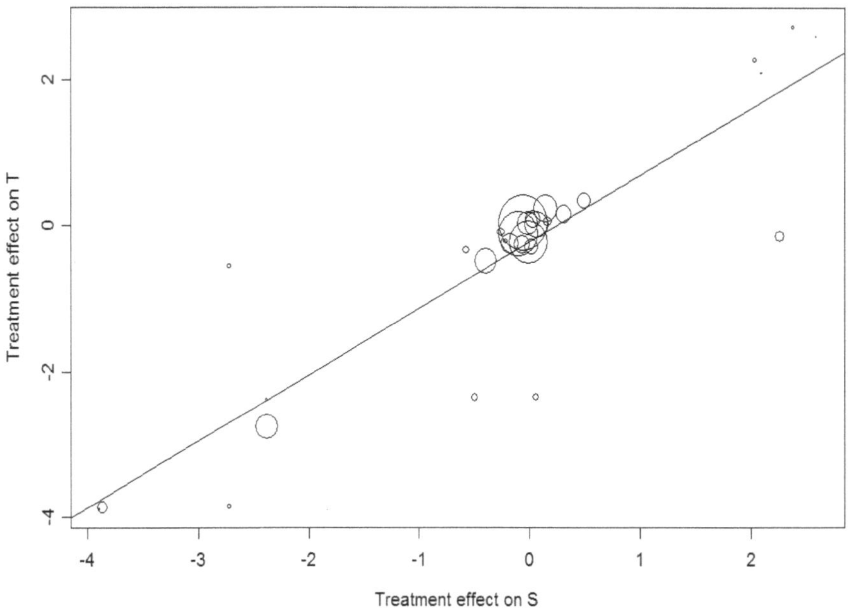

FIGURE 10.2. *Acute migraine data. Estimated treatment effects: S = photophobia, T = absence of pain relief.*

carry over measures of surrogacy R^2_{trial} and R^2_{indiv} in a natural way, under the assumption that the latent variables are normally distributed. This, in turn, dictates the use of a joint probit model for the surrogate and true endpoints.

The major difficulty rests in parameter estimation since, on the one hand, a direct likelihood approach would be computationally demanding and, on the other hand, standard approximate methods such as PQL may not be satisfactory because interest focuses on the random components of the model. Use of the MPL procedure is therefore attractive as it provides a net balance between computational burden and bias. Obviously, computational ease comes at a price, namely, some loss of efficiency compared to a full likelihood approach. Renard, Molenberghs, and Geys (2003) found a generally moderate (less than 20%) loss of efficiency relative to ML when the procedure was tested in simple models.

It is well-known that GLMMs are challenging models to fit and can pose numerous estimation problems. From our personal experience, it is not so uncommon for the PQL algorithm to exhibit numerical instability and fail to converge. The problem is even worse with PQL2 and/or more complicated models such as (10.3)–(10.4). MPL, however, tends to be more robust against convergence problems (Renard, Molenberghs, and Geys 2003), which gives an added advantage to this procedure.

Numerical problems should nevertheless be expected to occur frequently in the kind of applications sought here. In particular, such factors as the number of trials, between-trial variability, and trial size can be critical for improving convergence properties of the algorithm, just as they are for normally distributed endpoints. Also, with binary outcomes the two-stage approach does not always provide a valuable alternative to fitting model (10.3)–(10.4) because estimates cannot be obtained in small units where only positive or negative responses are recorded.

Finally, this methodology can easily be extended to deal with ordinal endpoints by extending the threshold model. An extension to mixed situations, where one endpoint is continuous and the other discrete, is also feasible.

11

Validation in the Case of Two Failure-time Endpoints

Tomasz Burzykowski and José Cortiñas Abrahantes

11.1 Introduction

In this chapter, we consider the case where both the surrogate and the true endpoints are failure-time variables. Such a setting is commonly encountered, for instance, in oncology, where time-to-progression or progression-free survival time are frequently used, for practical purposes, as a surrogate for survival time (Ellenberg and Hamilton 1989, Fleming 1994, Lohrisch and Piccart 2000). The validation of surrogates in this setting is complicated by several factors, like the presence of censoring and competing risks, or the absence of a unifying framework such as the multivariate normal distribution. The latter is common to, for example, the binary case (see Chapter 10). For all of these reasons, several authors attempted to develop methods for the assessment of the validity of surrogates aimed particularly at this setting. For instance, Chen *et al.* (1998) proposed an approach based on a stochastic model for survival and disease-free survival developed by Lagakos (1976). They used the model to develop a method allowing to verify the validity of Prentice's definition (Prentice 1989; see also Chapter 5 of this volume). They applied the method to assess the validity of disease-free survival as a surrogate for survival in adjuvant colorectal cancer trials. On the other hand, Burzykowski *et al.* (2001) developed a method based on an extension of the meta-analytic proposed by Buyse *et al.* (2000a). In view of the drawbacks of the approaches derived from Prentice's definition (see Chapter 5), as compared to the meta-analytic approach (summarized in Chapter 7), we will focus in this chapter on the methods based on the latter approach.

11.2 Meta-analytic Approach: The Two-stage Model

To extend the approach proposed by Buyse *et al.* (2000a) to the case where both the surrogate and the true endpoint are failure-time random variables, Burzykowski *et al.* (2001) proposed to replace the first-stage model (7.1)–(7.2) by a copula model (Genest and McKay 1986, Shih and Louis 1995a, Joe 1997, Nelsen 1999). More specifically, they assumed that the joint survival function of (S_{ij}, T_{ij}) can be written as:

$$F(s, t) = P(S_{ij} \geq s, T_{ij} \geq t) = C_\theta\{F_{Sij}(s), F_{Tij}(t)\}, \quad s, t \geq 0, \qquad (11.1)$$

where F_{Sij} and F_{Tij} denote marginal survival functions and C_θ is a copula, i.e., a bivariate distribution function on $[0, 1]^2$ with uniform margins. An excellent review of the theory of copulas is given by Nelsen (1999).

An attractive feature of model (11.1) is that the margins do not depend on the choice of the copula function. In principle, in model (11.1) any copula function can be used. For simplicity, Burzykowski *et al.* (2001) considered primarily one-parameter families; hence the use of a single parameter θ in (11.1). In practical applications, they considered the following three copula functions:

The Clayton copula Its intensive use in research and applications followed the paper by Clayton (1978), where it was proposed in the context of proportional frailty models. The copula function has got the following form:

$$C_\theta(u, v) = (u^{1-\theta} + v^{1-\theta} - 1)^{\frac{1}{1-\theta}}, \quad \theta > 1. \qquad (11.2)$$

It implies a positive association when $\theta > 1$; the strength of the association decreases with decreasing θ and reaches independence when $\theta \to 1$.

The Hougaard copula It was first discussed by Gumbel (1960). However, it has been a focus of interest following a paper by Hougaard (1986). The copula function is given by

$$C_\theta(u, v) = \exp[-\{(-\ln u)^{\frac{1}{\theta}} + (-\ln v)^{\frac{1}{\theta}}\}^\theta], \quad 0 < \theta < 1. \qquad (11.3)$$

It induces positive association among the failure-times; the strength of the association decreases with increasing θ and reaches independence when $\theta \to 1$.

The Plackett copula It is closely related to the Plackett family of bivariate distributions (Plackett 1965). The copula function is defined as follows:

$$C_\theta(u,v) = \begin{cases} \dfrac{1+(u+v)(\theta-1)-H_\theta(u,v)}{2(\theta-1)} & \text{if } \theta \neq 1 \\ uv & \text{otherwise} \end{cases} \tag{11.4}$$

where

$$H_\theta(u,v) = \sqrt{[1+(\theta-1)(u+v)]^2 + 4\theta(1-\theta)uv} \tag{11.5}$$

and $\theta \in [0, +\infty]$. Parameter θ has an interesting interpretation as the constant global cross-ratio (Dale 1986). A value of $\theta = 1$ corresponds to independence.

To model the effect of treatment on the marginal distributions of S_{ij} and T_{ij} in (11.1), Burzykowski *et al.* (2001) proposed to use the proportional hazards model:

$$F_{Sij}(s) = \exp\left\{-\int_0^s \lambda_{Si}(x)\exp(\alpha_i Z_{ij})dx\right\}, \tag{11.6}$$

$$F_{Tij}(t) = \exp\left\{-\int_0^t \lambda_{Ti}(x)\exp(\beta_i Z_{ij})dx\right\}, \tag{11.7}$$

where λ_{Si} and λ_{Ti} are trial-specific marginal baseline hazard functions and α_i and β_i are trial-specific effects of treatment Z on the endpoints in trial i. The hazard functions can be specified parametrically or can be left unspecified as in the classical model proposed by Cox (1972a). When the hazard functions are specified, estimates of the parameters for the joint model (11.1) and (11.6)–(11.7) can be obtained using the maximum likelihood method. Alternatively, the two-stage parametric procedure proposed by Shih and Louis (1995a) can be used, in which parameters of the marginal survival functions F_{Sij} and F_{Tij} are estimated first (assuming independence), and then θ is estimated conditional on the estimated values of the marginal parameters. When the hazard functions are left unspecified, a two-stage semi-parametric procedure of Shih and Louis (1995a), similar to the parametric version just described, can be applied.

At the second stage, Burzykowski *et al.* (2001) proposed to use the model:

$$\begin{pmatrix} \alpha_i \\ \beta_i \end{pmatrix} = \begin{pmatrix} \alpha \\ \beta \end{pmatrix} + \begin{pmatrix} a_i \\ b_i \end{pmatrix}, \tag{11.8}$$

where the second term on the right hand side of (11.8) is assumed to follow a zero-mean normal distribution with dispersion matrix

$$D = \begin{pmatrix} d_{aa} & d_{ab} \\ d_{ab} & d_{bb} \end{pmatrix}. \tag{11.9}$$

In principle, in a fully parametric setting, parameters related to the baseline hazards λ_{si} could be used as well.

Note that the first-stage model (11.1) with the marginal proportional hazard models (11.6)–(11.7) and the second-stage model (11.8) can be seen as an analogue of the fixed-effects model, given by (7.1)–(7.2) and (7.14) in Chapter 7. Recall that the latter model was developed based on a linear mixed-effects model including random intercepts independent of random treatment effects.

In view of using model (11.8) at the second stage of the two-stage approach, the quality of surrogate S at the trial level is assessed based on the coefficient of determination

$$R^2_{\text{trial(r)}} = \frac{d_{ab}^2}{d_{aa}d_{bb}}. \tag{11.10}$$

To assess the quality of the surrogate at the individual level, according to the approach proposed by Buyse *et al.* (2000a), a measure of association between S_{ij} and T_{ij}, calculated while adjusting the marginal distributions of the two endpoints for both the trial and treatment effects, is needed. For the case of two normally distributed endpoints, the natural measure was the correlation coefficient R^2_{indiv} (see equation (7.21), Chapter 7). It is important to note that in that case the coefficient remains constant after specifying trial-specific intercepts and treatment effects in (7.1)–(7.2).

For the case of the two failure-time endpoints the situation is different. First, non-linear association between the endpoints is more likely. Second, the correlation between S_{ij} and T_{ij} depends on the shape of the marginal baseline hazard functions. It follows that if the general form of (11.6)–(11.7) is assumed, there will be a separate correlation coefficient for each trial. Consequently, the correlation is not a good candidate for the required measure of the association between S_{ij} and T_{ij}. Instead, Burzykowski *et al.* (2001) proposed to use Kendall's τ (Wang and Wells 2000b), as it depends only on the copula function C_θ and is independent of the marginal distributions of S_{ij} and T_{ij} (Schweizer and Wolff 1981):

$$\tau = 4\int_0^1 \int_0^1 C_\theta(u, v) C_\theta(du, dv) - 1. \tag{11.11}$$

It describes the strength of the association between the two endpoints remaining after adjustment, through the marginal models (11.6)–(11.7), for trial- and treatment effects.

11.2.1 Bias in the Estimation of Measures of Surrogacy

Under model (11.8)–(11.9), $R^2_{\text{trial(r)}}$ given by (11.10) might be estimated by the square of the correlation coefficient between treatment effects α_i and β_i. As such, the square of the sample correlation coefficient is a biased estimator of the coefficient of determination (Lucke 1984). To reduce the bias, several adjusted estimators have been proposed (Fisher 1924, Wherry 1931, Olkin and Pratt 1958, Kendall and Stuart 1973, Lucke 1984). The adjusted estimators are successful in reducing the bias present in the squared sample correlation coefficient, but none of them has got uniformly minimum mean square error (MSE). Because all of them can yield negative estimates of the coefficient of determination, it has been proposed to use truncated versions of the estimators by taking the maximum of their value and zero.

A more fundamental issue, however, is related to the fact that, in practice, only estimates $\widehat{\alpha}_i$ and $\widehat{\beta}_i$, obtained from the first-stage copula model, are available. It is known that in general ignoring the measurement error when fitting regression models may lead to bias in the estimated coefficients of the models (Fuller 1987, Carroll, Ruppert, and Stefanski 1995). As noted by Burzykowski *et al.* (2001), irrespective of the choice of the estimator, the resulting estimate of $R^2_{\text{trial(r)}}$, obtained by treating the estimates $\widehat{\alpha}_i$ and $\widehat{\beta}_i$ as equal to the true, unobserved treatment effects, might therefore be biased. To see this more formally, assume that the estimated treatment effects $\widehat{\alpha}_i$ and $\widehat{\beta}_i$ follow the model:

$$\begin{pmatrix} \widehat{\alpha}_i \\ \widehat{\beta}_i \end{pmatrix} = \begin{pmatrix} \alpha_i \\ \beta_i \end{pmatrix} + \begin{pmatrix} \varepsilon_{ai} \\ \varepsilon_{bi} \end{pmatrix} \tag{11.12}$$

where the estimation errors ε_{ai} and ε_{bi} are normally distributed with mean zero and covariance matrix:

$$\Omega_i = \begin{pmatrix} \sigma_{aa,i} & \sigma_{ab,i} \\ \sigma_{ab,i} & \sigma_{bb,i} \end{pmatrix}, \tag{11.13}$$

and $(\alpha_i, \beta_i)^T$ follows model (11.8) with the dispersion matrix D given by (11.9). Consequently, $(\widehat{\alpha}_i, \widehat{\beta}_i)^T$ follows a normal distribution with mean $(\alpha, \beta)^T$ and dispersion matrix $D + \Omega_i$.

For the sake of illustration, let us assume for the time being that $\Omega_i = \Omega$ (this assumption will be relaxed in what follows), with

$$\Omega = \begin{pmatrix} \sigma_{aa} & \sigma_{ab} \\ \sigma_{ab} & \sigma_{bb} \end{pmatrix},$$

and denote by ρ the correlation based on Ω. The correlation between $\widehat{\alpha}_i$

and $\widehat{\beta}_i$ can then be written as:

$$\mathrm{Corr}(\widehat{\alpha}_i, \widehat{\beta}_i) = \frac{\mathrm{Corr}(\alpha_i, \beta_i)}{\sqrt{(1+\kappa_a)(1+\kappa_b)}} + \frac{\rho}{\sqrt{(1+\kappa_a^{-1})(1+\kappa_b^{-1})}}, \tag{11.14}$$

where $\kappa_a = \sigma_{aa}/d_{aa}$ and $\kappa_b = \sigma_{bb}/d_{bb}$ denote the reliability ratios for $\widehat{\alpha}_i$ and $\widehat{\beta}_i$. From (11.14) it follows that in the presence of independent estimation errors $R^2_{\mathrm{trial(r)}}$ will be underestimated, whereas for $\rho \neq 0$, $R^2_{\mathrm{trial(r)}}$ may be either under- or overestimated.

Additional insight might be gained under the assumption that $\kappa_a = \kappa_b = \kappa$. Then, (11.14) can be written as:

$$\mathrm{Corr}(\widehat{\alpha}_i, \widehat{\beta}_i) = \mathrm{Corr}(\alpha_i, \beta_i) + \frac{\kappa}{1+\kappa}\left[\rho - \mathrm{Corr}(\alpha_i, \beta_i)\right]. \tag{11.15}$$

It follows that if $\rho > \mathrm{Corr}(\alpha_i, \beta_i)$, then the coefficient $\mathrm{Corr}(\widehat{\alpha}_i, \widehat{\beta}_i)$ will overestimate $\mathrm{Corr}(\alpha_i, \beta_i)$. And conversely, if $\rho < \mathrm{Corr}(\alpha_i, \beta_i)$, then $\mathrm{Corr}(\widehat{\alpha}_i, \widehat{\beta}_i)$ will underestimate $\mathrm{Corr}(\alpha_i, \beta_i)$.

The aforementioned results were given by Burzykowski *et al.* (2001). It is worth mentioning that similar observations were made by Schaalje and Butts (1993). In fact, (11.14) is equivalent to their equation (2.10).

To adjust bias in the estimation of $R^2_{\mathrm{trial(r)}}$ for the measurement error in $\widehat{\alpha}_i$ and $\widehat{\beta}_i$, Burzykowski *et al.* (2001) considered an approach based on developments by van Houwelingen, Arends, and Stijnen (2002) (see also Section 7.4.2). More specifically, the dispersion matrix D, defined by (11.8), can be obtained by fitting the model resulting from (11.12)–(11.13) and (11.8)–(11.9) to the estimated pairs $(\widehat{\alpha}_i, \widehat{\beta}_i)$. To fit the model, the covariance matrices Ω_i, defined by (11.13), might be assumed known and equal to their estimates obtained from the bivariate copula model (11.1). An estimate $\widehat{R}^2_{\mathrm{trial(r)}}$ of $R^2_{\mathrm{trial(r)}}$ can then be obtained from the resulting estimate $\widehat{D}$ of D by means of the formula (11.10).

Alternatively, one might use the methods developed for the measurement error models with an error in the equation and unequal error variances (Fuller 1987). We will briefly summarize them here. Assume that the true unobserved trial-specific treatment effects follow the simple linear regression model

$$\beta_i = \gamma_0 + \gamma_1\alpha_i + \varepsilon_i, \tag{11.16}$$

where γ_0 and γ_1 are constant coefficients and ε_i is a random variable with mean 0 and variance σ. We will use γ to denote the vector $(\gamma_0, \gamma_1)^T$. Let the observed estimates $\widehat{\alpha}_i$ and $\widehat{\beta}_i$ follow model (11.12); the normality assumption is not crucial here. We will also assume that ε_i is independent of

$(\varepsilon_{ai}, \varepsilon_{bi})$. It follows that

$$\begin{aligned} \mathrm{Var}(\beta_i|\alpha_i) &= \sigma, & (11.17)\\ \mathrm{Var}(\beta_i) &= \gamma_1^2 d_{aa} + \sigma, & (11.18)\\ \mathrm{Var}(\widehat{\beta}_i|\widehat{\alpha}_i) &= \sigma + \sigma_{aa,i} - 2\gamma_i\sigma_{ab,i} + \gamma_1^2\sigma_{bb,i}, & (11.19)\\ \mathrm{Var}(\widehat{\alpha}_i) &= d_{aa} + \sigma_{aa,i}, & (11.20) \end{aligned}$$

where d_{aa} is an element of matrix D given in (11.9), while $\sigma_{aa,i}$, $\sigma_{ab,i}$ and $\sigma_{bb,i}$ are elements of matrix Ω_i given in (11.13). Using (11.17) and (11.18), the formula (11.10) can be re-written as

$$R^2_{\mathrm{trial(r)}} = \frac{\gamma_1^2 d_{aa}}{\gamma_1^2 d_{aa} + \sigma}. \tag{11.21}$$

From (11.19) it follows that, given an estimate of γ, $\tilde{\gamma}$ say, and maximum likelihood estimates $\widehat{\Omega}_i$ of matrices Ω_i, we can estimate σ by

$$\begin{aligned} \tilde{\sigma} &= \frac{1}{N-2}\sum_{i=1}^{N}\left(\widehat{\beta}_i - \tilde{\gamma}_0 - \tilde{\gamma}_1\widehat{\alpha}_i\right)^2 \\ &\quad -\sum_{i=1}^{N}\left(\widehat{\sigma}_{bb,i} - 2\tilde{\gamma}_1\widehat{\sigma}_{ab,i} + \tilde{\gamma}_1^2\widehat{\sigma}_{aa,i}\right). \end{aligned} \tag{11.22}$$

On the other hand, equation (11.20) suggests that d_{aa} can be estimated by

$$\tilde{d}_{aa} = S_{aa} - \sum_{i=1}^{N}\frac{\widehat{\sigma}_{aa,i}}{N}, \tag{11.23}$$

where

$$S_{aa} = \frac{1}{N-1}\sum_{i=1}^{N}\left(\widehat{\alpha}_i - \sum_{j=1}^{N}\frac{\widehat{\alpha}_j}{N}\right)^2$$

is the sample variance of the estimates $\widehat{\alpha}_i$.

The estimators $\tilde{\gamma}_1$, $\tilde{d}_{aa}$ and $\tilde{\sigma}$ can in turn be plugged in the formula (11.21) to obtain an estimator of trial-level R^2 adjusted for the measurement errors Ω_i.

One should note that none of the estimators given by (11.22) and (11.23) is guaranteed to be positive. If a negative estimate is obtained for one of them, the formula (11.21) produces an estimate of R^2 outside the [0,1] range. In such case the estimate has to be taken as non-defined.

Fuller (1987) suggests several possible estimators of γ. The unweighted method-of-moments-based estimator can be written as (Buonaccorsi 1995)

$$\tilde{\gamma}_1 = \frac{S_{ab} - \sum_{i=1}^{N} \widehat{\sigma}_{ab,i}/N}{S_{aa} - \sum_{i=1}^{N} \widehat{\sigma}_{aa,i}/N}, \tag{11.24}$$

$$\tilde{\gamma}_0 = \sum_{i=1}^{N} \frac{\widehat{\beta}_i}{N} - \tilde{\gamma}_1 \sum_{i=1}^{N} \frac{\widehat{\alpha}_i}{N}, \tag{11.25}$$

where

$$S_{ab} = \frac{1}{N-1} \sum_{i=1}^{N} \left[\left(\widehat{\beta}_i - \sum_{j=1}^{N} \frac{\widehat{\beta}_j}{N} \right) \left(\widehat{\alpha}_i - \sum_{j=1}^{N} \frac{\widehat{\alpha}_j}{N} \right) \right]$$

is the sample covariance of the estimates $\widehat{\alpha}_i$ and $\widehat{\beta}_i$. The estimator given by (11.24) and (11.25) can be modified to guarantee the existence of its finite mean and variance in small samples. Moreover, it can be used to construct a (weighted) generalized least squares (GLS) estimator. Fuller (1987) suggests that in almost all practical situations the weighted estimator should have a smaller variance than the unweighted one. Also, the weighted estimator can be adjusted to guarantee its finite moments in small samples. For all the estimators of γ, two asymptotic variance-covariance matrices can be considered, depending on whether the normality of random errors can be assumed or not (Fuller 1987, Section 3.1.2).

The estimator of $R^2_{\text{trial(r)}}$ based on formula (11.21) is easier to compute than the one based on the maximum likelihood estimate of the dispersion matrix D, $\widehat{D}$ say, obtained by fitting the model defined by (11.12)–(11.13) and (11.8)–(11.9) to the estimated pairs $(\widehat{\alpha}_i, \widehat{\beta}_i)$. In particular, the former estimator can be obtained in one step, while the latter requires an iterative procedure, for which convergence is not guaranteed. On the other hand, if the iterative procedure converges, it provides an estimate of the asymptotic variance-covariance of $\widehat{D}$, which allows to compute the variance of the estimate of $R^2_{\text{trial(r)}}$. Computation of the variance of the estimator based on the formula (11.21) would require resorting to bootstrap or simulation methods, as no analytical formula for it can be given.

The above methodology can easily be extended to the case where the second stage model (11.12) includes additional parameters, other than α_i, of the marginal model (11.6) for the surrogate endpoint.

11.2.2 Prediction of Treatment Effect on the True Endpoint

Assume we are interested in predicting treatment effect on a true endpoint based on treatment effect on a surrogate in a new trial $i = 0$. Burzykowski *et al.* (2001) argue that the prediction for β_0, under model (11.8)–(11.9), could be based on the simple linear regression model (11.16). It is important to recall that, in practice, only estimated treatment effects $\widehat{\alpha}_i$ and $\widehat{\beta}_i$ will be available. One should therefore consider using the methods appropriate for the prediction when both the dependent and independent variables in a simple linear regression model are subject to measurement error. It follows that, in principle, three strategies for computing the prediction might be followed (Buonaccorsi 1995):

1. Regress $\widehat{\beta}_i$ on $\widehat{\alpha}_i$ for $i = 1, \ldots, N$ in the meta-analytic data, and carry out the prediction for $i = 0$ as if there were no measurement error.
2. Regress $\widehat{\beta}_i$ on $\widehat{\alpha}_i$ for $i = 1, \ldots, N$ and, recognizing the measurement error in $\widehat{\beta}_i$, obtain a corrected estimate of the residual variance σ (see (11.16)) for purposes of computing the precision of the prediction.
3. Regress $\widehat{\beta}_i$ on $\widehat{\alpha}_i$ for $i = 1, \ldots, N$ adjusting for the measurement error in both $\widehat{\beta}_i$ and $\widehat{\alpha}_i$, and obtain estimates of γ_0, γ_1, and σ, defined in (11.16), for purposes of computing the prediction and its precision.

The first two options would require that $\widehat{\alpha}_0$ is a random selection from the same distribution that generated $\widehat{\alpha}_i$ for $i = 1, \ldots, N$ (Fuller 1987, p.75; Buonaccorsi 1995). Although in particular situations this condition may be fulfilled, it will usually not be the case, as different trials included in the analysis will differ with respect to sample size. Moreover, Schaalje and Butts (1993) note that, although ignoring the measurement error does not necessarily have to lead to predicted values much different from those that would be obtained if the measurement error were accounted for, it is likely to lead to substantially different estimates of the prediction variance. These authors therefore state that "the most compelling reason for not ignoring correlated measurement errors may be to obtain appropriate standard errors of prediction and prediction intervals."

In general, therefore, one should apply the third strategy and, following Buonaccorsi (1995), predict β_0 using

$$\widehat{\beta}_0 = \tilde{\gamma}_0 + \tilde{\gamma}_1 \widehat{\alpha}_0, \tag{11.26}$$

where $\tilde{\gamma}_0$ and $\tilde{\gamma}_1$ are estimates of γ_0 and γ_1 from model (11.16), obtained using (11.24) or one of its modifications (Fuller 1987), while $\widehat{\alpha_0}$ is obtained from the marginal proportional hazard model (11.6) fitted to the data on the surrogate in the new trial. Assuming negligible bias in $\widehat{\gamma}_0$, $\widehat{\gamma}_1$, the variance of the prediction error can be written (Buonaccorsi 1995) as

$$\begin{aligned} \text{Var}(\widehat{\beta}_0 - \beta_0) &= \sigma + \text{Var}(\tilde{\gamma}_0) + 2\alpha \text{Cov}(\tilde{\gamma}_0, \tilde{\gamma}_1) \\ & \quad + (\alpha^2 + d_{aa}) \text{Var}(\tilde{\gamma}_1) + E(\tilde{\gamma}_1^2 \sigma_{aa,0}), \end{aligned} \tag{11.27}$$

where σ is the residual variance defined in (11.16), α and d_{aa} are the mean and variance of α_0 specified in (11.8)–(11.9), and $\sigma_{aa,i}$ is the measurement error associated with $\widehat{\alpha}_0$ in (11.13). To estimate (11.27), one might use

$$\begin{aligned}\widehat{\text{Var}}(\widehat{\beta}_0 - \beta_0) &= \tilde{\sigma} + \widehat{\text{Var}}(\tilde{\gamma}_0) + 2\widehat{\alpha}_0\widehat{\text{Cov}}(\tilde{\gamma}_0, \tilde{\gamma}_1) \\ &\quad + (\widehat{\alpha}_0^2 - \widehat{\sigma}_{aa,0})\widehat{\text{Var}}(\tilde{\gamma}_1) + \tilde{\gamma}_1^2\widehat{\sigma}_{aa,0}, \qquad (11.28)\end{aligned}$$

with $\tilde{\sigma}$ defined by (11.22) and $\widehat{\sigma}_{aa,0}$ obtained from the marginal proportional hazards model (11.6) (Buonaccorsi 1995).

Note that the variance in (11.27) consists of five different contributions. The first one is related to the error in equation (11.16); the second, third and fourth are associated with the uncertainty about γ; and the fifth results from the error due to the estimation of treatment effect on the surrogate in the new trial. It is worth noting that, if prediction without adjusting for measurement error in treatment effects were considered, the fifth contribution to (11.27) would be equal to zero. The first one (residual variability), on the other hand, would in general be larger, as the variability in observed treatment effects due to the measurement error would not be removed. This suggests that, if the measurement (estimation) error for treatment effect on the surrogate in the new trial is small, the prediction based on (11.26) can be less variable than the one resulting from the use of an estimate of γ obtained without adjusting for the estimation of treatment effects.

Following Buonaccorsi (1995), it should be mentioned that some caution is needed in constructing the prediction intervals for β_0 using (11.26) and (11.28). Naively, one might treat $\widehat{\beta}_0$ as a normally distributed random variable with variance (11.28). However, the properties of the estimator of the variance (11.28) are not yet established and it is therefore not clear if the normality assumption is justified. As suggested by Buonaccorsi (1995), more research is needed in this area.

11.3 Analysis of Case Studies

Burzykowski *et al.* (2001) applied the proposed two-stage approach to two case studies, described in Sections 4.2.2 and 4.2.3. To construct the bivariate model at the first stage, the baseline hazard functions in (11.6)–(11.7) were assumed to arise from a Weibull distribution. For both datasets the Clayton, Hougaard, and Plackett models were considered, with copula functions given by (11.2), (11.3) and (11.4)–(11.5), respectively.

In principle, one might also consider a version of (11.6)–(11.7) with common (across centers/trials) baseline hazard functions. In fact, Burzykowski *et al.* (2001) did consider this option. One might regard it as a construction similar to the reduced fixed-effects model, given by (7.16)–(7.17) and (7.14), presented in Chapter 7. Recall that the latter model was developed based on a linear mixed-effects model including only random treatment effects.

However, the common baseline-hazards model should be treated with caution, as in this case treatment effects become nonorthogonal across the trials and their values (and the association) depend on the coding of the treatment covariate (Burzykowski 2001). In principle, therefore, the use of this model is not recommended.

Maximum likelihood parameter estimates for the copula models were obtained using the Newton-Raphson procedure with numerical second order derivatives implemented in SAS-IML 6.12 as routine NLPNRR (SAS Institute Inc. 1995). Standard errors of the parameters were calculated using the inverse of the observed matrix of second derivatives. The standard error of $\widehat{\tau}$ was computed from the variance of $\widehat{\theta}$ using the delta method. Thus, for the Clayton model:

$$\text{Var}(\widehat{\tau}) \approx \frac{4 \cdot \text{Var}(\widehat{\theta})}{(\widehat{\theta}+1)^4},$$

as for this model $\tau = (\theta - 1)/(\theta + 1)$. On the other hand, for the Hougaard model $\tau = 1 - \theta$, so

$$\text{Var}(\widehat{\tau}) = \text{Var}(\widehat{\theta}).$$

For the Plackett copula there is no closed-form expression linking τ and θ. Thus, in this case, $\widehat{\tau}$ and its variance were computed directly from (11.11) using numerical integration, according to the 9-interior-points rule for bidimensional integrals on a square based (see Section 25.4.62 in Abramowitz and Stegun 1972). For a square of size h^2 the rule gives the approximation error of h^6. To apply the method, the $[0, 1] \times [0, 1]$ unit square was subdivided into squares of size 0.01^2. The variance of $\widehat{\tau}$ was computed from the variance of $\widehat{\theta}$ using the delta method, with derivatives w.r.t. θ computed under the integral sign.

At the second stage, model (11.8)–(11.9) was used. Effectively, it implied ignoring the information about the parameters related to the marginal Weibull model for S in modeling the relationship between α_i and β_i.

11.3.1 Advanced Ovarian Cancer: Four Clinical Trials

These data were described in Section 4.2.2. Center was used as the unit of analysis. Thus, the term "trial-specific" should be understood as meaning "center-specific" when results of the analysis of the case studies throughout

TABLE 11.1. *Advanced ovarian cancer. Results of the trial- and individual-level surrogacy analysis.*

Model	Individual-level	Trial-level $R^2_{\text{trial(r)}}$	
	τ	Unadjusted	F
Clayton	0.87 [0.86, 0.88]	0.87 [0.80, 0.95]	0.94
Hougaard	0.85 [0.84, 0.86]	0.88 [0.81, 0.95]	0.83
Plackett	0.87 [0.86, 0.87]	0.87 [0.78, 0.95]	0.77

NOTE: F, adjusted estimates of $R^2_{trial(r)}$ obtained by using the estimator of γ given by (11.24)–(11.25) (Fuller 1987); 95% confidence intervals in brackets (not available for F).

this chapter. The analysis was restricted to centers with at least 3 patients on each treatment arm. This constraint was adopted to ensure estimability of the joint copula models, as they require the estimation of six marginal parameters related to the marginal distributions of T and S for each trial i. In general, the minimum for the estimability of the marginal parameters would require at least three patients per center, with at least one observed failure and at least one patient in each treatment group. As a result, data for 39 centers (including the two smaller trials) were used, with a total sample size of 1153 patients.

Table 11.1 presents the results of the analysis. For all models two values of $R^2_{\text{trial(r)}}$ are given, both unadjusted and adjusted. The former was not adjusted for the measurement error in $\widehat{\alpha}_i$ and $\widehat{\beta}_i$ and obtained by calculating the correlation coefficient for pairs $(\widehat{\alpha}_i, \widehat{\beta}_i)$. The adjusted estimate was computed using the method based on the developments by Fuller (1987), as described in Section 11.2.1. The alternative adjusted estimates, resulting form the approach based on the results developed by van Houwelingen, Arends, and Stijnen (2002), could not be obtained due to convergence problems. The problems are due to the magnitude of the measurement error present in the estimates of treatment effects. For example, when the estimated error is simply halved, the alternative adjusted estimates can be computed.

Figure 11.1 shows a plot of the treatment effects on the true endpoint (survival) by the treatment effects on the surrogate endpoint (progression-free survival), corresponding to the three models considered in the analysis. The effects are strongly correlated. The results shown in Table 11.1 confirm this conclusion. The unadjusted estimates suggest values of $R^2_{\text{trial(r)}}$ around 0.90. The estimates of $R^2_{\text{trial(r)}}$ adjusted for the measurement error using the approach by Fuller (1987) show somewhat more variability, ranging from 0.77 to 0.94.

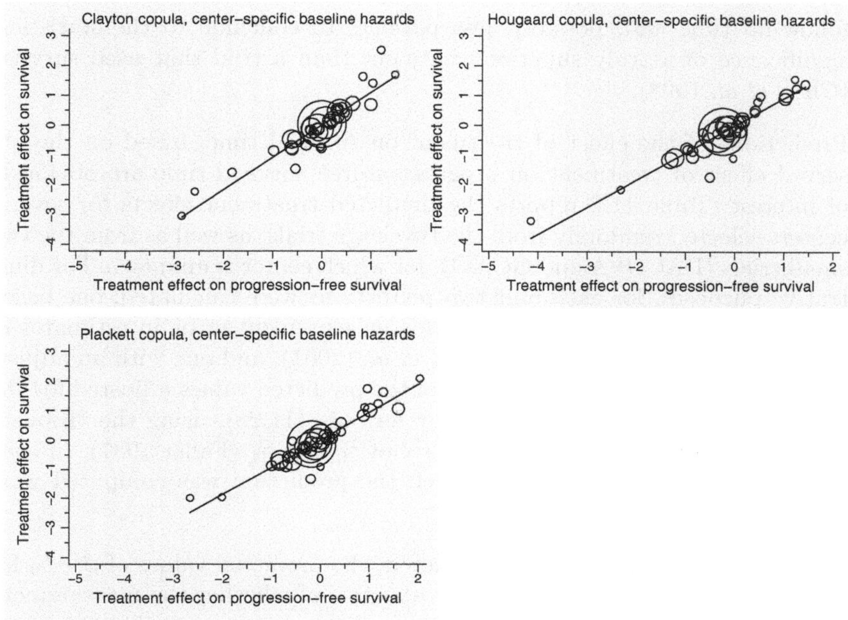

FIGURE 11.1. *Advanced ovarian cancer. Treatment effects on the true endpoint (survival time) versus treatment effects on the surrogate endpoint (progression-free survival time) for all units of analysis. The size of each point is proportional to the number of patients in the corresponding unit. The straight lines are predictions from a (weighted by sample size) simple linear regression model.*

It may be of interest to compare these results to those obtained by Buyse *et al.* (2000a) (see also Chapter 7, Section 7.5.3) by ignoring censoring and assuming normal distribution for the logarithm of both endpoints. These results were based on data for 1192 patients included into the meta-analysis (excluding two individuals lost to follow up after randomization). In the analysis of the trial-level surrogacy, unadjusted $R^2_{\text{trial(r)}} = 0.94$ (standard error 0.02). This value is somewhat higher than the unadjusted estimates presented in Table 11.1. The values of Kendall's τ shown in Table 11.1 are close to 0.85 for all the models.

Although interpretation of the value of the coefficients of determination and Kendall's τ is subjective, based on the unadjusted estimates presented in Table 11.1, Burzykowski *et al.* (2001) found it plausible to conclude that progression-free survival might be a valid surrogate for survival in advanced ovarian cancer for treatments of the type used in the trials analyzed. The effect of treatment can be observed earlier if progression-free survival is used instead of survival, although in this particular example the difference is small. A trial that records progression-free survival might require less follow-up time and, possibly, less patients to conclude to the statistical significance of a truly superior treatment than a trial that used survival (Chen *et al.* 1998).

Predictions of the effect of treatment on survival time, based on the observed effect of treatment on progression-free survival time are obviously of interest. Table 11.2 reports the predicted treatment effects for several centers selected randomly from the two large trials, as well as from the two small trials (DACOVA and GONO), for which center is unknown. For illustrative purposes, for each unit two predictions were calculated: one based on (11.8)–(11.9) without adjusting for measurement error in estimates of treatment effects, as in Burzykowski *et al.* (2001), and one with an adjustment (see Section 11.2.2). Variance of the predicted values adjusted for the measurement error was estimated by formula (11.28), using the "robust" estimate of variance-covariance matrix of $\widehat{\gamma}_0$ and $\widehat{\gamma}_1$ (Fuller 1987). In each case, the data for the unit for which the prediction was computed were excluded from fitting the model.

For each of the three copulas considered, the predicted values of $\beta + b_0$ for a particular unit are quite close, irrespective of whether the measurement error in estimated treatment effects was adjusted for or not. The predicted values obtained using the Plackett model are located between those predicted under the Clayton and Hougaard models. For the Hougaard and Plackett copulas the values obtained with the adjustment for measurement error are a bit more shrunken toward 0 than the values obtained without the adjustment. For the Clayton copula the converse can be observed. The predicted values, at least for the Hougaard and Plackett copulas, agree reasonably well with the effects estimated from the data, although in certain cases (for Center 8, for instance) they differ by approximately 50%.

As the differences between point estimates and predictions are expected, the prediction error is obviously of interest. From Table 11.2 it can be seen that ignoring the measurement error in treatment effects leads, at least for the smaller centers, to substantially underestimated standard errors of the predicted values. However, for DACOVA and GONO trials, the reverse can be observed. The reason for this difference lies in the magnitude of the standard error of the estimate of α_0, as suggested at the end of Section 11.2.2. For the smaller centers, the standard error is much larger and it becomes the dominant contribution to the variance (11.27) of the prediction adjusted for the measurement error. On the other hand, for the DACOVA and GONO trials the standard error is much smaller and, combined with residual variability σ, which is smaller than the one obtained for a simple linear regression based on observed pairs $(\widehat{\beta}_i,\widehat{\alpha}_i)$, results in the smaller prediction variance.

TABLE 11.2. *Advanced ovarian cancer. Predictions of treatment effect on survival based on the estimated effect on progression-free survival.*

Unit	N	$\widehat{\alpha}_0$	$\widehat{E}(\beta+b_0\|a_0)$			$\widehat{\beta+b_0}$
			Clayton	Hougaard	Plackett	
Center 6	17	1.40 (0.64)	1.59 (0.38) 1.73 (0.82)	1.26 (0.35) 1.15 (0.61)	1.38 (0.34) 1.35 (0.71)	1.14 (0.74)
Center 8	10	-1.00 (0.93)	-1.04 (0.35) -1.10 (1.07)	-0.85 (0.27) -0.80 (0.78)	-0.90 (0.28) -0.84 (0.84)	-1.43 (1.06)
Center 37	12	-0.82 (0.68)	-0.89 (0.38) -0.96 (0.84)	-0.73 (0.34) -0.69 (0.62)	-0.77 (0.35) -0.73 (0.67)	-0.55 (0.78)
Center 49	40	-1.14 (0.46)	-1.23 (0.38) -1.32 (0.60)	-1.02 (0.35) -0.95 (0.47)	-1.07 (0.35) -1.01 (0.52)	-1.06 (0.48)
Center 55	31	-1.13 (0.47)	-1.22 (0.38) -1.31 (0.61)	-1.01 (0.35) -0.95 (0.48)	-1.06 (0.35) -1.00 (0.53)	-1.13 (0.49)
Center 102	21	1.24 (0.64)	1.38 (0.39) 1.48 (0.80)	1.12 (0.35) 1.01 (0.61)	1.18 (0.35) 1.10 (0.67)	0.92 (0.78)
GONO	125	-0.24 (0.20)	-0.24 (0.38) -0.25 (0.31)	-0.21 (0.34) -0.20 (0.31)	-0.21 (0.34) -0.20 (0.33)	-0.16 (0.23)
DACOVA	274	-0.26 (0.13)	-0.27 (0.38) -0.28 (0.26)	-0.23 (0.34) -0.23 (0.28)	-0.24 (0.34) -0.23 (0.31)	-0.21 (0.14)

NOTE: N is the number of patients per unit. $\widehat{\alpha}_0$ and $\widehat{\beta+b_0}$ are treatment effects on progression-free survival and survival, respectively, estimated from the data; $\widehat{E}(\beta+b_0|a_0)$ is the predicted effect of treatment on survival, given its effect upon progression-free survival (for each center, first line: simple regression; second line: regression corrected for measurement error). Standard errors are given in parenthesis.

11.3.2 Advanced Colorectal Cancer: Two Clinical Trials

These data were described in Section 4.2.3. Center was used as the unit of analysis. Similar to the advanced ovarian cancer study presented in the previous section, in the analysis of the advanced colorectal cancer data only centers with at least 3 patients on each treatment arm were considered. As a result, data for 48 centers were used, with the sample size amounting to 642 patients. For comparability purposes, the common marginal hazard functions version of (11.6)–(11.7) was applied to the same dataset.

Table 11.3 shows results obtained for the analysis. Figure 11.2 presents a plot of the treatment effects on the true endpoint (survival time) by the treatment effects on the surrogate endpoint (progression-free survival time), corresponding to the models considered in the analysis. The picture is very much different from that obtained for the ovarian cancer study. For all models, the association of the trial-specific treatment effects is low.

TABLE 11.3. *Corfu study in advanced colorectal cancer. Results of the trial- and individual-level surrogacy analysis.*

Model	Individual-level	Trial-level $R^2_{\mathrm{trial(r)}}$	
	τ	Unadjusted	F
Clayton	0.603 [0.589, 0.617]	0.46 [0.25, 0.68]	0.54
Hougaard	0.632 [0.597, 0.667]	0.53 [0.34, 0.72]	0.64
Plackett	0.662 [0.652, 0.671]	0.43 [0.21, 0.65]	0.37

NOTE: F, adjusted estimates of $R^2_{trial(r)}$ obtained by using the estimator of γ given by (11.24)–(11.25) (Fuller 1987); 95% confidence intervals in brackets (not available for F).

The unadjusted estimates of $R^2_{\mathrm{trial(r)}}$ lie around 0.45. Again, due to the convergence problems, the estimates adjusted for the measurement error using the approach of van Houwelingen, Arends, and Stijnen (2002) could not be obtained. The estimates adjusted for the measurement error using the approach by Fuller (1987) range from 0.37 to 0.64.

An interesting question is whether accounting for known important prognostic factors in the marginal models (11.6)–(11.7) might change the results of the analysis presented in Table 11.3. For the patients in the advanced colorectal dataset, additional information about their performance status (PS) at baseline was available. PS is an important prognostic factor in cancer. It measures the overall ability of a patient to perform daily self-care and work activities. It is a categorical variable with the categories ranging from 0 to 4, indicating the increasing level of restrictions experienced in this ability. In the advanced colorectal dataset, 27.2% of patients had PS= 0 ("no restrictions"), 57.6% had PS= 1 ("restricted, but ambulatory and able to carry out light work") and 15.1% had PS= 2 ("ambulatory and capable of all self-care but unable to carry out any work; up and about more than 50% of waking hours"). To investigate whether taking into account the information about PS would change the results of the analysis, all models from Table 11.3 were re-fitted with PS included as a continuous covariate in the marginal models (11.6)–(11.7). Results are shown in Table 11.4. The estimated values of Kendall's τ are very close to their counterparts in Table 11.3. The estimates of $R^2_{\mathrm{trial(r)}}$ are slightly increased, as compared to their values from Table 11.3. A truly remarkable change can be seen for the one adjusted for the measurement error using the approach of Fuller (1987) for the Plackett copula, which increased from 0.64 to 0.80. Overall, however, the estimates presented in Table 11.4 do not offer convincing evidence for an increased individual- or trial-level association.

To summarize, the results suggest that progression-free survival time is neither trial-level nor individual-level valid. It should probably not be used

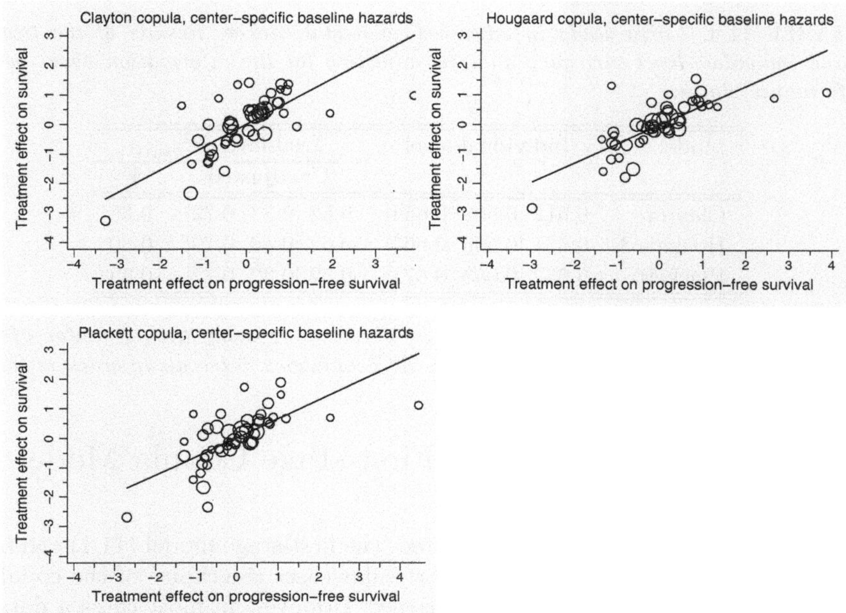

FIGURE 11.2. *Corfu study in advanced colorectal cancer. Treatment effects on the true endpoint (survival time) versus treatment effects on the surrogate endpoint (progression-free survival time) for all units of analysis. The size of each point is proportional to the number of patients in the corresponding unit. The straight lines are predictions from a simple linear regression model, that has been weighted by sample size.*

as a surrogate for survival in colorectal cancer for treatments of the type used in the trials analyzed.

The marked difference between this example in colorectal cancer and the previous one in ovarian cancer underscores the difficulty of making general claims about surrogate endpoints. In both examples, the average time between progression and death is about six months (see Figures 4.3 and 4.4), yet in colorectal cancer progression-free survival is not nearly as good a surrogate for survival as in ovarian cancer. This may be due to the fact that in advanced colorectal cancer, progression occurs early (median time to progression of about 6 months) and is often followed by aggressive second-line therapies that may themselves have an impact on survival. In the presence of effective second-line therapies, progression-free survival might be expected to be a poor surrogate for survival because of the "dilution" of the effect of first-line therapy upon the final endpoint (Prentice 1989). The examples analyzed illustrate that generally the validity of a particular endpoint as a surrogate may depend both on the treatment and the disease under consideration.

TABLE 11.4. *Corfu study in advanced colorectal cancer. Results of the trial- and individual-level surrogacy analysis adjusting for the information about performance status.*

Model	Individual-level	Trial-level $R^2_{\mathrm{trial(r)}}$	
	τ	Unadjusted	F
Clayton	0.612 [0.569, 0.654]	0.52 [0.33, 0.72]	0.66
Hougaard	0.631 [0.596, 0.665]	0.62 [0.46, 0.79]	0.80
Plackett	0.662 [0.653, 0.671]	0.52 [0.32, 0.72]	0.39

NOTE: F, adjusted estimates of $R^2_{trial(r)}$ obtained by using the estimator of γ given by (11.24)–(11.25) (Fuller 1987); 95% confidence intervals in brackets (not available for F).

11.4 The Choice of the First-stage Copula Model

As Burzykowski *et al.* (2001) suggested, the first-stage model (11.1) can be based on any copula function. In particular cases the choice of the copula can be motivated by previous experience. However, in most cases a data-driven choice will be necessary. In this section, we will discuss and illustrate several possible approaches.

Akaike's (1978) information criterion (AIC) and Schwarz's (1978) Bayesian criterion (SBC) are useful for comparing non-nested models with different numbers of parameters; the model with the largest value of AIC or SBC is considered best. They are both defined as $\log(L) - h(q)$, where $\log(L)$ is the log of the likelihood for a particular model and $h(n, q)$ is a function of the sample size n and the number of the parameters q in the model. For AIC, $h(n, q) \equiv q$, while for SBC, $h(n, q) \equiv q \ln(n)/2$.

Table 11.5 presents numbers of parameters q, log-likelihoods, and AIC values for the models considered in the analysis of advanced ovarian and colorectal cancer studies. For the advanced ovarian cancer data, the largest value of the criterion is observed for the model based on the Plackett copula. For the advanced colorectal data the largest value is observed for the Hougaard copula.

A method providing a check on whether a model provides adequate description of data at hand is to fit a larger model, for which the model of interest is a special case. The family of copulas generated by the two-parameter Power Variance Function (PVF) distributions includes the Clayton and Hougaard copulas as special cases (Hougaard 2000). Consequently, the model using the copula generated by a PVF distribution can be used to construct a likelihood ratio test of the hypothesis that the simpler Clayton or Hougaard copula models, which only use a single parameter to describe the associ-

TABLE 11.5. *Advanced ovarian cancer and Corfu study in advanced colorectal cancer. Likelihood-based characteristics for the copula models.*

Model	Ovarian cancer				Colorectal cancer			
	q	$\ln(L)$	AIC	χ^2	q	$\ln(L)$	AIC	χ^2
Plackett	235	-2760.8	-2995.8	-	289	-501.8	-790.8	-
Clayton	235	-2966.2	-3201.2	280.8	289	-549.1	-838.1	135.4
Hougaard	235	-2825.9	-3060.9	0.2	289	-481.4	-770.4	0
PVF	236	-2825.8	-3061.8	-	290	-481.4	-771.4	-

NOTE: q: number of parameters in the model; χ^2: likelihood-ratio test relative to the PVF model.

ation structure, are providing acceptable fit. Unfortunately, this method cannot be used for the Plackett model.

To illustrate the method, the model using a PVF copula was fitted to both advanced ovarian and colorectal cancer datasets. The number of parameters in the model, log-likelihood, and AIC are presented in Table 11.5. The table includes also the values of the likelihood-ratio test statistics comparing the fit of the Clayton and Hougaard models with that obtained using the PVF copula. Note that the parameters for the Clayton and the Hougaard copulas lie on the boundary of the parameter space for the PVF copula. By analogy to the linear mixed models case (Stram and Lee 1994, 1995, Verbeke and Molenberghs 2000, 2003), one should be careful in using χ^2_1 as the asymptotic distribution of the likelihood-ratio test statistic in this situation.

With due caution, however, it can be concluded that the large values of the likelihood-ratio test statistic presented in Table 11.5 indicate that, in both datasets, the fit of the PVF model was much better as compared to the Clayton model. On the other hand, the difference for the Hougaard model was much smaller. In both datasets, the difference in fit between the model based on the Hougaard copula and the PVF model was negligible.

The choice of the copula model could also be guided by an assessment of the overall goodness-of-fit. For the Clayton copula, several methods for such an assessment are available. Shih and Louis (1995a) proposed a graphical method based on the plot of the estimated Pearson's correlation coefficient for martingale residuals based on a copula model. Shih and Louis (1995b) proposed another graphical method based on the plot of the average of cluster-specific posterior expectations of the frailty distribution *versus* time. Shih (1998) developed an overall test based on estimators of Kendall's τ. Glidden (1999) proposed a method based on a weighted sum of the cluster-specific posterior expectations of the frailty.

Under the assumption that an uncensored sample of bivariate failure-times is available, Genest and Rivest (1993) developed a method of checking goodness-of-fit applicable to any one-parameter bivariate Archimedean family of copulas (see, e.g., Nelsen 1999). This family includes the Clayton and the Hougaard copulas as special cases. Their approach was based on the non-parametric estimation of a function that uniquely defines the Archimedean copula. Recently, Wang and Wells (2000a) have extended the ideas of Genest and Rivest to the case of a censored sample of bivariate failure-time observations. Burzykowski (2001) applied the approach proposed by Wang and Wells (2000a) to assess the fit of the Clayton and Hougaard copulas to the advanced ovarian and colorectal cancer datasets. Separate analyses were performed for each treatment arm within each dataset. The results indicated that, for the advanced ovarian cancer data, neither the Clayton nor the Hougaard copula provided a reasonable fit. This conclusion corresponds to the result obtained using the AIC (see Table 11.5), that suggested the choice of the Plackett copula. For the advanced colorectal cancer data, the Wang and Wells (2000a) approach indicated that the Hougaard copula offered a reasonable description of the data. This conclusion is also in accordance with the one obtained using AIC (see Table 11.5).

Recently, for a broad class of copulas, Andersen *et al.* (2004) have proposed a class of tests of the hypothesis that the copula is in parametric family, with unspecified association parameter, based on bivariate right censored data. Also Durrleman, Nikeghbali, and Roncalli (2004) have developed procedures for the selection of an "optimal" copula, using the empirical copula and copula approximations. These methods could be applied to choose the appropriate copula function for model (11.1).

11.5 A Simulation Study

In this section, results of simulations investigating small-sample properties of the two-stage model based on the copula approach, proposed by Burzykowski *et al.* (2001), are briefly reported. In these simulations, the bias and variability for different estimators of individual-level and trial-level association were investigated. Also, numerical properties (convergence) of algorithms used for the computation of the estimators were evaluated. A full description of the simulations was reported by Burzykowski (2001).

11.5.1 Parameter Settings

In the simulation study, data for N independent randomized clinical trials ($N = 10, 20$) with n ($n = 50, 100, 200$) patients each were generated. Combinations of the assumed values of N and n implied total sample sizes of 500, 1000, 2000, and 4000, corresponding to the sizes encountered in meta-analyses in oncology. Within each trial a 1:1 randomization to one of two treatments was assumed. For each of the N trials, pairs of (possibly censored) failure-times S_{ij} and T_{ij} for n patients were generated. The times were assumed to have the joint survival function defined by the Clayton copula (see equation (11.2)). Parameter θ of the copula was assumed to equal 3 and 9, resulting in Kendall's τ of 0.5 and 0.9, respectively, for the association between S_{ij} and T_{ij}. Marginally, S_{ij} and T_{ij} were assumed to be exponentially distributed. Conditionally on Z_{ij}, the marginal survivor functions $F_{S_{ij}}$ and $F_{T_{ij}}$ for S_{ij} and T_{ij}, respectively, were defined as

$$F_{S_{ij}}(s_{ij}) = \exp\{-s_{ij}\lambda_S \exp[a_{0,i} + (\alpha + a_{1,i})Z_{ij}]\}, \tag{11.29}$$

$$F_{T_{ij}}(t_{ij}) = \exp\{-t_{ij}\lambda_T \exp[b_{0,i} + (\beta + b_{1,i})Z_{ij}]\}, \tag{11.30}$$

where λ_S and λ_T were fixed baseline hazards, α and β were fixed treatment effects, and trial-specific random effects $(a_{0,i}, b_{0,i}, a_{1,i}, a_{1,i})$ followed a zero-mean normal distribution with the variance-covariance matrix

$$D = \sigma \begin{pmatrix} 1 & \rho & 0 & 0 \\ & 1 & 0 & 0 \\ & & 1 & \rho \\ & & & 1 \end{pmatrix}. \tag{11.31}$$

Three censoring schemes were considered:

No censoring: In this case, no censoring was applied.

Homogeneous: Independent homogenous censoring of S_{ij} and T_{ij} (Hougaard 2000). This censoring scheme corresponds to the most typical situation in randomized clinical trials, where the end of follow-up terminates simultaneously observation of all patient's characteristics.

Time-to-progression (TTP): On top of the independent homogeneous censoring, T_{ij}-dependent censoring of S_{ij} was applied. As a result, the observed value of S_{ij} could not be higher then the observed value of T_{ij}. In oncology, this set-up corresponds to S_{ij} being, for example, time-to-progression and T_{ij} being survival time.

The parameters for the independent homogeneous censoring were set so that around 50% (30%) or 67% (50%) censored observations on T (S) were generated.

The simulations were performed using SAS Version 6.12. The following values of the fixed parameters were used:

$\lambda_T =$ 0.69 (median $T_{ij} = 1$) and $\lambda_S = 1.39$ (median $S_{ij} = 0.54$), corresponding to the situation when the information about the surrogate can be obtained earlier than about the true endpoint;

$(\alpha, \beta) =$ (0,0), i.e., no treatment effect on S and T, or $(-0.4, -0.4)$, i.e., a 33% reduction in the failure rate for S and T;

$\sigma =$ 0.1 and 0.2; these values implied that in 95% of simulated trials, the baseline hazards and treatment effects would vary, as compared to the mean values, by factors ranging between 82%–122% (for $\sigma = 0.1$) and 67%–149% (for $\sigma = 0.2$);

$\rho =$ $\sqrt{0.5}$ and $\sqrt{0.9}$, resulting in trial-level R^2 of 0.5 and 0.9, respectively.

For each resulting combination of the parameter values, 500 independent samples were generated. In each sample, maximum likelihood estimates of the parameters were obtained, assuming the fixed-effects representation of (11.29)–(11.30):

$$F_{S_{ij}}(s_{ij}) = \exp[-s_{ij}\lambda_{Si}\exp(\alpha_i Z_{ij})], \qquad (11.32)$$

$$F_{T_{ij}}(t_{ij}) = \exp[-t_{ij}\lambda_{Ti}\exp(\beta_i Z_{ij})]. \qquad (11.33)$$

The estimates of Kendall's τ and their standard errors were computed from the estimates of the copula parameter θ using the relationship $\tau = (\theta - 1)/(\theta + 1)$. To estimate $R^2_{\text{trial(r)}}$, trial-specific treatment effects α_i and β_i, defined in (11.32)–(11.33), were assumed to follow the simple linear regression model

$$\beta_i = \gamma_0 + \gamma_1 \alpha_i + \varepsilon_i, \qquad (11.34)$$

with ε_i distributed according to a zero-mean normal distribution with variance σ_0. In particular, two strategies of estimating $R^2_{\text{trial(r)}}$ were used. In the first one, the estimation error present in the estimates of treatment effects α_i and β_i was ignored. The resulting "unadjusted" estimator, the square of the sample correlation coefficient, R_{unadj} say, of the estimated treatment effects, will be denoted by R^2_{unadj}. In the second strategy, the estimation error was adjusted for, using the methods described in Section 11.2.1. In particular, three different "adjusted" estimates were considered: one based on the developments by van Houwelingen, Arends, and Stijnen (2000) and two based on Fuller's unweighted estimator of the coefficients of the regression line (11.34), without and with the adjustment for finite moments (see equation (11.24) and the related discussion in Section 11.2.1).

It should be noted that the marginal models (11.29)–(11.30) imply the following regression equation for the trial-specific treatment effects α_i and β_i from the fixed-effects representation (11.32)–(11.33):

$$E(\beta_i|\alpha_i) = (\beta - \rho\alpha) + \rho\alpha_i. \tag{11.35}$$

If $\alpha = \beta$, the intercept (in parentheses) at the right hand of (11.35) equals $\beta(1-\rho)$. It follows that for $\rho \neq 1$ and $\alpha = \beta \neq 0$ it is different from 0 and the regression line does not pass through the origin. Clearly, this is the case for the chosen values of $\alpha = \beta = -0.4$. Admittedly, this choice is not the most preferable from the surrogate endpoint validation point of view, as a zero intercept would be expected for a "good" surrogate endpoint S (Daniels and Hughes 1997). It did assure the comparability of the simulated percentages of censored observations with the zero-treatment-effect situation, though, and was therefore deemed sufficient for the purpose of assessment of the influence of the treatment effect on the estimation of individual- and trial-level measures of association.

11.5.2 Summary Conclusions

The results for the "homogeneous" and "TTP" censoring schemes were quite similar. Moreover, the presence of treatment effect did not substantially influence the bias in the estimation of the individual- and trial-level association. No major problems with the convergence of the algorithm fitting the bivariate Clayton copula model were observed. Non-convergence, if any, was observed exclusively for $\tau = 0.9$. The percentage of samples for which non-convergence occurred never exceeded 1.4% (7 cases out of 500).

For the individual-level association, as measured by Kendall's τ, the simulations suggest a small positive bias for both censoring schemes. The was bias below 1% for $\tau = 0.9$, while for $\tau = 0.5$ it was generally below 4%. Though relatively small, the bias was statistically significantly different from zero. It is worth mentioning that a similar finding was reported by Shih and Louis (1995a), who observed a small positive bias for their estimator of θ. From a practical point of view, estimates of the parameters describing the strength of the individual-level association, obtained by using the two-stage approach to validate surrogate endpoints, might be considered as upper-bounds for the true values of the parameters.

For $\tau = 0.5$, under both censoring schemes, the mean "model-based" standard error of τ (the mean, over the simulated samples, of the estimates of standard error obtained from the model) was approximately 50% larger than the "empirical" error (standard error based on the estimates of τ obtained for the simulated samples). For $\tau = 0.9$, both mean errors were approximately equal.

In general, for the unadjusted estimator of the trial-level R^2, the simulations showed a positive bias under no censoring (except of the case of $\tau = 0.5$ and $R^2 = 0.9$) and a negative bias under censoring (except for the case of $\tau = 0.9$ and $R^2 = 0.5$). The changes of the sign of the bias could be explained by the amount of the correlation of measurement errors in the estimated treatment effects for the surrogate and true endpoints (Burzykowski 2001). Results similar to those observed under no censoring, for the case of two normally distributed endpoints, were noted by Tibaldi *et al.* (2003).

For $n = 200$, with $\tau = 0.9$ or no censoring, the absolute bias of R^2_{unadj} was below 10%, irrespectively of the censoring and other parameters. For $\tau = 0.5$, when censoring was present, the bias was substantial (around 25–30%) even with $n = 200$. As the bias generally decreased with increasing n, it might be conjectured that it should be possible to reduce the bias further with a higher sample size n. It should be noted, though, that even in the cases when the bias was relatively small, it was usually statistically significantly different from zero.

In practice, one might expect surrogate endpoints to exhibit substantial association with true endpoints at individual level. It follows that, with a sample size of 100–200 patients per trial, the use of R^2_{unadj} to estimate the strength of the trial-level association might yield reasonable results. The estimated value of Kendall's τ can be used as an indicator of the possible magnitude of the bias in the estimation.

A seemingly attractive alternative to R^2_{unadj} is the use of the adjusted estimators, which take into account the error associated with the estimation of trial-specific treatment effects. The simulations indicated, though, that the use of the estimators can be very much complicated by the problems with obtaining admissible estimates. The limitation seemed somewhat less severe for the estimators based on Fuller's unweighted estimator of the coefficients of the regression line (11.34) than for the estimator based on the developments by van Houwelingen, Arends, and Stijnen (2000). Nevertheless, when the use of the adjusted estimators would be most advantageous, that is, for $\tau = 0.5$, non-convergence rates for all the estimators, for the considered configurations of the simulation parameters, were generally high. This effectively precludes their use in practice.

In the simulations, both the bias in the estimation of the trial-level R^2 and the non-convergence rates for the adjusted estimators of R^2 decreased with increasing variability of the trial-specific random treatment effects σ, increasing number of trials N and increasing number of patients per trial n. This indicates that they both depend on the observed amount of heterogeneity in trial-specific treatment effects (which is related to σ and N) and on the amount of the error associated with the estimation of the effects (which is related to n and the censoring). It may be concluded that, from the point of view of the assessment of the trial-level surrogacy, it is important to have data from a large number of large sample-size trials, exhibiting substantial variability in their treatment effects. Interestingly, the last requirement distinguishes the meta-analytic approach to the validation of surrogate endpoints from "ordinary" meta-analyses, where heterogeneity is considered rather a disadvantage from the inferential point of view (Thompson 1994).

11.6 Alternatives to the Two-stage Modeling

The method proposed by Burzykowski *et al.* (2001) allows to extend the approach of validation of surrogate endpoints developed by Buyse *et al.* (2000a) to the important case of two failure-time endpoints. An important issue related to the assessment of the estimated values of $R^2_{\text{trial(r)}}$ is the possibility of bias induced by using the two-stage model and estimation of treatment effects. To account for the bias, two methods of estimating the coefficient of determination can considered (see Section 11.2.1): one based on the model proposed by van Houwelingen, Arends, and Stijnen (2000), and one based on the measurement error modelling developed by Fuller (1987). However, the use of the methods is complicated by problems with non-convergence of their numerical algorithms.

An optimal solution to the bias problem would be the use of a full mixed-effects model with random intercepts and random treatment effects. Such a model might replace the two-stage model (11.1)–(11.8) and allow for a full generalization of the method proposed by Buyse *et al.* (2000a). To this aim, one could consider a model in which the hazard functions for the surrogate and true endpoints for individual j in trial i would be assumed to take the following form:

$$\lambda_{Sij}(s_{ij}) = \lambda_{0S}(s_{ij}) \exp^{m_{S_i}+(\alpha_i+a_i)Z_{ij}+\varepsilon_{ij}}, \quad (11.36)$$

$$\lambda_{Tij}(t_{ij}) = \lambda_{0T}(t_{ij}) \exp^{m_{T_i}+(\beta_i+b_i)Z_{ij}+\varepsilon_{ij}}, \quad (11.37)$$

where $\lambda_S(s)$ and $\lambda_T(t)$ are the baseline hazard functions for S and T, respectively, α_i and β_i are trial-specific fixed effects of treatment Z_{ij}, $(m_{Si}, m_{Ti}, a_i, b_i)^T$ is a vector of trial-specific random effects, assumed to be mean-zero normally distributed, and ε_{ij} are individual random effects, also assumed to be mean-zero normally distributed. Alternatively, model (11.36)–(11.37) can be written as

$$\log \lambda_{Sij}(s_{ij}) = \log \lambda_{0S}(s_{ij}) + m_{S_i} + (\alpha_i + a_i)Z_{ij} + \varepsilon_{ij}, \quad (11.38)$$

$$\log \lambda_{Tij}(t_{ij}) = \log \lambda_{0T}(t_{ij}) + m_{T_i} + (\beta_i + b_i)Z_{ij} + \varepsilon_{ij}. \quad (11.39)$$

In this form, it can be seen as a linear mixed-effects model on the log-hazard scale, with a similar structure as model (7.6)–(7.7), originally proposed by Buyse *et al.* (2000a) for the case of normally distributed surrogate and true endpoints. Note that the role of the random effects ε_{ij} is to induce association at the individual level. It is not absolutely necessary that they are normally distributed; any other mean-zero distribution (e.g., log-gamma) might be used.

Model (11.36)–(11.37) is an example of a multivariate frailty model. Multivariate frailty models are a topic of intensive research. The key problem related to their use is the difficulty in fitting them, especially in the semi-parametric proportional hazard setting. Within the frequentist framework, a few successful implementations were formulated using REML estimation (McGilchrist and Aisbett 1991, McGilchrist 1993), the Laplace approximation to the marginal likelihood function (Ripatti and Palmgren 2000), and EM algorithm with either Gibbs sampling (Vaida and Xu 2000, Ripatti, Larsen, and Palmgren 2002) or the Laplace approximation (Cortiñas and Burzykowski 2004) applied in the expectation step. The computational complexity of all the estimating approaches is high, though. In particular, none of them can effectively deal with model (11.36)–(11.37) with individual-level random effects.

Alternatively, the use of the estimation approach developed for the multilevel modeling by Goldstein (1995), could be considered. The methodology can be adapted to the multivariate failure-time setting. An advantage would be the availability of the software (MLwiN). Unfortunately, the estimation methods are also not straightforward and can produce biased results in the presence of censoring (Yang *et al.* 1999). In fact, all attempts to use this methodology in the examples considered in this chapter failed.

It is worth pointing out that, although the structure of model (11.36)–(11.37) offers a natural way to assess the validity of a surrogate at the trial-level, it is much less suitable for the evaluation of the individual-level validity. In fact, when the model is used in a semi-parametric setting (with unspecified baseline hazards), no individual-level measure of association between the surrogate and true endpoints can be constructed. Thus, from a practical point of view, one would use model (11.36)–(11.37) to assess only the trial-level validity of a surrogate.

However, if one is willing to resign from the assessment of the individual-level validity of a surrogate, use of other, simpler modelling approaches become possible. For instance, marginal models fitted using generalized estimating equations might be considered (Wei, Lin, and Weissfeld 1992, Gail *et al.* 2000). An interesting question is whether the use of marginal models (e.g., Cox models with fixed trial-specific treatment effects), fitted separately for each endpoint (i.e., not adjusting for the association between the surrogate and true endpoints at the individual level), might be also a plausible strategy. Simulation results obtained for the case of normally distributed endpoints indicate that such a strategy might actually work (Tibaldi *et al.* 2003). The question was investigated by Cortiñas (2004). In the next section we will shortly summarize results of his research.

11.7 Simplified Modeling Strategies

Just as discussed for the Gaussian case in Section 8.3, Cortiñas (2004) considered the following three modelling strategies, in which the individual level association is ignored.

Marginal Models with Fixed Effects (MFE). A Cox proportional hazards model was fitted separately for each trial and also for each endpoint:

$$\lambda_{Sij}(s_{ij}) = \lambda_{Si}(s_{ij})e^{\alpha_i Z_{ij}}, \tag{11.40}$$

$$\lambda_{Tij}(t_{ij}) = \lambda_{Ti}(t_{ij})e^{\beta_i Z_{ij}}, \tag{11.41}$$

where α_i, and β_i are trial-specific treatment effects. At the second stage the determination coefficient $R^2_{\text{trial(r)}}$ was computed from the regression of $\widehat{\beta}_i$ on $\widehat{\alpha}_i$.

A Stratified PH Model with Random Treatment Effects (SRTE). In this model, stratified baseline hazards were used to account for the between-trial variability in baseline hazards, and trial-specific random treatment effects were assumed:

$$\lambda_{Sij}(s_{ij}) = \lambda_{Si}(s_{ij})e^{(\alpha+a_i)Z_{ij}}, \tag{11.42}$$

$$\lambda_{Tij}(t_{ij}) = \lambda_{Ti}(t_{ij})e^{(\beta+b_i)Z_{ij}}, \tag{11.43}$$

where α and β are fixed treatment effects, while a_i and b_i are trial-specific random effects assumed to be zero-mean normally distributed with variance-covariance matrix

$$\begin{pmatrix} d_{aa} & d_{ab} \\ d_{ab} & d_{bb} \end{pmatrix}. \tag{11.44}$$

The trial-level validity of surrogate S was evaluated using the square of the correlation coefficient based on the estimated covariance matrix (11.44).

TABLE 11.6. *The mean relative bias (in %) for the estimates of $R^2_{trial(r)}$ for the copula approach proposed by Burzykowski* et al. *(2001) and the simplified strategies under no treatment effect ($\alpha = \beta = 0$), for various number of trials N and patients per trial n. In parentheses: the mean model-based and empirical (first and second number, respectively) standard error.*

N	n_i	Copula	MFE	SRTE	RITE
		$\tau = 0.5$, $\rho^2 = R^2_{\text{trial(r)}} = 0.5$			
		No censoring			
10	50	-0.2(0.225;0.228)	-0.5(0.236;0.220)	-3.4(0.226;0.219)	0.6(0.230;0.218)
	100	1.4(0.224;0.226)	-7.6(0.241;0.223)	-1.5(0.212;0.209)	-1.5(0.218;0.214)
	200	1.7(0.225;0.220)	-9.7(0.240;0.226)	-0.3(0.211;0.210)	-0.3(0.214;0.210)
20	50	5.5(0.154;0.164)	-1.0(0.161;0.166)	-2.7(0.169;0.156)	-1.7(0.162;0.157)
	100	2.6(0.158;0.156)	-8.7(0.165;0.169)	-0.6(0.151;0.145)	-0.6(0.149;0.146)
	200	0.9(0.158;0.168)	-12.5(0.167;0.170)	-0.3(0.141;0.135)	-0.2(0.137;0.134)
		Homogeneous censoring 50%/30% (T/S)			
10	50	-12.6(0.228;0.233)	-4.7(0.235;0.235)	-4.9(0.247;0.239)	-4.3(0.256;0.243)
	100	-7.2(0.228;0.235)	-4.1(0.239;0.227)	-3.3(0.229;0.222)	-2.1(0.228;0.221)
	200	-1.9(0.228;0.225)	-10.4(0.240;0.222)	-4.1(0.229;0.223)	-2.6(0.225;0.221)
20	50	-19.1(0.167;0.167)	-4.6(0.164;0.161)	-5.7(0.161;0.154)	-3.7(0.164;0.157)
	100	-9.7(0.163;0.169)	-6.0(0.164;0.166)	-2.9(0.154;0.148)	-1.8(0.151;0.147)
	200	-5.4(0.163;0.162)	-12.1(0.167;0.163)	-2.5(0.147;0.142)	-1.7(0.144;0.141)
		$\tau = 0.9$, $R^2_{\text{trial(r)}} = \rho^2 = 0.9$			
		No censoring			
10	50	0.7(0.065;0.065)	-1.8(0.094;0.085)	2.1(0.091;0.076)	-1.3(0.076;0.064)
	100	-0.7(0.073;0.082)	-1.7(0.092;0.079)	-0.7(0.078;0.068)	-0.7(0.074;0.067)
	200	-0.2(0.071;0.068)	-4.1(0.105;0.086)	-0.6(0.069;0.065)	-0.2(0.073;0.069)
20	50	1.0(0.042;0.045)	-1.1(0.054;0.054)	-0.4(0.056;0.043)	-0.2(0.049;0.044)
	100	0.3(0.045;0.044)	-1.4(0.055;0.049)	-0.7(0.046;0.037)	-0.6(0.043;0.039)
	200	-0.2(0.046;0.049)	-3.4(0.063;0.060)	-0.2(0.041;0.039)	-0.1(0.042;0.039)
		Homogeneous censoring 50%/30% (T/S)			
10	50	-3.1(0.086;0.096)	-10.2(0.139;0.128)	-8.5(0.123;0.106)	-7.9(0.113;0.101)
	100	-1.4(0.077;0.079)	-9.3(0.135;0.120)	-8.6(0.116;0.108)	-7.6(0.111;0.104)
	200	-1.1(0.075;0.086)	-10.5(0.140;0.139)	-8.4(0.140;0.134)	-7.3(0.137;0.133)
20	50	-2.8(0.054;0.089)	-9.6(0.085;0.086)	-8.8(0.083;0.069)	-6.8(0.076;0.068)
	100	-1.0(0.049;0.053)	-9.1(0.084;0.083)	-7.8(0.078;0.070)	-6.4(0.073;0.068)
	200	-1.0(0.049;0.050)	-8.9(0.083;0.080)	-7.3(0.080;0.075)	-6.1(0.079;0.075)

Random Intercepts and Treatment Effects (RITE). In this model, trial-specific random intercepts and treatment effects were specified:

$$\lambda_{Sij}(s_{ij}) = \lambda_{Si}(s_{ij})e^{m_{S_i}+\alpha Z_{ij}+a_i Z_{ij}}, \tag{11.45}$$

$$\lambda_{Tij}(t_{ij}) = \lambda_{Ti}(t_{ij})e^{m_{T_i}+\beta Z_{ij}+b_i Z_{ij}}, \tag{11.46}$$

where $(m_{S_i}, m_{T_i}, a_i, b_i)^T$ is a vector of random effects, assumed to be

TABLE 11.7. *The mean relative bias (in %) for the estimates of* $R^2_{trial(r)}$ *for the copula approach proposed by Burzykowski* et al. *(2001) and the simplified strategies under no treatment effect* ($\alpha = \beta = 0$)*, for various number of trials N and patients per trial n. In parentheses: the mean model-based and empirical (first and second number, respectively) standard error.*

N	n_i	Copula	MFE	SRTE	RITE
		$\tau = 0.5$, $\rho^2 = R^2_{\text{trial(r)}} = 0.9$			
		No censoring			
10	50	-8.5(0.114;0.119)	-30.7(0.211;0.201)	-30.9(0.187;0.179)	-28.1(0.181;0.171)
	100	-4.8(0.096;0.094)	-27.5(0.201;0.186)	-25.4(0.173;0.159)	-23.3(0.168;0.159)
	200	-3.7(0.088;0.105)	-24.4(0.191;0.186)	-17.6(0.122;0.121)	-15.2(0.126;0.119)
20	50	-8.0(0.074;0.078)	-30.3(0.140;0.143)	-31.5(0.135;0.125)	-31.1(0.131;0.125)
	100	-4.8(0.063;0.065)	-27.3(0.133;0.135)	-23.2(0.113;0.105)	-21.7(0.106;0.103)
	200	-2.6(0.055;0.057)	-24.5(0.128;0.120)	-16.1(0.076;0.071)	-14.4(0.074;0.069)
		Homogeneous censoring 50%/30% (T/S)			
10	50	-32.7(0.202;0.206)	-36.9(0.224;0.217)	-36.6(0.215;0.200)	-34.5(0.213;0.202)
	100	-20.8(0.166;0.173)	-31.1(0.213;0.199)	-31.0(0.187;0.178)	-30.7(0.184;0.175)
	200	-12.2(0.131;0.140)	-28.3(0.203;0.191)	-27.3(0.167;0.158)	-25.5(0.162;0.154)
20	50	-33.4(0.141;0.151)	-36.2(0.151;0.148)	-36.4(0.148;0.135)	-34.2(0.140;0.134)
	100	-20.0(0.111;0.107)	-31.0(0.141;0.140)	-30.4(0.122;0.115)	-29.0(0.119;0.114)
	200	-12.4(0.089;0.092)	-28.3(0.136;0.124)	-26.3(0.099;0.093)	-24.6(0.098;0.092)
		$\tau = 0.9$, $\rho^2 = R^2_{\text{trial(r)}} = 0.5$			
		No censoring			
10	50	16.2(0.211;0.209)	71.7(0.110;0.096)	72.8(0.086;0.079)	71.2(0.084;0.071)
	100	6.9(0.225;0.217)	66.7(0.123;0.108)	72.5(0.107;0.089)	71.0(0.096;0.087)
	200	3.9(0.224;0.217)	55.7(0.153;0.125)	60.6(0.091;0.087)	59.4(0.095;0.091)
20	50	10.2(0.150;0.161)	73.0(0.064;0.061)	75.4(0.055;0.047)	73.5(0.055;0.049)
	100	5.3(0.156;0.155)	67.9(0.074;0.068)	68.9(0.059;0.049)	67.8(0.053;0.050)
	200	0.8(0.159;0.153)	57.0(0.095;0.089)	57.1(0.058;0.055)	56.7(0.060;0.057)
		Homogeneous censoring 50%/30% (T/S)			
10	50	16.6(0.209;0.215)	60.8(0.141;0.127)	58.3(0.123;0.106)	55.8(0.116;0.101)
	100	10.5(0.215;0.220)	61.5(0.139;0.125)	57.5(0.126;0.111)	55.2(0.115;0.108)
	200	5.1(0.220;0.225)	56.8(0.150;0.146)	48.9(0.149;0.140)	47.3(0.145;0.139)
20	50	16.1(0.147;0.138)	61.7(0.087;0.084)	60.2(0.081;0.069)	58.4(0.075;0.068)
	100	10.1(0.151;0.156)	61.5(0.088;0.090)	53.6(0.080;0.071)	50.2(0.077;0.071)
	200	4.6(0.156;0.159)	59.9(0.090;0.088)	49.1(0.085;0.079)	44.9(0.084;0.079)

zero-mean normally distributed with variance-covariance matrix

$$D = \begin{pmatrix} d_{SS} & d_{ST} & d_{Sa} & d_{Sb} \\ d_{ST} & d_{TT} & d_{Ta} & d_{Tb} \\ d_{Sa} & d_{Ta} & d_{aa} & d_{ab} \\ d_{Sb} & d_{Sa} & d_{ab} & d_{bb} \end{pmatrix}. \tag{11.47}$$

The association at the trial-level was evaluated using the determination coefficient $R^2_{\text{trial(r)}}$ computed using the estimated components of matrix (11.47).

The models were fitted using SAS PHREG procedure for MFE approach and the EM algorithm with the Laplace approximation at the E-step (Cortiñas and Burzykowski 2004) for the SRTE and RITE approaches. The performance of the simplified strategies was compared with the copula approach developed by Burzykowski *et al.* (2001) in a simulation study. The simulations were conducted using a similar configuration of the parameters as in Burzykowski (2001) (see Section 11.5.1).

The results of the simulations indicated that the presence of a treatment effect did not have much influence on the relative bias of the estimation of $R^2_{\mathrm{trial(r)}}$ for any of the simplified strategies. Tables 11.6 and 11.7 show the simulation results, assuming no treatment effect, for various combinations the number of trials N, number of patients per trial n, individual-level τ and $R^2_{\mathrm{trial(r)}} = \rho^2 = 0.5$. None and moderate (50% censored observations for T, 30% for S) censoring schemes are presented. Note that for the copula approach, the results are based on 500 datasets, while for the simplified strategies they are based on 250 datasets.

A few general conclusions can be drawn. Under censoring, the absolute relative bias is slightly higher as compare to no censoring. For MFE, model-based estimates of the standard error of $R^2_{\mathrm{trial(r)}}$ overestimate the empirical standard errors. The other approaches yield comparable model-based and empirical standard errors of the estimates of $R^2_{\mathrm{trial(r)}}$.

For $\tau = 0.5$ and $\rho^2 = 0.5$ (see Table 11.6), RITE approach yields the smallest absolute relative bias, followed by SRTE approach, whereas the largest bias is observed for MFE approach. Interestingly, for the latter the bias seems to increase with the size of the trial. It can also be noted that the estimators obtained for RITE and SRTE approaches show a similar empirical variability, with the method proposed by Burzykowski *et al.* (2001) and MFE approach expressing a larger variability. For the other settings of (τ, ρ^2), the smallest absolute relative bias is observed in general for the copula approach proposed by Burzykowski *et al.* (2001), while the MFE approach yields estimates with the largest absolute value of relative bias. It is worth noting that the three simplified strategies produce substantially biased estimates of $R^2_{\mathrm{trial(r)}}$ when the association at the individual level (measured by τ) and the association at the trial level (measured by ρ^2) are different (see Table 11.7). In these cases, the copula approach is giving markedly better results. It is interesting to note that for a fixed value of τ, only moderate changes in the magnitude of the variability of the estimates produced by the simplified strategies are observed for different values of ρ^2. This suggests that, when the individual-level association is ignored in the fitting process, the value of τ determines the magnitude of the variability of the estimates.

From the evaluation of the relative bias one can conclude that the use of the simplified strategies does not yield reasonable results. This is in contrast to the case of normally distributed data considered in Section 7.4.2. There may be several reasons for that. For instance, Cortiñas (2004) found that ignoring the individual-level association in the simplified models leads to severe bias in the estimated cumulative baseline hazard functions. This bias can result in distorted estimates of the mean structure parameters and, consequently, in biased estimation of the trial-level association. It may be especially relevant for the MFE approach since, in this method, the strength of the trial-level association is estimated from the estimates of the fixed treatment effects. Also, as reported by Cortiñas *et al.* (2004; see also Chapter 8) ignoring a level when fitting a hierarchical model results affects the estimates of the strength of the association at the higher level. Similar effects can be present in the estimates obtained for STRE and RITE approaches. More investigation is needed to arrive at a more precise explanation of the differences in the relative bias observed in Tables 11.6 and 11.7.

11.8 Discussion

As discussed earlier, from a practical point of view, it is unrealistic to expect perfect surrogacy. Consequently, an application of the method developed by Buyse *et al.* (2000a) requires the specification of a threshold allowing for an assessment of the proximity to 1 of the value of association measures such as Kendall's τ or the coefficients of determination $R^2_{\text{trial(r)}}$ and R^2_{indiv}. On purely theoretical grounds, however, it is difficult to propose such a threshold. Any other choice is necessarily subjective. Preferably, it should be guided by practical experience in using the definition of validity of a surrogate proposed by Buyse *et al.* (2000a). For obvious reasons, such an experience thus far is very limited. Taking the above into account, observed values of $R^2_{\text{trial(r)}}$ around 0.9 have been judged as "sufficiently close to 1," while those around 0.5 as "not close to 1."

One might argue whether the estimates and intervals for $R^2_{\text{trial(r)}}$ presented in Table 11.1 constitute enough evidence to consider progression-free survival a valid surrogate for survival in advanced ovarian cancer. However, even if it is judged insufficient, from Table 11.3 it is clear that for advanced colorectal cancer there is even less evidence. This possibility of assessment of strength of evidence for validity of a surrogate can be seen as an advantage of the method proposed by Buyse *et al.* (2000a).

The method proposed by Burzykowski *et al.* (2001) allows to extend the approach of validation of surrogate endpoints developed by Buyse *et al.*

(2000a) to the case of two failure-time endpoints. It is worth noting that the proposed method can be also used in the case of an uncensored continuous surrogate with an arbitrary marginal distribution (for example, normal). The only necessary adjustment to the developments presented in Section 11.2 would be the choice of the marginal model corresponding to (11.6).

A practical issue related to the use of the copula approach is the need for a relatively complex numerical implementation, for which no standard software exists. From this point of view, the possibility of using a simplified modelling strategy (e.g., marginal Cox models) would be an attractive solution. Unfortunately, the preliminary results obtained by Cortiñas (2004) suggest that, in contrast to the findings of Tibaldi *et al.* (2003), this may not be a valid option. This topic requires certainly more research.

An important limitation of the copula models and, in fact, of all the models mentioned in this chapter, is that the two endpoints are treated symmetrically. In general, this need not be the case, as is clear from the examples analyzed: progression-free survival time cannot be longer than survival time. Obviously, this calls for caution in interpreting the results on the validity of progression-free survival as a surrogate for survival time presented in this chapter. Note, however, that the results presented in Section 11.4 suggest that, at least for the advanced colorectal cancer example, the Hougaard copula might provide a reasonable description of the data. To overcome the problem, it would be of interest to develop an approach allowing for a non-symmetrical treatment of the endpoints, for example using a conditional survival type model (Arnold 1995). Alternatively, the method of estimation of copula models when one of the failure-time variables might be censored by the other, recently proposed by Wang (2003), might be considered. As the method was developed in a one-sample setting, it would need an extension allowing for adjustment for covariates, though.

12

An Ordinal Surrogate for a Survival True Endpoint

Tomasz Burzykowski

12.1 Introduction

In this chapter, we consider the case where the surrogate is an ordinal or binary variable, whereas the true endpoint is a failure time. As the basic paradigm, we will consider the use of the shrinkage of tumor mass, also called a "tumor response," as a surrogate for survival time in cancer research.

The most meaningful and the most objectively measured endpoint used to evaluate new cancer treatments is overall survival time. However, it does require a long observation time and as such may not be optimal for a fast assessment of therapeutic advances. The Food and Drug Administration (FDA) has stated in its recommendations for accelerated approval of investigational cancer treatments, that "for many cancer therapies it is appropriate to utilize objective evidence of tumor shrinkage as a basis for approval, allowing additional evidence of increased survival and/or improved quality of life associated with that therapy to be demonstrated later" (Food and Drug Administration 1996). As a matter of fact, tumor response has long been the cornerstone of the development of cytotoxic therapies for solid tumors, even though the effect of a tumor response upon the patient's survival has often been questioned (Anderson, Cain, and Gelber 1983, Oye and Shapiro 1984, Ellenberg and Hamilton 1989, Buyse and Piedbois 1996, Lohrisch and Piccart 2000).

Due to the widespread use of tumor response to evaluate new cancer treatments, the question about the validity of the use of tumor response as a surrogate for survival did attract some attention. In the attempts to address the issue, different statistical approaches were used. For instance, A'Hern, Ebbs, and Baum (1988) analyzed summary data for 50 published chemotherapy trials in advanced breast cancer. They used a weighted linear regression model to investigate the association between the odds ratio, that summarized the difference in response rates in pairs of arms within the same study, and its corresponding ratio of median survival times. Torri *et al.* (1992) pointed out to several limitations of the model used by A'Hern, Ebbs, and Baum (1988) and proposed to use an "errors in variables" model, aiming at the evaluation of the association between the odds of tumor response and the median survival. They applied the model to summary data from 26 published randomized clinical trials in chemotherapy-treated patients with advanced ovarian cancer. Chen *et al.* (2000) used a Bayesian model to investigate the relationship between response rates and the median survival observed in Phase II studies with the median survival observed in subsequent Phase III studies. They applied the method to summary data for nine pairs of Phase II-Phase III studies in extensive-stage small-cell lung cancer.

It is interesting to note that all the aforementioned attempts to address the issue of the validity of tumor response as a surrogate for survival in cancer clinical trials used meta-analytic data. Unfortunately, they all suffered from various drawbacks. For instance, they all used summary data from published studies. Consequently, they were subject to publication bias. More importantly, however, they did not explicitly focus on the precision of the prediction of the treatment effect on the true endpoint (survival) from the effect on the surrogate (tumor response). As argued in Chapters 7 and 9, the precision of the prediction is the key issue in the assessment of the validity of a surrogate endpoint.

In this chapter, therefore, we will describe an approach that addresses this key issue. In particular, we will review an extension of the meta-analytic approach of Buyse *et al.* (2000a) (see also Chapter 7) developed by Burzykowski, Molenberghs, and Buyse (2004). This extension builds upon the developments by Molenberghs, Geys, and Buyse (2001) and uses the copula models described in Chapter 11. It has been used to study the validity of tumor response as a surrogate for survival in assessing the benefits of various treatment regimens for advanced colorectal cancer (Buyse *et al.* 2000b, Burzykowski, Molenberghs, and Buyse 2004). For this purpose, the data from four meta-analyses of advanced colorectal cancer trials (Section 4.2.4) were used.

12.2 A Meta-analytic Approach: The Two-stage Model

Assume that the true endpoint T is a failure-time random variable and the surrogate S is a categorical variable with K ordered categories, i.e., an ordinal variable (Agresti 1990). For each of $j = 1, \ldots, n_i$ patients from trial i $(i = 1, \ldots, N)$ we thus have quadruplets $(X_{ij}, \Delta_{ij}, S_{ij}, Z_{ij})$, where X_{ij} is a possibly censored version of survival time T_{ij} and Δ_{ij} is the censoring indicator assuming value of 1 for observed failures and 0 otherwise.

To extend the approach proposed by Buyse *et al.* (2000a) to the aforementioned setting, Burzykowski, Molenberghs, and Buyse (2004) proposed to replace the first-stage model (7.1)–(7.2) by a bivariate copula model (Genest and McKay 1986, Shih and Louis 1995a, Joe 1997, Nelsen 1999) for the true endpoint T_{ij} and a latent continuous variable $\tilde{S}_{ij}$ underlying the surrogate endpoint S_{ij}. Specifically, to model S_{ij} they proposed the proportional odds model:

$$\text{logit}\{P(S_{ij} \leq k \mid Z_{ij})\} = \gamma_{ik} + \alpha_i Z_{ij}. \tag{12.1}$$

The model be interpreted as assuming a logistic distribution for the latent variable $\tilde{S}_{ij}$. The value of the marginal cumulative distribution function of $\tilde{S}_{ij}$, given $Z_{ij} = z$, will be denoted by $F_{\tilde{S}_{ij}}(s; z)$. Note that, in the case of a binary surrogate S_{ij}, model (12.1) is equivalent to logistic regression model.

It is worth noting that estimation of model (12.1) requires that in each trial all response levels are observed. In practice, it often happens that in some trials not all levels are observed. To adapt model (12.1) for such a case, it can be rewritten as follows:

$$\text{logit}\{P(S_{ij} \leq k \mid Z_{ij})\} = \eta_k^0 + \eta_i + \eta_{ik} + \alpha_i Z_{ij}, \tag{12.2}$$

where, for identifiability purposes, one might specify that, for example,

$$\eta_1 = \eta_{11} = \ldots = \eta_{1,K-1} = 0.$$

If, for a particular trial, i_0 say, not all levels of S are observed, one might use model (12.2) with the terms $\eta_{i_0 1}, \ldots, \eta_{i_0, K-1}$ constrained to 0. As a special case, the following model might be considered:

$$\text{logit}\{P(S_{ij} \leq k \mid Z_{ij})\} = \eta_k^0 + \eta_i + \alpha_i Z_{ij}. \tag{12.3}$$

The model assumes a fixed set of cutpoints $\eta_1^0, \ldots, \eta_{K-1}^0$, but allows for trial-specific shifts η_i of the set.

To model the effect of treatment Z_{ij} on the marginal distribution of T_{ij}, Burzykowski, Molenberghs, and Buyse (2004) proposed to use the proportional hazard model:

$$\lambda_{ij}(t \mid Z_{ij}) = \lambda_i(t) \exp(\beta_i Z_{ij}), \tag{12.4}$$

where β_i are trial-specific effects of treatment Z and $\lambda_i(t)$ is a trial-specific baseline hazard function. The marginal cumulative distribution function of T_{ij}, following model (12.4) with $Z_{ij} = z$, will be denoted by $F_{T_{ij}}(t; z)$.

To specify fully a bivariate model corresponding to (7.1)–(7.2), it is assumed that the joint cumulative distribution of T_{ij} and $\tilde{S}_{ij}$, given $Z_{ij} = z$, is generated by a one-parameter copula function C_θ:

$$F_{T_{ij},\tilde{S}_{ij}}(t, s; z) = C_\theta[F_{T_{ij}}(t; z), F_{\tilde{S}_{ij}}(s; z), \theta]. \tag{12.5}$$

C_θ is a distribution function on $[0,1]^2$ with $\theta \in I\!R^1$ (Genest and McKay 1986, Shih and Louis 1995a, Nelsen 1999), describing the association between $\tilde{S}_{ij}$ and T_{ij}. An attractive feature of model (12.5) is that the marginal models (the proportional odds and proportional hazards models in our particular case) and the association model can be selected without constraining each other.

Using the joint distribution function (12.5), with proportional hazard model (12.4) and proportional odds model (12.1) (or a suitable modification) as marginal models, it is possible to construct the likelihood function for the observed data $(X_{ij} = x_{ij}, \Delta_{ij} = \delta_{ij}, S_{ij} = s_{ij}, Z_{ij} = z_{ij})$. Namely, the bivariate density $g_{ij}(t, k; z)$ for T_{ij} and S_{ij}, given $Z_{ij} = z$, can be specified by taking

$$g_{ij}(t, k; z) = \frac{\partial F_{T_{ij},\tilde{S}_{ij}}(t, \gamma_{ik}; z)}{\partial t} - \frac{\partial F_{T_{ij},\tilde{S}_{ij}}(t, \gamma_{i(k-1)}; z)}{\partial t}.$$

Consequently, one can define

$$\begin{aligned} G_{ij}(t, k; z) &\equiv P(T_{ij} \geq t, S_{ij} = k \mid Z_{ij} = z) \\ &= [F_{\tilde{S}_{ij}}(\gamma_{ik}; z) - F_{\tilde{S}_{ij}}(\gamma_{i(k-1)}; z)] \\ &\quad -[F_{T_{ij},\tilde{S}_{ij}}(t, \gamma_{ik}; z) - F_{T_{ij},\tilde{S}_{ij}}(t, \gamma_{i(k-1)}; z)]. \end{aligned}$$

As a result, for the observed data $(X_{ij} = x_{ij}, \Delta_{ij} = \delta_{ij}, S_{ij} = s_{ij}, Z_{ij} = z_{ij})$, the log-likelihood can be expressed as:

$$\sum_{i,j} [\delta_{ij} \log g_{ij}(x_{ij}, s_{ij}; z_{ij}) + (1 - \delta_{ij}) \log G_{ij}(x_{ij}, s_{ij}; z_{ij})]. \tag{12.6}$$

At the first stage, Burzykowski, Molenberghs, and Buyse (2004) proposed to use the likelihood function to obtain an estimate of θ and estimates of trial-specific treatment effects α_i and β_i on the surrogate and the true endpoint, respectively. At the second stage, they suggested to use the trial-level model:

$$\begin{pmatrix} \eta_i \\ \alpha_i \\ \beta_i \end{pmatrix} = \begin{pmatrix} \eta \\ \alpha \\ \beta \end{pmatrix} + \begin{pmatrix} e_i \\ a_i \\ b_i \end{pmatrix}, \tag{12.7}$$

with η_i obtained from models (12.2) or (12.3). The second term on the right-hand side of (12.7) is assumed to follow a zero-mean normal distribution with dispersion matrix

$$D = \begin{pmatrix} d_{ee} & d_{ea} & d_{eb} \\ & d_{aa} & d_{ab} \\ & & d_{bb} \end{pmatrix}.$$

The quality of surrogate S at the trial level can be assessed based on the coefficient of determination:

$$R^2_{\text{trial}(\alpha,\,\eta)} = \frac{\begin{pmatrix} d_{eb} \\ d_{ab} \end{pmatrix}^T \begin{pmatrix} d_{ee} & d_{ea} \\ d_{ea} & d_{aa} \end{pmatrix}^{-1} \begin{pmatrix} d_{eb} \\ d_{ab} \end{pmatrix}}{d_{bb}}. \tag{12.8}$$

The index "trial(α, η)" in $R^2_{\text{trial}(\alpha,\,\eta)}$ indicates that the coefficient pertains to the distribution of β_i conditional on the set of trial-specific parameters including α_i and η_i.

In principle, if the unrestricted marginal model (12.1) is used at the first stage, one might consider taking into account the information about the cutpoints $\gamma_{i1}, \ldots, \gamma_{i(K-1)}$. A simple solution would be to replace η_i in (12.7) with vector $(\gamma_{i1}, \ldots, \gamma_{i(K-1)})^T$. From a formal point of view, however, in this case the assumption of normality would have to be modified to reflect the ordering of γ_{ij}'s.

Alternatively, if the information in the cutpoints can be ignored, the use of a simple linear regression model could be considered:

$$\begin{pmatrix} \alpha_i \\ \beta_i \end{pmatrix} = \begin{pmatrix} \alpha \\ \beta \end{pmatrix} + \begin{pmatrix} a_i \\ b_i \end{pmatrix} \tag{12.9}$$

with dispersion matrix

$$D_\alpha = \begin{pmatrix} d_{aa} & d_{ab} \\ & d_{bb} \end{pmatrix}. \tag{12.10}$$

In that case coefficient of determination $R^2_{\text{trial}(\alpha,\,\eta)}$ reduces to

$$R^2_{\text{trial}(\alpha)} = \frac{d^2_{ab}}{d_{aa} d_{bb}}, \tag{12.11}$$

the square of the correlation between α_i and β_i. It can be noted here that, using (12.8) and (12.11), one can write

$$\begin{aligned} R^2_{\text{trial}(\alpha,\,\eta)} &= \frac{R^2_{\text{trial}(\alpha)}}{1 - \text{Corr}^2(\eta_i, \alpha_i)} \\ &\quad + \text{Corr}(\eta_i, \beta_i) \frac{\text{Corr}(\eta_i, \beta_i) - 2\text{Corr}(\alpha_i, \beta_i)\text{Corr}(\eta_i, \alpha_i)}{1 - \text{Corr}^2(\eta_i, \alpha_i)}. \end{aligned} \tag{12.12}$$

It follows that, formally, $R^2_{\mathtt{trial}(\alpha,\,\eta)} = R^2_{\mathtt{trial}(\alpha)}$ if

$$\mathrm{Corr}(\eta_i, \alpha_i) = \mathrm{Corr}(\eta_i, \beta_i) = 0.$$

To use $R^2_{\mathtt{trial}(\alpha)}$ and model (12.9) instead of $R^2_{\mathtt{trial}(\alpha,\,\eta)}$ and (12.7), one would thus require that treatment effects on true and surrogate endpoints should be uncorrelated with the baseline distribution (for $Z = 0$) of S. The use of $R^2_{\mathtt{trial}(\alpha)}$ might give different results than the use of $R^2_{\mathtt{trial}(\alpha,\,\eta)}$, e.g., in the presence of treatment/surrogate interaction.

To assess the quality at the individual level, a measure of association between S_{ij} and T_{ij} is needed. A natural candidate is θ, as its value modifies the form of the copula function and, consequently, influences the strength of the association between $\tilde{S}_{ij}$ and T_{ij}. A drawback of θ is that, for different copula functions, it may assume values from different domains. To overcome this difficulty, the use of Kendall's τ or Spearman's ρ may be considered (Burzykowski *et al.* 2001; see also Section 11.2). Both measures are transformations of θ and can be interpreted similarly to a correlation coefficient, irrespective of the copula function (Nelsen 1999). Alternatively, it may be possible to choose a copula such that θ has got a meaningful interpretation. This option will be discussed next.

In principle, different copula functions can be used for the bivariate distribution (12.5). Burzykowski, Molenberghs, and Buyse (2004) proposed to use the bivariate Plackett copula (Plackett 1965, Mardia 1970, Dale 1986, Nelsen 1999). This particular choice was motivated by the fact that, for the Plackett copula, the association parameter θ takes the form of a (constant) global odds ratio. Specifically, in the current setting (for $k = 1, \ldots, K-1$ and $t > 0$):

$$\begin{aligned} \theta &= \frac{P(T_{ij} > t,\, S_{ij} > k)\, P(T_{ij} \le t,\, S_{ij} \le k)}{P(T_{ij} > t,\, S_{ij} \le k)\, P(T_{ij} \le t,\, S_{ij} > k)} \\ &= \frac{P(T_{ij} > t \mid S_{ij} > k)}{P(T_{ij} \le t \mid S_{ij} > k)} \left\{ \frac{P(T_{ij} > t \mid S_{ij} \le k)}{P(T_{ij} \le t \mid S_{ij} \le k)} \right\}^{-1}. \end{aligned} \tag{12.13}$$

Thus, θ is naturally interpreted as the (constant) ratio of the odds for surviving beyond time t given response higher than k to the odds of surviving beyond time t given response at most k. For a binary surrogate, it is just the odds ratio for responders versus non-responders (assuming $k = 2$ indicates response).

12.3 Analysis of Case Study

The two-stage approach described in the previous section was applied to the advanced colorectal cancer data, introduced in Section 4.2.4 and analyzed before (Buyse *et al.* 2000c, Burzykowski, Molenberghs, and Buyse 2004). Four-category tumor response is considered as a potential surrogate for survival time. It is contrasted with a binary version.

12.3.1 Descriptive Analysis

The data came from the four meta-analyses of 28 advanced colorectal cancer trials introduced in Section 4.2.4. Several of the 28 trials were multi-armed. In total, 33 randomized comparisons were considered in the four meta-analyses. Individual-patient data were available for 27 of the comparisons (in 24 studies). From now on, we will refer to each of the comparison as a separate "trial."

Table 12.1 presents summary data for the trials included in the analysis. In particular, for each trial and each treatment arm the table contains the median survival time (in months) and the distribution of the four tumor response categories: complete response (CR), partial response (PR), stable disease (SD), and progressive disease (PD) (World Health Organization 1979). Also, the observed percentage for the binary response (CR+PR) is given. The first column of Table 12.1 contains the labels used to identify the trials in the papers by the Advanced Colorectal Cancer Meta-Analysis Project (1992, 1994) and Meta-Analysis Group In Cancer (1996, 1998) describing the four meta-analyses; we refer to these papers for additional details regarding the original publications of results of the trials.

From Table 12.1 it can be seen that the trials varied quite considerably in sample size. The total size ranged from 15 ("City of Hope, HAI *versus* ST") to 382 ("GITSG") patients. The last two rows of the table indicate that, overall, CR was rarely observed. Nevertheless, CR and PR were observed more frequently for experimental FU (3.2% and 19.2%, respectively) than for FU bolus (2.1% and 9.6%, respectively). Consequently, the response rate, i.e., the combined percentage of CR and PR, was higher for experimental FU (22.4% *versus* 11.7% for FU bolus). This conclusion applies also to all but three ("NCOG", "GOIRC", "RPCI, 5FU+M") individual trials. Similarly, the median survival time was slightly longer for experimental FU (9.8 months) than for FU bolus (8.9 months). This pattern can be consistently seen for all but eight individual trials.

Table 12.2 presents estimates of odds for binary response (CR+PR *versus*

TABLE 12.1. *Meta-analyses in advanced colorectal cancer. Summary data for 27 analyzed trials.*

Trial	Treatment	*N*	Tumor response (%)					Median
			CR	PR	SD	PD	(CR+PR)	survival
Advanced Colorectal Cancer Meta-Analysis Project (1992)								
GITSG	5FU+L	269	1.5	20.1	0.0	78.4	21.6	11.3
	ST	113	0.0	10.6	0.0	89.4	10.6	10.7
NCOG	5FU+L	107	5.6	12.1	62.6	19.6	17.7	10.5
	ST	55	9.1	9.1	65.4	16.4	18.2	11.4
GOIRC	5FU+L	91	3.3	9.9	36.3	50.5	13.2	12.4
	ST	90	6.7	8.9	31.1	53.3	15.6	14.5
GISCAD	5FU+L	91	5.5	15.4	31.9	47.2	19.9	13.0
	ST	89	3.4	6.7	31.5	58.4	10.1	13.0
Genova	5FU+L	75	6.7	14.7	36.0	42.7	21.4	11.0
	ST	73	2.7	5.5	52.0	39.7	8.2	11.0
Toronto	5FU+L	66	0.0	31.8	0.0	68.2	31.8	12.0
	ST	64	0.0	6.2	0.0	93.7	6.2	9.6
City of Hope	5FU+L	39	2.6	35.9	35.9	25.6	38.7	14.2
	ST	40	0.0	12.5	47.5	40.0	12.5	12.7
RPCI	5FU+L	30	3.3	36.7	23.3	36.7	40.2	11.0
	ST	23	0.0	8.7	4.3	87.0	8.7	11.1
Bologna	5FU+L	34	0.0	26.5	32.3	41.2	26.5	10.1
	ST	30	0.0	3.3	56.7	40.0	3.3	7.5
Advanced Colorectal Cancer Meta-Analysis Project (1994)								
EORTC	5FU+M	152	2.6	15.1	38.2	44.1	17.7	12.1
	ST	154	2.6	9.1	31.2	57.1	11.7	8.9
RPCI	5FU+M	23	0.0	4.3	13.0	82.6	4.3	10.3
	ST	23	0.0	8.7	4.3	87.0	8.7	11.1
NGTAG	5FU+M+L	122	2.5	13.9	39.3	44.3	16.4	8.1
	ST	127	0.0	2.4	43.4	54.3	2.4	6.0
AIO	5FU+M+L	86	4.6	18.6	33.7	43.0	23.2	10.7
	ST	78	2.6	14.1	46.1	37.2	16.7	13.7
NCOG	5FU+M+L	103	5.8	12.6	65.0	16.5	18.4	12.3
	ST	55	9.1	9.1	65.4	16.4	18.2	11.4
GOCS	5FU+M+L	64	1.6	25.0	32.8	40.6	26.6	11.9
	ST	61	0.0	11.5	22.9	65.6	11.5	8.9
Mar del Plata	5FU+M+L	28	3.6	14.3	7.1	75.0	17.9	0.7
	ST	33	0.0	0.0	57.6	42.4	0.0	1.0
Spain	5FU+M+L	26	3.8	19.2	53.8	23.1	23.0	13.2
	ST	33	3.0	12.1	51.5	33.3	15.1	8.6
Meta-Analysis Group In Cancer (1996)								
MSKCC	HAI	43	0.0	48.8	37.2	13.9	48.8	18.3
	ST	48	0.0	16.7	33.3	50.0	16.7	14.5
NCCTG	HAI	39	2.6	38.5	33.3	25.6	41.1	12.8
	ST	35	0.0	17.1	57.1	25.7	17.1	11.0
NCI	HAI	32	3.1	37.5	3.1	56.2	40.6	16.9
	ST	32	3.1	12.5	0.0	84.4	15.6	11.6
City of Hope	HAI	9	0.0	77.8	0.0	22.2	77.8	22.9
	ST	6	0.0	50.0	0.0	50.0	50.0	23.0
Meta-Analysis Group In Cancer (1998)								
SWOG	CII	174	2.9	10.3	19.5	67.2	13.2	15.0
	ST	182	2.7	9.9	30.2	57.1	12.6	13.9
ECOG	CII	162	4.9	22.8	8.6	63.6	27.7	13.0
	ST	162	3.1	14.2	5.6	77.2	17.3	10.5
NCIC	CII	95	1.0	10.5	36.8	51.6	11.5	10.1
	ST	90	1.1	5.6	32.2	61.1	6.7	9.3
France	CII	77	3.9	22.1	41.6	32.5	26.0	8.5
	ST	78	0.0	12.8	39.7	47.4	12.8	9.8
MAOP	CII	88	4.5	25.0	69.3	1.1	29.5	10.6
	ST	85	0.0	9.4	89.4	1.2	9.4	11.2
Jerusalem	CII	11	0.0	9.1	18.2	72.7	9.1	8.6
	ST	15	0.0	6.7	60.0	33.3	6.7	12.0
Total	EX	2136	3.2	19.2	29.9	47.7	22.4	9.8
	ST	1874	2.1	9.6	34.1	54.2	11.7	8.9

NOTE: ST - control treatment (bolus 5FU/FUDR); EX - experimental treatment (M - methotrexate; L - leucovorin; HAI - FUDR by hepatic arterial infusion; CII - 5FU by continuous intravenous infusion). N - sample size. Median survival time (in months) estimated from the Kaplan-Meier survival curve.

TABLE 12.2. *Meta-analyses in advanced colorectal cancer. Summary results for binary tumor response and survival for 27 analyzed trials.*

Trial	Odds ratio [95% C.I.]	Hazard ratio [95% C.I.]
Advanced Colorectal Cancer Meta-Analysis Project (1992)		
GITSG	2.31 [1.19, 4.50]	0.88 [0.70, 1.12]
NCOG	0.97 [0.42, 2.26]	1.22 [0.86, 1.72]
GOIRC	0.82 [0.36, 1.90]	1.23 [0.88, 1.72]
GISCAD	2.34 [1.00, 5.51]	1.09 [0.76, 1.56]
Genova	3.03 [1.11, 8.24]	0.90 [0.65, 1.25]
Toronto	7.00 [2.24, 21.82]	0.78 [0.54, 1.13]
City of Hope	4.37 [1.40, 13.65]	0.78 [0.50, 1.23]
RPCI	7.00 [1.38, 35.51]	1.13 [0.65, 1.98]
Bologna	10.44 [1.23, 88.21]	0.74 [0.43, 1.28]
Advanced Colorectal Cancer Meta-Analysis Project (1994)		
EORTC	1.63 [0.86, 3.11]	0.79 [0.62, 1.02]
RPCI	0.48 [0.04, 5.66]	1.28 [0.71, 2.30]
NGTAG	8.10 [2.34, 28.05]	0.76 [0.59, 0.98]
AIO	1.51 [0.70, 3.30]	1.03 [0.75, 1.40]
NCOG	1.02 [0.44, 2.37]	0.89 [0.63, 1.26]
GOCS	2.79 [1.06, 7.31]	0.78 [0.54, 1.12]
Mar del Plata	15.68 [0.83, 297.4]*	0.98 [0.58, 1.67]
Spain	1.68 [0.45, 6.28]	1.17 [0.62, 2.24]
Meta-Analysis Group In Cancer (1996)		
MSKCC	4.77 [1.81, 12.54]	0.77 [0.51, 1.17]
NCCTG	3.36 [1.13, 9.96]	0.95 [0.60, 1.50]
NCI	3.69 [1.13, 12.10]	0.81 [0.46, 1.40]
City of Hope	3.50 [0.37, 32.97]	0.91 [0.31, 2.66]
Meta-Analysis Group In Cancer (1998)		
SWOG	1.05 [0.57, 1.96]	0.93 [0.75, 1.15]
ECOG	1.84 [1.08, 3.14]	0.89 [0.71, 1.12]
NCIC	1.83 [0.65, 5.18]	0.80 [0.59, 1.07]
France	2.39 [1.03, 5.51]	0.86 [0.62, 1.19]
MAOP	4.04 [1.71, 9.54]	0.83 [0.58, 1.20]
Jerusalem	1.40 [0.08, 25.14]	1.29 [0.57, 2.91]
Overall	2.19 [1.84, 2.61]	0.90 [0.84, 0.96]

NOTE: Observed odds ratios for response for experimental FU versus *5FU bolus, with 95% confidence intervals (C.I.) based on the Mantel-Haenszel test (* - using Gart's (1966) logit estimate with 0.5 correction for zero cells). Hazard ratios for experimental FU* versus *5FU bolus estimated using a proportional hazard model, with 95% confidence intervals based on Wald's test. Overall odds ratio estimated using trial-adjusted Mantel-Haenszel estimator. Overall hazard ratio estimated using a trial-stratified proportional hazard model.*

SD+PD) and relative mortality hazard for experimental FU *versus* FU bolus. Overall, the odds were approximately double for the experimental treatment, with a simultaneous 10% reduction of the risk of death.

Figure 4.5 in Chapter 4 shows survival curves by treatment within tumor response categories. As it has been mentioned in Section 4.2.4 of Chapter 4, there is no statistically significant difference between experimental FU and bolus FU in any tumor response category, which confirms that the overall survival benefit in favor of experimental FU is due to the higher tumor response rates obtained with experimental FU as compared to bolus FU. This observation suggests that tumor response might be a valid surrogate for survival according to Prentice's definition (1989).

In what follows, the true endpoint T is survival time, defined as the time from randomization to death from any cause. In the analyzed set of data, most patients have died (3591 out of 4010 patients, i.e., 89.5%). The surrogate endpoint S is tumor response, defined either as a binary variable with $S = 2$ for CR or PR and $S = 1$ for SD or PD, or as a categorical variable with $S = 4, 3, 2, 1$ for CR, PR, SD and PD, respectively. The binary indicator for treatment (Z) is set to 0 for FU bolus and to 1 for experimental FU.

12.3.2 Analysis of Four-category Tumor Response

The bivariate model (12.5) was defined using the Plackett copula. For survival, proportional hazards model (12.4) was used, with Weibull trial-specific baseline hazard functions. tumor response was modeled using a constrained version of proportional odds model (12.2). More specifically, for those trials, for which not all levels of tumor response were observed (see Table 12.1), all coefficients η_{ik} were constrained to zero.

Under these assumptions, the likelihood function for the observed data. given in equation (12.6), is fully specified. Maximum likelihood parameter estimates can be obtained using the Newton-Raphson algorithm. In the example analyzed, the algorithm with numerical second order derivatives, as implemented in SAS-IML 6.12 (and higher versions) in the form of a standard routine NLPNRR (SAS Institute Inc. 1995), was used (Burzykowski, Molenberghs, and Buyse 2004).

It should be noted that θ, as defined by (12.13), involves comparison of survival times of patients classified according to tumor response. It is well known that such a comparison is likely to be length-biased, because response to treatment is not observed instantaneously. As a result, patients who enjoy long survival times are more likely to be responders than non-

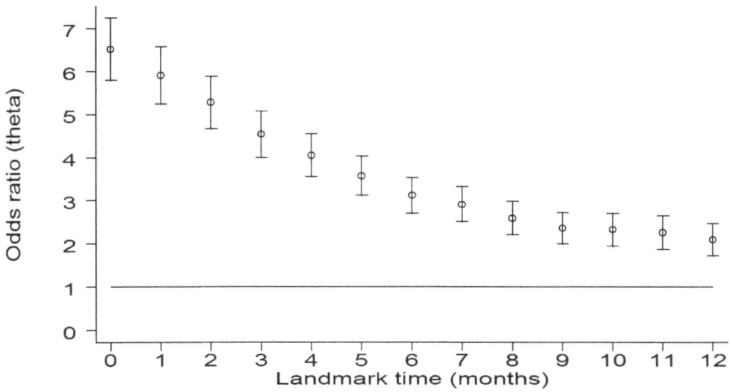

FIGURE 12.1. *Meta-analyses in advanced colorectal cancer. Estimated individual-level association parameter (θ), with 95% confidence interval limits, by landmark time.*

responders, and therefore the survival of responders is likely to be biased upwards compared to that of non-responders.

There are several methods that can be used to correct for length bias in such a comparison. One of them is a landmark analysis (Anderson *et al.* 1983). In a landmark analysis, only patients alive at an arbitrary, pre-specified, landmark time are considered, and their response status is assessed at the landmark time. In this way, response is no longer time-dependent, and no bias affects the comparison of responders and non-responders.

To use any of the methods correcting for length bias, information on the time to response has to be available for individual patients. As no such information was available in the advanced colorectal cancer data analyzed, Burzykowski, Molenberghs, and Buyse (2004) used an approximate solution, which consisted of excluding patients dying before the landmark time and assuming that all recorded responses had occurred before the landmark. By way of a sensitivity analysis, they conducted the analysis based on the bivariate model (12.1)–(12.5) for landmark times ranging from 0 (no correction) to 6 months. Of highest interest, however, is the range between 3 and 6 months. This is because tumor response is usually assessed 3 to 6 months after the beginning of chemotherapy. In fact, this was the case for most of the trials analyzed, for which information on the response assessment scheme could be obtained from the original publication of results.

Figure 12.1 shows a plot of estimates of θ for different landmark times up to 12 months for the four-category tumor response. Here, the zero value corresponds to the analysis without any correction for length bias. As expected, the estimates decrease, approaching a value of 2 around 10–12 months. The dependence of θ on the landmark time clearly illustrates the need for length-bias correction. It should be underscored that this need is not due to the particular choice of the method of analysis, but rather to the nature of the endpoints considered. In fact, a correction for length-bias would most likely have to be considered in any analysis of the validity of tumor response as a surrogate for survival.

Importantly, lower 95% confidence limits for θ at all landmark times in Figure 12.1 are greater than 1.7. It might therefore be concluded that length bias, if any, does not induce an association, but rather affects the magnitude of an existing one. Moreover, as already mentioned, the landmark times between 3 and 6 months are of the most interest. For these time points, estimates of θ remain between 3 and 4.6, with lower 95% C.I. limits above 2.5. They indicate that the odds for surviving beyond time t for, e.g., responders (partial or complete) were at least 2.5 times higher than the odds for non-responders (patients with a stable or progressive disease). This suggests that, even after taking into account possible length bias, there remains a considerable association between tumor response and survival time at the level of individual.

The upper part of Table 12.3 ("without adjustment for PS") presents estimates of θ, $R^2_{\text{trial}(\alpha,\,\eta)}$ and $R^2_{\text{trial}(\alpha)}$ for the analysis with no adjustment for length bias (landmark 0) and for landmark times between 3 and 6 months. The estimates of $R^2_{\text{trial}(\alpha,\,\eta)}$ and $R^2_{\text{trial}(\alpha)}$ were obtained using models (12.7) and (12.9), respectively. The 95% confidence intervals for $R^2_{\text{trial}(\alpha,\,\eta)}$ and $R^2_{\text{trial}(\alpha)}$ were obtained by finding such values of these parameters, for which the corresponding estimates were equal to 2.5% and 97.5% quantiles of the cumulative distribution function of R^2 (Fisher 1928, Algina 1999). The distribution function was computed using the algorithm proposed by Ding (1996).

The estimates of $R^2_{\text{trial}(\alpha,\,\eta)}$ presented in the upper part of Table 12.3 are only slightly higher than those of $R^2_{\text{trial}(\alpha)}$. Thus, one might conclude that not much would be gained in the precision of the prediction if instead of the model (12.9), the more complex model (12.7) were used to predict the treatment effect on survival.

Overall, the estimates are low and do not exceed 20%. The weak association between the estimated trial-specific treatment effects for survival and tumor response can be observed in Figure 12.2, which presents the plot of the effects for the analysis using the landmark time of 3 months. The size of each point is proportional to the number of patients in the corresponding trial. The straight line presents predictions from model (12.9). The estimated slope of the regression line is equal to 0.12 (standard error 0.06). (Note that, according to the parameterization used in model (12.1)–(12.5), $\beta_i > 0$

TABLE 12.3. *Meta-analyses in advanced colorectal cancer. Four-category tumor response: individual-level association (θ) and trial-level association (R^2), for different landmark times (in months).*

	Individual-level	Trial-level			
Time	θ	$R^2_{\text{trial}(\alpha,\,\eta)}$	$R^2_{\text{trial}(\alpha)}$	HAS	F
		Without adjustment for PS			
0	6.78 [6.01, 7.55]	0.16 [0, 0.42]	0.16 [0, 0.42]	⋆	⋆
3	4.59 [4.04, 5.15]	0.15 [0, 0.41]	0.15 [0, 0.41]	0.59 [−0.16, 1.35]	0.54
4	4.07 [3.56, 4.57]	0.10 [0, 0.34]	0.10 [0, 0.34]	0.53 [−0.34, 1.40]	0.35
5	3.56 [3.10, 4.03]	0.06 [0, 0.28]	0.05 [0, 0.26]	0.36 [−0.69, 1.41]	0.10
6	3.09 [2.67, 3.51]	0.08 [0, 0.31]	0.06 [0, 0.28]	0.44 [−0.44, 1.33]	0.08
		With adjustment for PS			
0	6.50 [5.75, 7.25]	0.22 [0, 0.49]	0.20 [0, 0.49]	0.19 [−0.49, 0.87]	0.40
3	4.52 [3.96, 5.07]	0.16 [0, 0.42]	0.16 [0, 0.45]	0.39 [−0.22, 1.01]	0.32
4	4.00 [3.49, 4.51]	0.11 [0, 0.35]	0.11 [0, 0.39]	0.34 [−0.30, 0.99]	0.21
5	3.50 [3.04, 3.96]	0.07 [0, 0.29]	0.06 [0, 0.32]	0.17 [−0.41, 0.77]	0.06
6	3.03 [2.62, 3.45]	0.08 [0, 0.31]	0.06 [0, 0.33]	0.27 [−0.35, 0.90]	0.06

NOTE: HAS, adjusted estimates of $R^2_{trial(\alpha)}$ based on the approach by van Houwelingen, Arends, and Stijnen (2002) (see Chapter 11, Section 11.2.1); F, adjusted estimates of $R^2_{trial(\alpha)}$ using the adjusted weighted estimator of γ given by (11.24)–(11.25). In the cases marked by ⋆, the estimates could not be obtained due to numerical problems. 95% confidence intervals in brackets (not available for F).

and $\alpha_i > 0$ indicate increases in the hazard of death and in the odds of non-response, respectively, for the experimental treatment.) The line passes very close to the origin. In fact, the estimated intercept is equal to -0.02 (standard error 0.06) and is not significantly different from zero. This suggests a simple multiplicative association between treatment effects for survival and tumor response. Daniels and Hughes (1997) consider this as one of the conditions for a good surrogate. Buyse and Molenberghs (1998) require it for prediction based on relative effect RE estimated from a single trial.

Based on the estimates of $R^2_{\text{trial}(\alpha,\,\eta)}$ and $R^2_{\text{trial}(\alpha)}$ from the upper part of Table 12.3, Burzykowski, Molenberghs, and Buyse (2004) suggested that four-category tumor response is a weak surrogate for survival at the trial level, in that it does not permit to reliably predict treatment effects on survival. On the other hand, by considering the estimates of θ, they concluded in favor of a strong association between tumor response and survival time for individual patients, after adjusting for treatment effects.

However, as argued in Section 11.2.1, the estimates of $R^2_{\text{trial}(\alpha,\,\eta)}$ and $R^2_{\text{trial}(\alpha)}$ presented in Table 12.3, are likely biased, as they ignore the error due to the use of the estimated treatment effects. Therefore, the last two columns

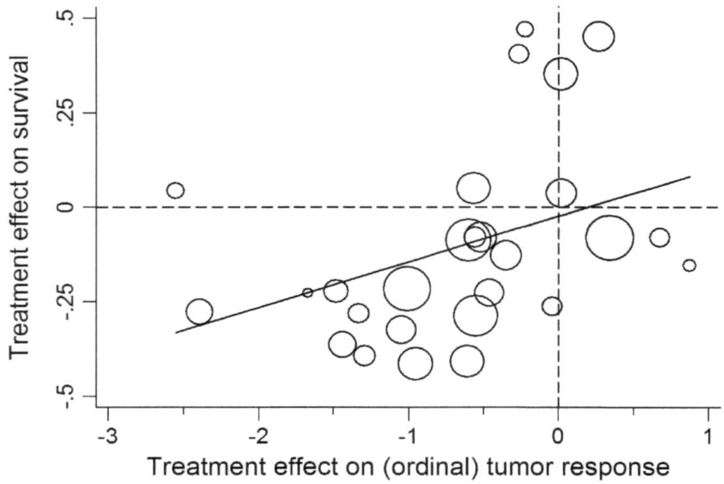

FIGURE 12.2. *Meta-analyses in advanced colorectal cancer. Estimated trial-specific treatment effects on survival versus treatment effects on four-category tumor response.*

of Table 12.3 (marked as "HAS" and "F") contain the estimates of $R^2_{\text{trial}(\alpha)}$ adjusted for the estimation error using the approach of van Houwelingen, Arends, and Stijnen (2002) and using the measurement error models developed by Fuller (1987). The confidence intervals for HAS estimates were obtained as HAS $\pm$ 2SE, where SE was the standard error computed by the delta method from the standard errors of the variance components involved in $R^2_{\text{trial}(\alpha)}$ (see equation (12.11)).

One can see that the estimates adjusted for the estimation error are higher then their unadjusted counterparts. Therefore, they seem to suggest a stronger association. Unfortunately, they are not very informative, as their precision is very low, what can be seen from the wide confidence intervals for HAS estimates.

Also here, as was done in Chapter 11 (page 178), one might wonder whether taking into account information about prognostic factors would influence the estimates of trial-level R^2 shown in the upper part of Table 12.3. The data collected for the patients included in the four meta-analyses of advanced colorectal cancer trials contained information about performance status (PS) at randomization. Overall, 41.3% of patients had PS$=0$, 43.5% had PS$=1$ and 13.7% had PS$=2$ (1.5% had missing information on PS). To investigate the extent to which taking into account the information about PS would change the estimates shown in the upper part of Table 12.3, the two-stage analysis was repeated with PS included as a continuous covariate in the marginal models (12.2) and (12.4). The patients with missing

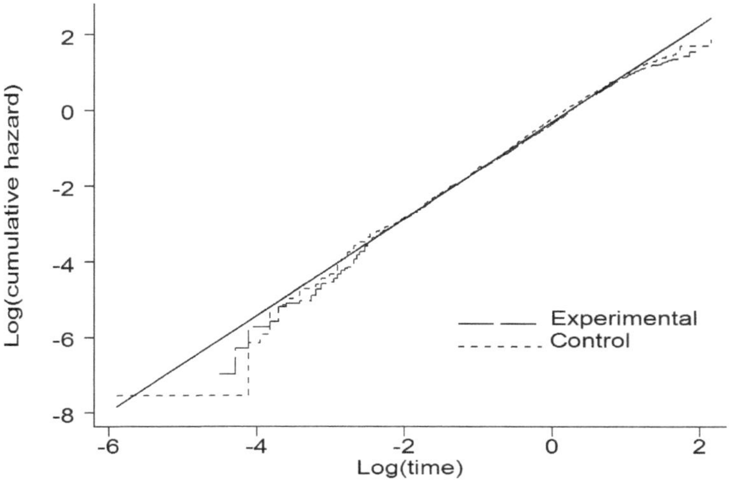

FIGURE 12.3. *Meta-analyses in advanced colorectal cancer. Estimated (stepped curves) and predicted (straight curves) cumulative hazard functions by treatment group.*

PS status were excluded from the analysis. The results are shown in the lower part of Table 12.3. The 95% confidence intervals for $R^2_{\text{trial}(\alpha)}$ were computed in the same way as those in Table 12.3. It can be seen that, as compared to the upper part of Table 12.3, the individual-level association remains essentially unchanged. The unadjusted trial-level estimates of R^2 increase only slightly. The adjusted estimates (HAS and F) are higher, but again they are not very informative. Altogether, the results from Table 12.3 indicate no substantial increase of the individual or trial-level association after adjusting for PS.

An important issue is the suitability of the assumed form of the model. Burzykowski, Molenberghs, and Buyse (2004) conducted a limited investigation of the issue. For instance, Figure 12.3 shows logarithms of Nelson-Aalen (Nelson 1972, Aalen 1978) estimates of cumulative hazard for the experimental and control treatment groups with predictions based on simple linear regression model. The plots look reasonably linear, justifying the choice of the Weibull distribution for survival.

Additionally, the assumed bivariate Plackett copula model was fitted using a separate association parameter θ for each trial. The analysis was performed for the landmark time of 3 months. It led to the log-likelihood of -6759.15. The log-likelihood for the model corresponding to the first line in the second row in Table 12.3 was equal to -6781.86. The resulting difference in deviances is -2(-22.71)=45.42 on 26 degrees of freedom. It suggests ($p = 0.010$) that there might be somewhat more variability in individual-level association between the trials than allowed in the model used to obtain the results presented in Table 12.3.

A separate issue is the verification of the assumed form of the copula function. To this end, some method allowing for a comparison of the goodness-of-fit of models based on different copula functions, including the Plackett copula, would be needed. At present, however, no such method is known.

12.3.3 Analysis of Binary Tumor Response

In clinical practice, tumor response is very often used as a binary variable, with patients with complete or partial response considered responders and patients with stable or progressive disease considered non-responders. It is therefore of interest to investigate validity of binary tumor response as a surrogate for survival. The methodology developed can be applied in this case as well. Table 12.4 presents the corresponding estimates of θ and $R^2_{\text{trial}(\alpha)}$ by landmark time for the analysis without and with the adjustment for PS, obtained by Burzykowski, Molenberghs, and Buyse (2004). The 95% confidence intervals for $R^2_{\text{trial}(\alpha)}$ were computed in the same way as those in Table 12.3. Note that, for binary response, proportional odds models (12.1)–(12.3) are equivalent to a logistic regression model. In the computations, model (12.2) was used. In one of the smallest trials, "Mar del Plata" (see Table 12.1), no tumor responses in the control arm were observed at all. This precluded the estimation of the trial-specific treatment effect on the surrogate. Therefore, this trial was removed from the analysis presented in Table 12.4.

The estimates of $R^2_{\text{trial}(\alpha,\,\eta)}$ and $R^2_{\text{trial}(\alpha)}$ presented in Table 12.4 do not exceed 50%, irrespectively of the landmark time and the adjustment for the information about PS. They suggest that no more than 50% of the variability in treatment effect on survival could be explained through treatment effect on binary tumor response. The weak association between the estimated trial-specific treatment effects for survival and binary tumor response can be observed in Figure 12.4, which presents the plot of the effects for the analysis with the landmark time set to 3 months and without adjustment for PS. The estimated intercept and slope of the straight line, containing the predictions from model (12.9), are equal to, respectively, 0.10 (standard error 0.06) and 0.22 (standard error 0.05). It follows that, similar to the case of four-category response, a simple multiplicative association between treatment effects for survival and binary tumor response can be inferred.

Based on these results Burzykowski, Molenberghs, and Buyse (2004) concluded that, though somewhat better than four-category response, binary tumor response would also be a poor surrogate for survival at the trial level. On the other hand, they suggested that the estimates of θ presented

TABLE 12.4. *Meta-analyses in advanced colorectal cancer. Binary tumor response: individual-level association (θ) and trial-level associations ($R^2_{trial(\alpha,\,\eta)}$ and $R^2_{trial(\alpha)}$), for different landmark times (in months).*

Time	Individual-level θ	Trial-level $R^2_{\text{trial}(\alpha,\,\eta)}$	Trial-level $R^2_{\text{trial}(\alpha)}$
	Without adjustment for PS		
0	4.91 [4.16, 5.67]	0.46 [0.12, 0.69]	0.44 [0.13, 0.69]
3	3.62 [3.07, 4.17]	0.47 [0.13, 0.70]	0.44 [0.13, 0.69]
4	3.29 [2.78, 3.80]	0.41 [0.08, 0.65]	0.37 [0.08, 0.64]
5	3.01 [2.54, 3.48]	0.36 [0.04, 0.61]	0.32 [0.05, 0.60]
6	2.71 [2.28, 3.14]	0.31 [0.02, 0.58]	0.29 [0.03, 0.57]
	With adjustment for PS		
0	4.78 [4.04, 5.53]	0.47 [0.13, 0.70]	0.46 [0.15, 0.71]
3	3.57 [3.02, 4.13]	0.49 [0.15, 0.71]	0.46 [0.15, 0.71]
4	3.25 [2.74, 3.76]	0.44 [0.10, 0.67]	0.41 [0.11, 0.67]
5	2.97 [2.50, 3.45]	0.39 [0.06, 0.64]	0.35 [0.07, 0.63]
6	2.68 [2.25, 3.12]	0.35 [0.04, 0.61]	0.32 [0.05, 0.60]

NOTE: 95% confidence intervals in square brackets.

in Table 12.4 would indicate a considerable association between binary tumor response and survival time for individual patients, after adjusting for treatment effects.

As was the case in Table 12.3, one could argue that the estimates of $R^2_{\text{trial}(\alpha,\,\eta)}$ and $R^2_{\text{trial}(\alpha)}$ presented in Table 12.4 are likely to biased due to ignoring the error associated with the estimation of treatment effects. Unfortunately, the computation of the adjusted estimates of $R^2_{\text{trial}(\alpha)}$ for the binary tumor response does not yield any meaningful results. More specifically, no valid estimates are obtained for any of the cases showed in Table 12.4 using the adjustment based on the measurement error models developed by Fuller (1987). On the other hand, the adjusted estimator based on the approach of van Houwelingen, Arends, and Stijnen (2002) yields valid point estimates only for the PS-adjusted analysis for landmark times of 5 and 6 months. However, the obtained values (0.93 and 0.96, respectively) are estimated too imprecisely (standard error of 0.51 and 0.52, respectively) to be meaningful. Thus, the conclusions drawn by Burzykowski, Molenberghs, and Buyse (2004) based on the unadjusted estimates cannot be verified using the adjusted estimates.

The problems with computing the adjusted estimates for Table 12.4 are most likely due to the larger estimation error of treatment effects on the

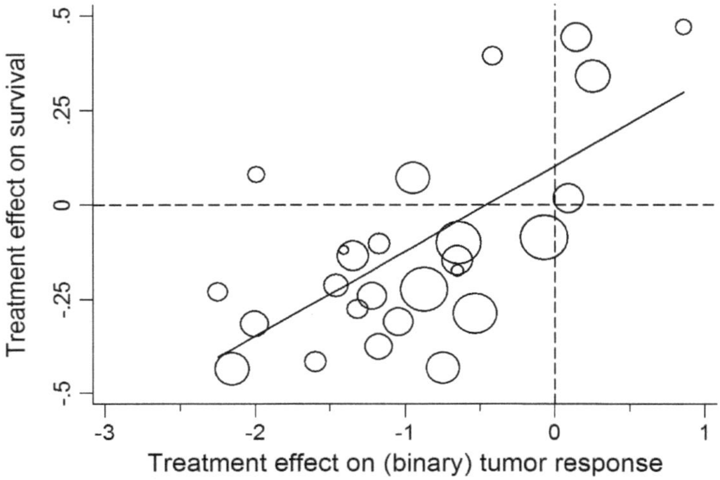

FIGURE 12.4. *Meta-analyses in advanced colorectal cancer. Estimated trial-specific treatment effects on survival versus treatment effects on binary tumor response.*

binary tumor response, as compared to the four-category response. For instance, in the case of the analysis for the landmark time of 3 months without the adjustment for PS, the estimated standard error for the trial-specific treatment effect on the binary response was on average higher by 48% (range: -3% to 152%) than the error for the four-category response. At the same time, the standard error of the trial-specific treatment effect on survival was basically the same in both analyses: the mean relative difference was 1% (range: -1% to 3%). The higher precision of the estimation of the treatment effects on the four-category tumor response can be attributed to the higher amount of the information provided in that case by the data (four-categories versus two for the binary response).

To provide evidence that the assumed parametric form, applied within the bivariate Plackett copula model, was appropriate, Burzykowski, Buyse, and Molenberghs (2004) fitted a model separately for each treatment arm in each trial, adjusting for length-bias by using landmark time of 3 months. Each model used four parameters: one for association (θ), one for the intercept in the marginal logistic regression for tumor response, and two for the Weibull model for survival. This led to a log-likelihood of -4973.0. The log-likelihood for the model corresponding to the second line in the first part of Table 12.4 was equal to -5019.0. Consequently, the difference in deviances was $-2 \times -46.0 = 92.0$ on $208 - 131 = 77$ degrees of freedom, and it was not significant ($p = 0.117$). The use of the reduced model (assuming a common copula parameter for all trials) to obtain the results presented in Table 12.4 thus seemed justified.

It is worth noting here that the results of the "Mar del Plata" trial, which was excluded from the analysis, indicated a large effect of the experimental treatment on the surrogate with virtually no effect on the true endpoint. Figure 12.4 allows to infer that adding a point corresponding to the raw treatment estimates for the excluded trial (based on the odds ratio and hazard ratio from Table 12.1) might rather decrease, than increase, the value of $R^2_{\text{trial}(\alpha)}$ presented in the first row of Table 12.4. The bias resulting from the exclusion of the data of the "Mar del Plata" trial from the analysis, if any, is thus most likely positive. Consequently, the weak association observed at the trial level for the binary response model might, in fact, be overestimated.

To investigate the effect of the "Mar del Plata" trial on the results in the analysis of binary tumor response, Burzykowski, Molenberghs, and Buyse (2004) proposed including the trial into the analysis (unadjusted for length bias and PS), with an assumed fixed value of treatment effect on tumor response. The following values of the effect, in terms of the logarithm of the odds ratio of response in favor of the "experimental" treatment, were considered: -6, -3, -1, 0, 1, 3, and 6. Note that the value of 3 is close to the logarithm (2.75) of the crude estimate of the odds ratio (15.68) presented in Table 12.1 for "Mar del Plata" trial. As a result, the following estimates of $R^2_{\text{trial}(\alpha)}$ were obtained: 0.28, 0.38, 0.44, 0.45, 0.44, 0.36, and 0.20, respectively. The observed differences between the coefficients of determination were entirely due to the changes in treatment estimates for the "Mar del Plata" trial: the estimates for the remaining trials essentially did not change. These results indicated that the exclusion of the trial from the analysis presented in Table 12.4 led to an overestimation of the trial-level R^2, as conjectured in the previous paragraph.

The increase in the strength of the trial-level association for binary tumor response, observed at least for the unadjusted estimates, might raise a question whether using a different dichotomization of the response categories might yield even a bigger increase. To verify this possibility, Burzykowski, Molenberghs, and Buyse (2004) performed two additional analyses (without adjusting for length bias or PS). In the first analysis, tumor response was defined as complete response, with partial response, stable disease or progressive disease regarded a failure (CR *versus* PR+SD+PD; it should be noted that, due to a small number of complete responses, the analysis was based on 12 trials only). In the second analysis, the response was defined as complete response, partial response or stable disease, with progressive disease treated as a failure (CR+PR+SD *versus* PD). Table 12.5 presents the results of the analyses, along with the corresponding result from Table 12.4 for the conventional dichotomization (complete or partial response *versus* stable or progressive disease). It can be seen that the estimates of $R^2_{\text{trial}(\alpha)}$ for the two alternative dichotomizations are much lower than the

TABLE 12.5. *Meta-analyses in advanced colorectal cancer. Tumor response, different definitions: individual-level (θ) and trial-level ($R^2_{trial(\alpha)}$) associations.*

Response	θ	$R^2_{\text{trial}(\alpha)}$
Four-category	6.78 [6.01, 7.55]	0.16 [0.00, 0.42]
Binary:		
CR *versus* PR+SD+PD	7.59 [4.71, 10.5]	0.08 [0.00, 0.51]
CR+PR *versus* SD+PD	4.91 [4.16, 5.67]	0.44 [0.13, 0.69]
CR+PR+SD *versus* PD	8.32 [7.17, 9.47]	0.04 [0.00, 0.28]

NOTE: 95% confidence intervals in square brackets.

estimate obtained for the conventional binary tumor response.

Table 12.5 also includes the corresponding result from Table 12.3 for the original, four-category, response. The strength of the trial-level association for the conventionally defined binary tumor response (CR+PR *versus* SD+PD) is remarkably higher than the strength for the other two binary responses or for the four-category response. This is an interesting observation from a practical (clinical) point of view. It is not straightforward to explain this difference. A possible reason might be that, for example, the categorizations other than CR+PR *versus* SD+PD, are clinically more difficult to establish and lead to more complicated models, than can be described by proportional odds. This might also be the reason why for the four-category response some inadequacies of the constant-association model were observed, while for the conventional binary response the model seemed satisfactory.

It is worth adding that for none of the cases presented in Table 12.5, an estimate of $R^2_{\text{trial}(\alpha)}$ adjusted for the error in estimation of trial-specific treatment effects could be computed.

12.4 Discussion

The method of validation for ordinal endpoints to be surrogates for failure-time true endpoints, proposed by Burzykowski, Molenberghs, and Buyse (2004) and summarized in this chapter, assumes the use of meta-analytic data. In this respect, it is consistent with the approaches developed by other authors in earlier attempts to validate tumor response as a surrogate for survival in cancer clinical trials (A'Hern, Ebbs, and Baum 1988, Torri *et al.* 1992, Chen *et al.* 2000). On the other hand, by building on the methodology developed by Buyse *et al.* (2000a), unlike in the other approaches, it focuses on the quality of the prediction of the treatment effect at the trial level, which, as argued earlier in this volume (Chapter 7), is central to the problem of surrogate marker validation.

By using copulas, the proposed approach allows for a wide range of possible models that can be formulated. For instance, it is possible to choose various association structures through the choice of various forms of copula functions. Moreover, the chosen copula can be combined with various models for the marginal distributions for the categorical/binary and survival variables, including (semi-parametric) proportional hazards and proportional odds models. In principle, the choice of a copula might be guided by adequacy of fit of the bivariate model (12.5) to the data at hand. Though methods for assessing the fit of such models in the setting considered in this chapter are not available yet, a possible solution might be, e.g., an adaptation of the method of checking goodness-of-fit of Archimedean copulas to bivariate survival data, proposed recently by Wang and Wells (2000a). This is an important topic for future research.

The analyses performed by Buyse *et al.* (2000b) and Burzykowski, Molenberghs, and Buyse (2004), as summarized and amended in the previous section, illustrate several issues, interesting both from a point of view of the validation of tumor response as a surrogate for survival in cancer clinical trials, as well as from a general point of view of the use of the proposed approach.

In the analyses, a subjective assessment was required as to what values of R^2 or θ are "high" enough for the candidate surrogate to be deemed acceptable. On purely theoretical grounds, it is difficult to propose a threshold. Any other choice is necessarily subjective. Preferably, it should be guided by practical experience in using the definition of validity of a surrogate proposed by Buyse *et al.* (2000a). For obvious reasons, such an experience thus far is very limited. Taking the above into account, observed values of $R^2_{\text{trial(r)}}$ below 0.5 have been judged as "not close to 1." Such subjectivity will be less of an issue if several endpoints are evaluated simultaneously as candidate surrogates for the same true endpoint.

An important problem, due to the nature of the endpoints considered (tumor response and survival), is an adjustment of the analysis for length bias. To this aim, Buyse *et al.* (2000b) and Burzykowski, Molenberghs, and Buyse (2004) used a form of a landmark analysis. They found that the strength of the individual-level and trial-level association depended on the landmark time; irrespectively of the landmark time, however, the individual-level association remained substantial, while the trial-level association was low. The dependence clearly points to the need for the adjustment for length bias. This need is a feature related to the question asked (about the association between tumor response and survival) and will appear irrespective of the method of the analysis.

The difference between the unadjusted and adjusted (HAS and F) estimates of the trial-level coefficient of determination, presented in Table 12.4, clearly points to the need to account in the analysis for the error in the estimation of treatment effects. The higher values observed for the adjusted estimates suggest that the conclusions regarding limited trial-level validity of tumor response as a surrogate for survival in advanced colorectal trial, drawn by Buyse *et al.* (2000b) and Burzykowski, Molenberghs, and Buyse (2004) based on the unadjusted estimates, may need to be treated with caution. Unfortunately, due to the low precision of the former estimates, a more definitive statement regarding the validity of tumor response cannot be reached.

The low precision of the adjusted estimates may look surprising, especially as a relatively large, meta-analytic set of data was used. It is worth mentioning here, however, that the response rate, especially for the "standard" arms, was low (see Table 12.1). Thus, although the overall sample size (4010 patients) may look respectable, the effective sample (especially for the binary response) is much lower. The low response rate also implies a large estimation error for trials with a small sample size. Treatment estimates for such trials are very "noisy" and may therefore cause problems with estimating the variability of the (unobserved) trial-specific random effects. From Table 12.1 one can observe that quite a few trials included in the analyzed data had a low sample size (e.g., 11 had less than 100 patients).

In this respect it is worth noting here that the meta-analytic approach to the validation of surrogate endpoints, as any meta-analysis, simply uses the data from previously organized clinical trials. One might expect that the trials will be powered for true endpoint. Of course, the resulting sample sizes, and the treatment estimation errors, will vary, reflecting different assumptions made at the trials' design stage. Thus, the problem with the presence of small trials may in practice occur quite commonly. Moreover, the sizes may appear to be too low from a point of view of the information provided for a surrogate endpoint. The case study analyzed illustrates this point very well.

The need to account for the error in the estimation of treatment effects is due to the two-stage modelling proposed by Burzykowski, Molenberghs, and Buyse (2004). This need might disappear if, for example, a genuine mixed-effects model could be formulated, which would allow for the simultaneous estimation of the fixed effects, the individual-level association and the parameters of the distribution of the random trial-specific treatment effects. At this moment, however, no such model is available.

Finally, it should be pointed out that if one is less interested in the individual-level surrogacy, simpler modeling approaches become possible. For instance, marginal models fitted using generalized estimating equations might be considered (Gail *et al.* 2000; see also Chapter 9).

13

A Combination of Longitudinal and Survival Endpoints

Didier Renard

13.1 Introduction

Interest in methods for joint modeling of longitudinal and survival time data has developed considerably in recent years (see, e.g., Pawitan and Self 1993, DeGruttola and Tu 1994, Taylor, Cumberland, and Sy 1994, Faucett and Thomas 1996, Lavalley and De Gruttola 1996, Hogan and Laird 1997a, 1997b, Wulfsohn and Tsiatis 1997, Henderson, Diggle, and Dobson 2000, Xu and Zeger 2001b). This problem frequently occurs in biomedical and public health studies where participants are followed over time. In such studies, measurements on a number of outcomes are obtained at different occasions throughout the study and times to key clinical events are recorded as well.

In randomized clinical trials, the main question is often whether the treatment under study has a beneficial effect on the time to some clinical outcome, the endpoint of primary interest. When the time elapsed between randomization and this event is long or the event is rare, it may be desirable to find a substitute for the clinical endpoint that is less distant in time or more frequently observed. This can result in shorter trial duration and make a potentially useful treatment available earlier to a wider range of patients. For example, in AIDS research, the number of CD4 T-lymphocytes and RNA viral load have been used as surrogate endpoints for time to disease progression or death (Brookmeyer and Gail 1994).

A number of researchers have used joint modeling methods to exploit longitudinal markers as surrogates for survival. Tsiatis, DeGruttola, and Wulfsohn (1995), for instance, propose a model for the relationship of survival to longitudinal data measured with error and, using Prentice criteria, examine whether CD4 counts may serve as a useful surrogate marker for survival in patients with AIDS. Xu and Zeger (2001a) investigate the issue of evaluating multiple surrogate endpoints and discuss a joint latent model for a time to clinical event and for repeated measures over time on multiple biomarkers that are potential surrogates. In addition, they propose two complementary measures to assess the relative benefit of using multiple surrogates as opposed to a single one. Another aspect of the problem, discussed by Henderson, Diggle, and Dobson (2002), is the identification of longitudinal markers for survival. These authors focus on the use of longitudinal marker trajectories as individual-level surrogates for survival. They derive a score test of association between the longitudinal marker and survival outcome and propose a measure to judge marker effectiveness in helping predict survival.

In this chapter, we extend the methodology developed in Chapter 7 for a combination of longitudinal and survival endpoints, as discussed by Renard *et al.* (2002). Technically, a joint model for longitudinal measurements and event time data is required, and we adopt the formulation of Henderson, Diggle, and Dobson (2000) here. Their approach assumes standard models for the longitudinal and survival time data and postulates a latent bivariate Gaussian process inducing stochastic dependence between the measurement and event processes. The joint model is presented in the next section, which also shows how the surrogacy measures $R^2_{\text{trial(f)}}$ and R^2_{indiv} can be carried over within this modeling framework. In Section 13.3, we apply the methodology to a set of two randomized clinical trials in advanced prostate cancer where we seek to evaluate the usefulness of prostate-specific antigen (PSA) level as a surrogate for survival.

13.2 Joint Modeling Approach

13.2.1 Model and Notation

We first describe the approach of Henderson, Diggle, and Dobson (2000) for joint modeling of longitudinal measurements and event time data. We follow their notation and consider a set of N grouping units (trial, center, etc.) where subjects within the ith unit are being followed for some time τ_i. The jth subject in unit i provides a set of measurements $\{y_{ijk} : k = 1, \ldots, n_{ij}\}$ at times $\{t_{ijk} : k = 1, \ldots, n_{ij}\}$, together with the realization of a counting process $\{N_{ij}(u) : 0 \leq u \leq \tau_i\}$ for the time-to-event endpoint and a zero-one process $\{H_{ij}(u) : 0 \leq u \leq \tau_i\}$ indicating whether a subject is at risk of experiencing an event at time u.

A central feature of the model is to postulate an unobserved (latent) zero-mean bivariate Gaussian process, $W_{ij}(t) = \{W_{1ij}(t), W_{2ij}(t)\}$, to describe the association between the longitudinal measurement and event processes.

The measurement and intensity models are linked as follows:

1. The sequence of measurements $\{y_{ijk} : k = 1, \ldots, n_{ij}\}$ of a subject is modeled using a standard linear mixed model, possibly allowing for a serially correlated component:

$$Y_{ijk} = \mu_{ij}(t_{ijk}) + W_{1ij}(t_{ijk}) + \varepsilon_{ijk}, \tag{13.1}$$

   where $\mu_{ij}(t_{ijk})$ describes the mean response profile and

$$\varepsilon_{ijk} \sim N(0, \sigma_e^2)$$

   is a sequence of mutually independent measurement errors. We will let $\boldsymbol{\alpha}_i$ denote the vector of parameters for the trial-specific treatment effects used in modeling the mean response profile. Examples will be given in what follows.

2. The event intensity process is modeled using a semi-parametric model

$$\lambda_{ij}(t) = H_{ij}(t)\lambda_0(t)\exp\{\beta_i Z_{ij} + W_{2ij}(t)\}, \tag{13.2}$$

   where the form of $\lambda_0(t)$ is left unspecified. The parameters β_i represent trial-specific treatment effects on the hazard function.

The specification of W_{1ij} and W_{2ij} can take different forms. For example, suppressing the indices for notational simplicity, we can assume

$$W_1(t) = U_1 + U_2 t,$$

with (U_1, U_2) being normally distributed with mean zero and covariance matrix G, to specify a model with random intercept and random slope for the longitudinal marker. For $W_2(t)$ we can include distinct effects for the initial value (U_1), the slope (U_2), and the current value ($U_1 + U_2 t$) of W_1, that is,

$$W_2(t) = \gamma_1 U_1 + \gamma_2 U_2 + \gamma_3 (U_1 + U_2 t).$$

Inclusion of a frailty component, orthogonal to the measurement process, is also possible.

Following Henderson, Diggle, and Dobson (2000), the preferred method of estimation for the above model is the EM algorithm. The procedure involves iterating between the following two steps until convergence is achieved:

1. E-step: determine expected values, conditional on the observed data, of all functionals of the random effects $h(U)$ appearing in the complete data log-likelihood using current parameter estimates;

2. M-step: maximize the complete data log-likelihood with each function $h(U)$ replaced by its corresponding expectation.

When a serially correlated component is included in the process $W_1(t)$, the authors suggest using a modification of the procedure which combines simplex and EM algorithms. However, this complicates somewhat the estimation procedure, and we restrict attention to models with random effects only in what follows.

13.2.2 Measures of Surrogacy

We now examine how surrogacy measures introduced in Chapter 7 can be carried over within the modeling framework described in the previous section.

The coefficient $R^2_{\text{trial(f)}}$ (or $R^2_{\text{trial(r)}}$) can be derived from its definition given in Chapter 7. Unlike model (7.6)–(7.7), which solely involves treatment effects, the longitudinal component will require, in general, a more complex specification to represent time evolution of the marker. For practical purposes, we will assume that the mean trajectory of the marker within each treatment group can be specified parsimoniously, as a low-order polynomial or a continuous piecewise linear function of time, for example. For the sake of illustration, suppose that the trajectory of the marker over time is quadratic; then $\mu_{ij}(t_{ijk})$ can be written

$$\mu_{ij}(t_{ijk}) = \mu_{0i} + \mu_{1i}t_{ijk} + \mu_{2i}t_{ijk}^2 + \alpha_{0i}Z_{ij} + \alpha_{1i}Z_{ij}t_{ijk} + \alpha_{2i}Z_{ij}t_{ijk}^2.$$

Evaluation of $R^2_{\text{trial(f)}}$ and $R^2_{\text{trial(r)}}$ at the second stage, after fitting model (13.1)–(13.2), is straightforward. For example, $R^2_{\text{trial(r)}}$ can be calculated as the coefficient of determination from the regression model

$$\widehat{\beta}_i = \lambda_0 + \lambda_1\widehat{\alpha}_{0i} + \lambda_2\widehat{\alpha}_{1i} + \lambda_3\widehat{\alpha}_{2i} + \varepsilon_i,$$

where the hat notation refers to estimated values.

At the individual level, it is natural to consider the association between W_1 and W_2. Stated otherwise, R^2_{indiv} will not refer to the direct association between the two endpoints but rather to the association between the two latent processes governing the longitudinal and event processes. This association is no longer summarized by a single number, however. It is now a time-dependent measure since the association between the marker and the event process can be defined relative to any time over the course of measurement of the marker. In fact, this can be extended even to the association between W_1 at some time t_1 and W_2, taken at a later time $t_2 \geq t_1$, which defines a surface describing the association between the latent processes. This feature can be important in selecting an optimal time at which the marker should be evaluated, either to enhance clinical judgment or even further, to predict the event time of interest.

To illustrate the derivation of $R^2_{\text{indiv}}(t)$, we continue with our previous example where it was assumed that $W_1(t) = U_1 + U_2 t$ and $W_2(t) = \gamma_1 U_1 + \gamma_2 U_2 + \gamma_3(U_1 + U_2 t)$. The correlation between $W_1(t)$ and $W_2(t)$, at any fixed time t, can easily be calculated since $W_1(t)$ and $W_2(t)$ have a joint normal distribution. Thus, if $(U_1, U_2) \sim N(0, G)$, we have:

$$\begin{aligned}\text{var}[W_1(t)] &= G_{11} + 2G_{12}t + G_{22}t^2, \\ \text{var}[W_2(t)] &= (\gamma_1^2 + 2\gamma_1\gamma_3)G_{11} + 2(\gamma_1\gamma_2 + \gamma_1\gamma_3 t + \gamma_2\gamma_3)G_{12} \\ &\quad +(\gamma_2^2 + 2\gamma_2\gamma_3 t)G_{22} + \gamma_3^2\text{var}[W_1(t)], \\ \text{cov}[W_1(t), W_2(t)] &= \gamma_1 G_{11} + (\gamma_2 + \gamma_1 t)G_{12} + \gamma_2 G_{22}t + \gamma_3\text{var}[W_1(t)],\end{aligned}$$

from which the (squared) correlation between $W_1(t)$ and $W_2(t)$ can be evaluated by plugging in estimates for γ_1, γ_2, G_{11}, G_{12}, and G_{22}. This function, that will be termed "model-based," is entirely based on the assumptions made in our model. A more heuristic estimate, which we will refer to as "empirical," could be derived along the same lines of development, except that sample estimators based on the expected U values obtained at the final step of the EM algorithm are substituted for the elements of G. Thus, G_{11} is replaced by $\widehat{\text{var}}\{\widehat{U}_{1i}\}$, G_{22} by $\widehat{\text{var}}\{\widehat{U}_{2i}\}$ and G_{12} by $\widehat{\text{cov}}\{\widehat{U}_{1i}, \widehat{U}_{2i}\}$.

It should be stressed that the "empirical" curve still depends heavily on the model specification. Thus, if we assume that $W_2(t) = \gamma W_1(t)$, R^2_{indiv} will be identically equal to one. As one departs from this basic model and further terms are added, a finer characterization of the curve is allowed in its admissible forms. We consequently recommend including a sufficiently large number of association parameters $\{\gamma_k\}$ in the model to avoid undue constraints on R^2_{indiv}.

13.3 Application to Advanced Prostate Cancer Data

We consider the data set introduced in Section 4.2.5. The goal is to investigate whether PSA level may serve as a suitable surrogate for survival in patients with advanced prostate cancer.

We will utilize pooled data and refer to control (CPA/flutamide) and experimental (liarozole) arms. In this analysis, we will use country as the grouping unit within each trial in order to have a sufficient number of patients in each unit. This yields a number of 19 units comprising between 3 and 69 patients. Two of these units were excluded from the analysis, however: in one of them ($n = 3$), subjects were accrued in only one treatment arm and no events were observed in the second ($n = 8$).

Figure 13.1 displays summaries of the data in terms of the basic entities connected through model (13.1)–(13.2). Smoothed PSA profiles were obtained using LOESS while smoothed estimates of the hazard rates were obtained following the method of Ramlau-Hansen (1983) with an Epanechnikov kernel function. The PSA profiles depicted in Figure 13.1 are rather flat, but this picture does not tell the entire story. In such cancer trials many patients are taken off study upon clinical progression or do not survive throughout the study period and this results in longitudinal sequences of largely varying length. To investigate this effect of "dropout," we grouped the data according to visits as planned in the protocol and we plotted the mean profiles for each dropout pattern. This is shown in Figure 13.2, where late-dropout patterns are not included because of the scarcity of data after 1.5 years. We can notice that patients who progressed early tend to have a higher initial PSA value and do not exhibit an early decline in their PSA level. The mean curved PSA profiles for subjects who progressed belatedly can be contrasted with the relatively flat curves displayed in Figure 13.1.

The first step in the analysis is to specify a parsimonious model that captures the evolution of the marker over time. A simplistic attempt could involve second-order polynomials, as suggested by patterns in Figure 13.2. We include random effects for each term (that is, intercept, t and t^2). To refine this initial choice, we can employ fractional polynomials (Royston and Altman 1994). A fractional polynomial is a linear combination of real-valued powers of X, where X represents some covariate (time in this case). More formally, a fractional polynomial $\phi(X; \boldsymbol{\beta}, \boldsymbol{p})$ of degree m can be defined as the function

$$\beta_0 + \sum_{j=1}^{m} \beta_j X^{(p_j)},$$

where the β_j are regression parameters and $\boldsymbol{p} = (p_1, \ldots, p_m)$ is a real-valued vector of powers with $p_1 < \ldots < p_m$ (this definition can be extended to handle equalities among power values). The notation $X^{(p)}$ denotes the Box-Tidwell power transformation

$$X^{(p)} = \begin{cases} X^p, & p \neq 0, \\ \ln X, & p = 0. \end{cases}$$

By definition, fractional polynomials extend the family of classical polynomials. A great advantage of fractional polynomials over standard polyno-

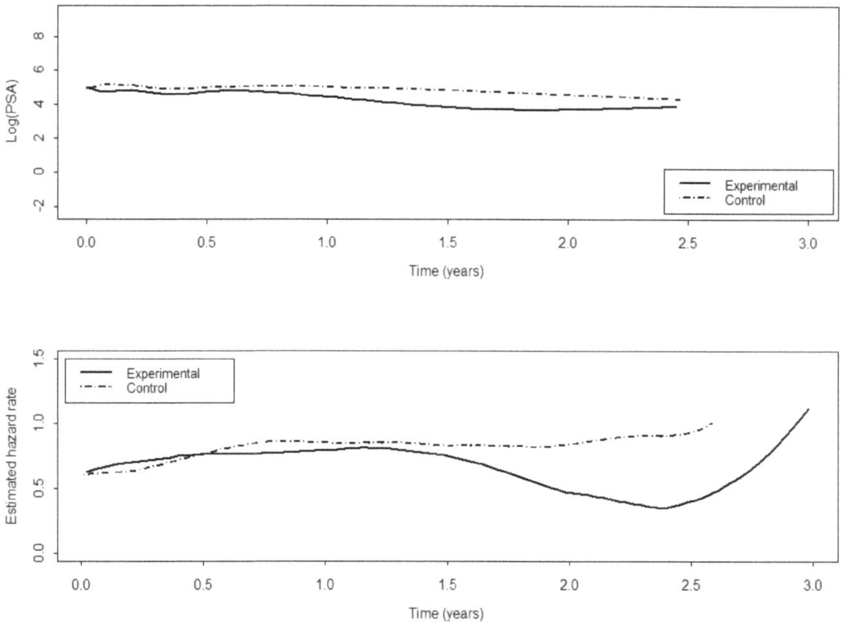

FIGURE 13.1. *Advanced prostate cancer study. Longitudinal and event time summaries for the combined liarozole trials. Top panel: smoothed PSA profiles; bottom panel: smoothed estimates of the hazard rates.*

mials is their providing a wide range of functional forms and their behavior near the extreme values is often more reasonable. Fractional polynomials are therefore useful for parsimonious parametric modeling.

Another advantage of fractional polynomials is that they are straightforward to fit. To determine the "best" value of m and $\boldsymbol{p}$, Royston and Altman (1994) propose restricting the power terms to a small predefined set of integer and non-integer values. More precisely, they suggest using $\mathcal{P} = \{-2, -1, -0.5, 0, 0.5, 1, 2, \dots, \max(3, m)\}$, and to select the power values associated to the model with the highest likelihood. As with conventional polynomials, the degree m of the fractional polynomial is selected either informally on *a priori* grounds or by increasing m until no noticeable improvement in model fit can be detected. Arguably, in many practical situation, $m = 2$ or $m = 3$ would be sufficient.

With longitudinal data, model specification involves modeling of both the mean and the covariance structures, and different strategies can be envisaged to incorporate fractional polynomials in the model. For example, a fixed covariance structure can be chosen for all fitted models, and the value

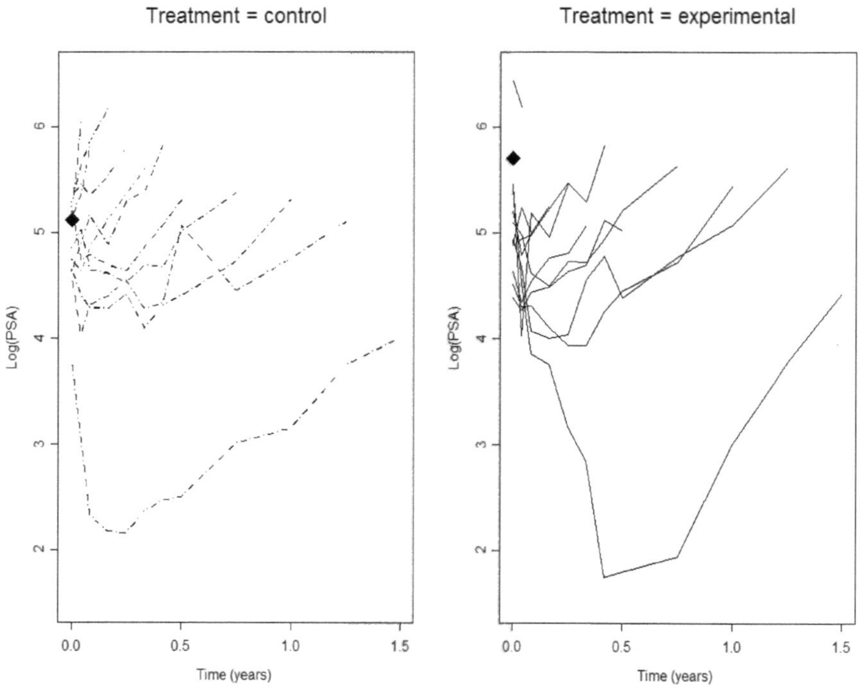

FIGURE 13.2. *Advanced prostate cancer study. Mean PSA profiles per "dropout" patterns (the black diamonds represent the mean PSA level of those patients who only have a baseline measurement).*

of $\boldsymbol{p}$ that provides the best model fit is then selected. An alternative is to update both the mean and the covariance structures for each fitted model. Thus, if the mean model assumes the form $\alpha_0 + \alpha_1 t^{p_1} + \alpha_2 t^{p_2}$, we may want to include (subject-specific) random effects to obtain a random-coefficient model $\alpha_{0j} + \alpha_{1j} t^{p_1} + \alpha_{2j} t^{p_2}$.

We follow the latter strategy here, with specific curves for each treatment group. The result of fitting a fractional polynomial of degree 2 gives $\boldsymbol{p} = (0.5, 1)$ for the prostate cancer data. Comparison of this model with the original (quadratic) model yields a large rise in likelihood.

The joint model we are going to fit is the following:

$$\begin{aligned} S_{ijk} &= \mu_{0i} + \mu_{1i} t_{ijk} + \mu_{2i} \sqrt{t_{ijk}} + (\alpha_{0i} + \alpha_{1i} t_{ijk} + \alpha_{2i} \sqrt{t_{ijk}}) Z_{ij} \\ &\quad + U_{0j} + U_{1j} t_{ijk} + U_{2j} \sqrt{t_{ijk}} + \varepsilon_{ijk} \qquad (13.3) \end{aligned}$$

and

$$\lambda_{ij}(t) = \lambda_0(t) \exp[\beta_i Z_{ij} + \gamma_0 U_{0j} + \gamma_1 U_{1j}$$

$$+\gamma_2 U_{2j} + \gamma_3 (U_{0j} + U_{1j} t + U_{2j} \sqrt{t})]. \qquad (13.4)$$

We can now evaluate trial- and individual-level surrogacy. With the relatively small number of units available, we focus on $R^2_{\text{trial(r)}}$ rather than on $R^2_{\text{trial(f)}}$. The coefficient of determination in the regression of $\{\widehat{\beta}_i\}$ on $\widehat{\boldsymbol{\alpha}}_i = \{\widehat{\alpha}_{0i}, \widehat{\alpha}_{1i}, \widehat{\alpha}_{2i}\}$ yields a value of 0.517. This mid-range value is probably too low to permit reliable prediction of treatment effects on survival, having observed the effect of treatment on the marker. Confidence limits on $R^2_{\text{trial(r)}}$ can be obtained from the cumulative distribution function of R^2 based on the assumption that the $\boldsymbol{\alpha}_i$'s and β_i's are normally distributed (Ding 1996, Algina 1999). In our example, the 95% confidence interval for $R^2_{\text{trial(r)}}$ is $[0.013, 0.748]$, thus showing that trial-level association is estimated rather imprecisely. This might be explained by the restricted number of grouping units and the mid-range value of $R^2_{\text{trial(r)}}$ (the confidence interval being more narrow for more extreme values of $R^2_{\text{trial(r)}}$).

Note that dependence between the marker and survival endpoint is a complicating assumption within our methodology. If interest centers on trial-level surrogacy alone, a naive approach would be to assume independence between the two outcomes, which greatly simplifies computations, as the two models can then be fitted separately. Tibaldi *et al.* (2003) explore this issue in the case of normally distributed endpoints and conclude that simplified computational methods perform quite well (see Section 7.4.2 for an account on this). Obviously, as one departs from the multivariate Gaussian framework, it is not at all clear whether such a simplistic approach works effectively well. Section 11.7 discussed simplified strategies when both the surrogate as well as the true endpoint are of a time-to-event type. For comparative purposes, we calculated $R^2_{\text{trial(r)}}$ by separately fitting models (13.3) and (13.4) with $\gamma_0 = \gamma_1 = \gamma_2 = \gamma_3 = 0$. This results in a value of $R^2_{\text{trial(r)}} = 0.291$, with 95% confidence interval $[0, 0.576]$, which is much lower than the one found above (although confidence limits should not be overlooked).

Figure 13.3a shows the model-based and empirical curves $R^2_{\text{indiv}}(t)$ for model (13.3)–(13.4). Both curves agree fairly well over the time range considered. They start from a relatively low level (~ 0.3), then raise sharply until a value of about 0.9 at year 1 and stabilize at that level thereafter. Although the interpretation of this plot holds, strictly speaking, at the level of the latent processes W_1 and W_2, this would suggest that, initially, PSA level bears relatively little information on a patient's future survival but as information on the marker is gathered over time (mostly within the first year of treatment), it achieves better predictive capability, with no further gain subsequently. The plot in the right panel (Figure 13.3b) shows the model-based and empirical curves for the original model (quadratic time evolution for the marker). In comparison with Figure 13.3a, the curves are similar

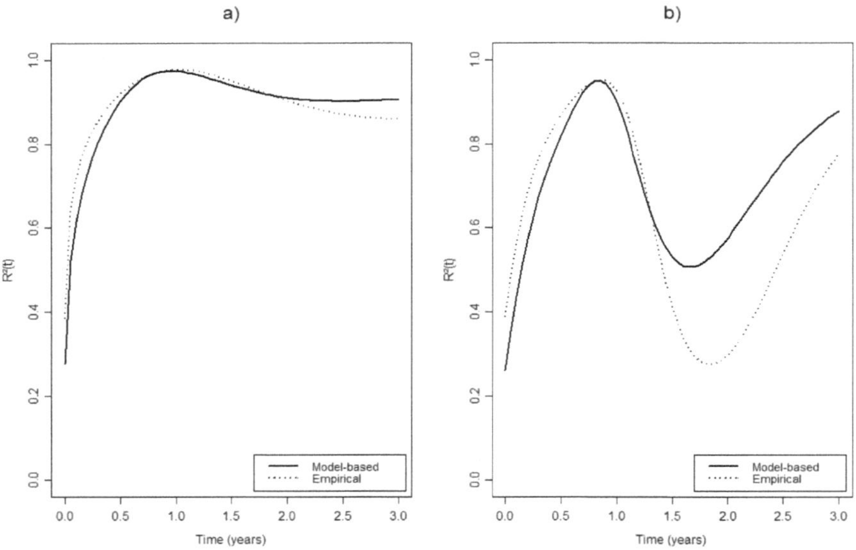

FIGURE 13.3. *Advanced prostate cancer study. Plots of the model-based and empirical* $R^2_{indiv}(t)$ *curves. Left panel: final model (t and* $\sqrt{t}$*). Right panel: quadratic model.*

until year 1, but then a dip can be observed. Also, both curves do not coincide very well. It is not clear whether this is caused by the inferior fit of the model, or by constraints imposed by the model itself, but this calls for caution when interpreting such plots. We do believe that they might shed some light on the basic intricacies between the marker and the survival endpoint under study, but they should not be over-interpreted as they may be strongly model-dependent.

As to the clinical interpretation of the above analysis, we have seen that PSA level and survival seem, as expected, strongly related, at least when a sufficiently large amount of information has been gathered on the marker. While bearing in mind that $R^2_{\text{trial(r)}}$ was estimated with rather large uncertainty, the value that was found stands mid-range in the unit interval and would prevent us from formulating any firm conclusion, had it been estimated more precisely. This points to an issue, not of the methodology, but rather of the biological nature of the marker. We may tentatively say, however, that PSA level has some value as a surrogate marker for survival, for the class of treatments considered in the two trials at least, but probably is not a very good one.

13.4 Discussion

A limiting feature of the modeling approach presented in Section 13.2 is the computational burden inherent to such complex models. This issue is exacerbated by the typical size of the meta-analytic data sets required for the validation exercise.

Another problem is associated with the use of the EM algorithm to fit the model, as it fails to provide precision estimates for the parameters. To obtain standard errors, Henderson, Diggle, and Dobson (2000) used a Monte-Carlo method by refitting the model to a number of simulated data sets generated using parameter values taken from the original analysis. Clearly, this procedure may be overly time-consuming here but it could help provide uncertainty measures around the $R^2_{\text{indiv}}(t)$ curve. Precision estimates would also be required if one wishes to correct for measurement error introduced by the fact that estimates of the $\boldsymbol{\alpha}_i$'s and the β_i's are effectively employed when estimating $R^2_{\text{trial(r)}}$.

14

Repeated Measures and Surrogate Endpoint Validation

Ariel Alonso Abad, Helena Geys, and Tony Vangeneugden

14.1 Introduction

In many practical applications, repeated measurements are encountered on either or both endpoints. In the previous chapters, the focus was on one or both of the endpoints to be of a univariate type. Going to a fully multivariate framework presents new challenges. The R^2 measures introduced in Chapter 7 are no longer applicable. In Chapter 7, the meta-analytic methodology has been based on the simplest cross-sectional case in which both the surrogate and the true endpoint are continuous and normally distributed. Subsequently, different variations to the theme were implemented for binary responses (Chapter 10), times to event (Chapter 11), and for the combination of a survival and a longitudinal endpoint (Chapter 13). In the cross-sectional cases, one assumes that only one potential surrogate is available and that treatment effect on both responses is a constant and hence can be characterized by a single parameter. These assumptions can fail when a patient is measured repeatedly over time. Extending the methodology to this setting opens some new conceptual problems.

In this chapter, we consider the setting where both the surrogate and the true endpoint are longitudinal. In such a situation, an additional challenge is to summarize surrogacy by means of simple measures. Technically, to this aim, a joint model for multivariate repeated measurements is required. Useful references on this topic include Galecki (1994), Sy, Taylor, and Cumberland (1997), and Jorgensen *et al.* (1999). In analogy to the cross-sectional setting considered by Buyse *et al.* (2000a), we will base the calculation of surrogacy measures on a two-stage approach rather than a full random-effects approach, which would take into account both the repeated measures as the multi-trial nature of the data, in order to reduce numerical complexity. Technically, we need (1) a model for bivariate longitudinal outcomes and (2) new measures that let us evaluate surrogacy when longitudinal data are available. Here, we will introduce a joint model for bivariate longitudinal outcomes along the ideas of Galecki (1994). An advantage of this approach is that it can be implemented easily within commonly available software programs.

14.2 The Model

Suppose we have data from $i = 1, \ldots, N$ trials in the ith of which $j = 1, \ldots, n_i$ subjects are enrolled. Assume further that ξ_{ijk} is the time corresponding to the kth occasion ($k = 1, \ldots, p_i$) when subject j in trial i was measured. Let T_{ijk} and S_{ijk} denote the associated true and surrogate endpoints, respectively, and let Z_{ij} be a binary indicator variable for treatment. Following the ideas of Galecki (1994), a specific joint model at the first stage for both responses can then be written as

$$\begin{cases} T_{ijk} & = & \mu_{T_i} + \beta_i Z_{ij} + g_{T_{ij}}(\xi_{ijk}) + \varepsilon_{T_{ijk}}, \\ S_{ijk} & = & \mu_{S_i} + \alpha_i Z_{ij} + g_{S_{ij}}(\xi_{ijk}) + \varepsilon_{S_{ijk}}, \end{cases} \tag{14.1}$$

where μ_{S_i} and μ_{T_i} are trial-specific intercepts, α_i, β_i are trial-specific effects of treatment Z_{ij} on the two endpoints, and $g_{T_{ij}}$ and $g_{S_{ij}}$ are trial and subject specific time functions. Note that even though in practice T_{ij} and S_{ij} are frequently measured at the same time points, model (14.1) would let us approach situations in which this condition does not hold.

In the case of univariate longitudinal endpoints, one can consider different types of covariance structures for T and S, including compound symmetry, auto-regressive, banded, factor-analytic, spatial, unstructured, etc. Here, however, we have repeated measurements on two outcome variables, the surrogate and the true endpoint. A possible joint covariance structure can then be based on the Kronecker product of (1) an unstructured variance-covariance matrix for the type of outcome and (2) a suitable covariance structure for the repeated measurements on an outcome. Note that, while in the setting defined in Chapter 7 the error variance-covariance matrix could be assumed constant over all trials (even though this was extended in Chapter 9), this assumption is no longer plausible in most practical longitudinal settings. That is because measurements could be taken at different time points within different trials, the number of measurements could be different in each trial, etc. Therefore, we should allow for different covariance structures over the different trials. To this aim, define the random vectors

$$\widetilde{\varepsilon}_{T_{ij}} = (\varepsilon_{T_{ij1}}, \ldots, \varepsilon_{T_{ijp_i}}),$$

$$\widetilde{\varepsilon}_{S_{ij}} = (\varepsilon_{S_{ij1}}, \ldots, \varepsilon_{S_{ijp_i}}),$$

and assume that they are jointly mean-zero multivariate normally distributed with variance-covariance matrix

$$\Sigma_i = \begin{pmatrix} \sigma_{TTi} & \sigma_{TSi} \\ \sigma_{TSi} & \sigma_{SSi} \end{pmatrix} \otimes R_i. \tag{14.2}$$

In the aforementioned formulation, R_i reflects a general correlation matrix for the repeated measurements of the responses. A frequent choice in practice would be the first-order auto-regressive structure (in case measures are equally spaced; otherwise, a spatial-type structure may be better)

$$R_i = \begin{pmatrix} 1 & \rho_i & \ldots & \rho_i^{p_i} \\ \vdots & \vdots & \vdots & \vdots \\ \rho_i^{p_i} & \rho_i^{p_i-1} & \ldots & 1 \end{pmatrix} \tag{14.3}$$

where p_i denotes the number of designed time points in trial i. It should be noted that if we only have one measurement per subject, time will disappear as a covariate on the right-hand side of (14.1) and $R_i = 1$. If it is also assumed that $\Sigma_i = \Sigma$, then our model reduces to the model proposed by Buyse *et al.* (2000a) and presented in Chapter 7.

As we will argue in what follows, the above model is, of course, not free from assumptions. It is therefore important to check the model assumptions in each specific example. However, the measures of surrogacy we will propose, also hold for other, more general covariance structures than the one defined in (14.2).

If treatment effect can be assumed constant over time, then the R^2_{trial} measured proposed by Buyse *et al.* (2000a) could still be useful to evaluate surrogacy at the trial level. However, at the individual level, R^2_{indiv} is no longer applicable and new concepts are needed.

14.3 Variance Reduction Factor

In general, the error vectors $\widetilde{\varepsilon}_{T_{ij}}$ and $\widetilde{\varepsilon}_{S_{ij}}$ follow a multivariate normal distribution with variance-covariance matrix

$$\Sigma_i = \begin{pmatrix} \Sigma_{TTi} & \Sigma_{TSi} \\ \Sigma_{TSi}^T & \Sigma_{SSi} \end{pmatrix},$$

where Σ_{TTi} and Σ_{SSi} are the variance-covariance matrices associated with the residual vectors $\widetilde{\varepsilon}_{T_{ij}}$ and $\widetilde{\varepsilon}_{S_{ij}}$, respectively, and Σ_{TSi} contains the covariances between the elements of $\widetilde{\varepsilon}_{T_{ij}}$ and the elements of $\widetilde{\varepsilon}_{S_{ij}}$. Hence, we allow for a different covariance structure in each clinical trial, thus leaving the possibility to tackle very general problems for which the assumption of homogeneous covariance structures over trials would be overly restrictive. Note that, under model (14.1), $\Sigma_{TTi} = \sigma_{TTi} R_i$, $\Sigma_{SSi} = \sigma_{SSi} R_i$, and $\Sigma_{TSi} = \sigma_{TSi} R_i$.

To validate a surrogate endpoint at the individual level in a univariate setting, Buyse *et al.* (2000a) suggested to look at the correlation between the surrogate and the true endpoint after adjustment for trial and treatment effects. Using multivariate ideas, Alonso *et al.* (2003) proposed the *Variance Reduction Factor* (VRF) to evaluate surrogacy at the individual level when repeated measurements are present. Essentially, they summarized the variability of the repeated measurements on the true endpoint by taking the sum, over all trials, of traces of the trial-specific variance-covariance matrices for the measurements. In a similar way, they summarized the conditional variability of the true-endpoint measurements, given the surrogate, by the sum of traces of the trial-specific conditional variance-covariance matrices. As a result, they quantified the relative reduction in the true endpoint variance after adjustment by the surrogate by

$$VRF_{\text{indiv}} = \frac{\sum_i [\text{tr}(\Sigma_{TTi}) - \text{tr}(\Sigma_{(T|S)i})]}{\sum_i \text{tr}(\Sigma_{TTi})}, \tag{14.4}$$

where $\Sigma_{(T|S)i} = \Sigma_{TTi} - \Sigma_{TSi}\Sigma_{SSi}^{-1}\Sigma_{TSi}^{T}$ denotes the conditional trial-specific variance-covariance matrix of $\widetilde{\varepsilon}_{T_{ij}}$ given $\widetilde{\varepsilon}_{S_{ij}}$. Intuitively, expression (14.4) quantifies how much of the total variability of the repeated measurements on the true endpoint is explained by adjusting for the treatment effects and the repeated measurements on the surrogate endpoint. In that respect, expression (14.4) fits into the general definition of the "proportion of variation of a dependent variable, Y, explained by a vector of covariates X" (PVE) in general regression models

$$PVE = \frac{\sum_i [D(Y_i) - D(Y_i|X_i)]}{\sum_i D(Y_i)},$$

where $D(Y_i)$ denotes a measure of distance of Y_i from a central location parameter of the estimated marginal distribution of Y, and $D(Y_i|X_i)$ denotes the same measure using the distribution of Y conditional on a given model and on the covariate vector for the ith observation (Schemper and Stare 1996).

One can further show that

1. VRF_{indiv} ranges between zero and one;

2. VRF_{indiv} equals zero if and only if the error terms of the true and surrogate endpoints are independent within each trial;

3. VRF_{indiv} equals one if and only if there exists a deterministic relationship between the error terms for the true and surrogate endpoints within each trial;

4. VRF_{indiv} reduces to R^2_{indiv}, defined by Buyse *et al.* (2000a) when the endpoints are measured only once.

If model (14.1) is considered, then VRF_{indiv} can be rewritten in terms of the trial-specific squared correlations $\rho^2_{TSi} = \sigma_{TSi}/(\sigma_{TTi}\sigma_{SSi})$ between surrogate and true endpoints at each time point:

$$VRF_{\text{indiv}} = \sum_i \left(\frac{p_i \sigma_{TTi}}{\sum_i p_i \sigma_{TTi}} \right) \rho^2_{TSi}. \tag{14.5}$$

The latter expression yields an appealing interpretation of VRF. Indeed, VRF is just a sum of different trial contributions, where each contribution is the product of the squared correlation between the surrogate and the true endpoint at each time point in that trial with the proportion of the total true endpoint variance that is accounted for by that trial.

As mentioned before, as soon as the treatment effect cannot be assumed constant over time, the trial-level measure of surrogacy defined by Buyse *et al.* (2000a) becomes inapplicable as well and other approaches are needed. In this case the treatment effect at the ith trial cannot be characterized by the scalars β_i and α_i, but by the p_i dimensional vectors $\widetilde{\beta}_i$ and $\widetilde{\alpha}_i$ (Verbyla 1999).

To overcome this difficulty, we can then define the variance reduction factor at the trial level (VRF_{trial}). Suppose that

$$\left(\widetilde{\beta}_i, \widetilde{\alpha}_i\right) \sim N\left[\left(\overline{\beta}_i, \overline{\alpha}_i\right), D_i\right],$$

with

$$D_i = \begin{pmatrix} D_{\beta\beta i} & D_{\beta\alpha i} \\ D^T_{\beta\alpha i} & D_{\alpha\alpha i} \end{pmatrix}.$$

Here, $(\overline{\beta}_i, \overline{\alpha}_i)$ is the $2p_i$-dimensional mean treatment effect vector for the ith trial. Note that a trial-specific variance-covariance matrix D_i is assumed as, for reasons explained earlier, it would be unrealistic to assume the same covariance structure across all the trials. Under these assumptions we can define, similarly to the individual level and with straightforward notations, VRF_{trial} as

$$VRF_{trial} = \frac{\sum_i \left[\text{tr}(D_{\beta\beta i}) - \text{tr}(D_{(\beta|\alpha)i})\right]}{\sum_i \text{tr}(D_{\beta\beta i})}. \tag{14.6}$$

The properties of VRF_{indiv} stated earlier can now be easily extended to VRF_{trial}. Moreover, in case of a single observation it can be shown that VRF_{trial} becomes equivalent to R^2_{trial} defined by Buyse *et al.* (2000a). The scope of the methodology presented above is not limited to the longitudinal framework. There are other settings in which the use of these tools can be appealing. For example, a lot of work on surrogate endpoint validation assumes only one potential surrogate is being evaluated. However, it is easy to conceive of situations where a treatment can affect a medical condition in a very complex way, thereby simultaneously acting on different factors. In such a case, it would make sense to presume that the prediction of the treatment effect on the true endpoint can be substantially improved by using information about the treatment effect on an entire set of possibly relevant variables at the same time.

To investigate this idea in more detail, let us assume that two potential surrogate endpoints are available. Following the development of the two-stage model proposed of Buyse *et al.* (2000a) (see also Chapter 7), we can postulate the following multivariate regression model at the first stage:

$$\begin{cases} T_{ij} &= \mu_{T_i} + \beta_i Z_{ij} + \varepsilon_{T_{ij}}, \\ S_{1ij} &= \mu_{S_{1i}} + \alpha_{1i} Z_{ij} + \varepsilon_{S_{1ij}}, \\ S_{2ij} &= \mu_{S_{2i}} + \alpha_{2i} Z_{ij} + \varepsilon_{S_{2ij}}, \end{cases} \tag{14.7}$$

where $\left(\varepsilon_{T_{ij}}, \varepsilon_{S_{1ij}}, \varepsilon_{S_{2ij}}\right) \sim N\left(0, \Sigma\right)$. At the second stage we will, by way of illustration, assume that $(\beta_i, \alpha_{1i}, \alpha_{2i}) \sim N\left[(\beta, \alpha_1, \alpha_2), D\right]$ with

$$D = \begin{pmatrix} 2\sigma + \vartheta & \sigma & \sigma \\ \sigma & \sigma & 0 \\ \sigma & 0 & \sigma \end{pmatrix}.$$

If we now apply the methodology described in Chapter 7 for each surrogate separately, it is easy to show that

$$R^2_{1,\text{trial}} = R^2_{2,\text{trial}} = \frac{\sigma}{2\sigma + \vartheta},$$

where $R^2_{\ell,\text{trial}}$ $(\ell = 1, 2)$ is the coefficient of determination corresponding to the use of surrogate S_ℓ. On the other hand, when both of the surrogates are considered jointly, we obtain

$$VRF_{\text{trial}} = \frac{2\sigma}{2\sigma + \vartheta}.$$

This leads us to a very interesting point about the new concept. Focusing on the population level, note that $\text{Var}(\beta_i|\alpha_{1i}, \alpha_{2i}) = \vartheta$ and hence it is clear that, for small values of ϑ, there is an almost deterministic relationship between β_i and $(\alpha_{1i}, \alpha_{2i})$. This will imply that we should be able to predict the treatment effect on the true endpoint with a high precision if the treatment effects on both surrogates S_1 and S_2 are known. However, these surrogates would poorly predict the treatment effect on the true endpoint if they were considered independently, as can be concluded from the expressions

$$\lim_{\vartheta \to 0} R^2_{1,\text{trial}}(\vartheta) = \lim_{\vartheta \to 0} R^2_{2,\text{trial}}(\vartheta) = 0.5.$$

On the other hand, VRF_{trial} clearly reflects that, in this setting, a very accurate prediction for the true endpoint treatment effect can be obtained if both endpoints are used jointly:

$$\lim_{\vartheta \to 0} VRF_{\text{trial}}(\vartheta) = 1.$$

This extreme situation is less likely to occur in practice, if only because we then have to account for measurement error due to finite sampling (Gail *et al.* 2000). Nevertheless, the previous example does illustrate that a lot might be gained if more than a single surrogate is used. In principle, any number of potential surrogates could be studied and even several endpoints and several surrogates could be analyzed together, in a multivariate fashion.

14.4 Validation from a Canonical Correlation Perspective

The original idea of Buyse *et al.* (2000a) of using a squared correlation coefficient (R^2_{indiv}) to summarize surrogacy at the individual level leads us to the concept of canonical correlations as a possible building block for multivariate extensions.

In this section, we will show that VRF can be incorporated into a much more general framework that allows interpretation in terms of the canonical correlations of the error vectors.

Assume that in trial i the repeated measurements for S and T are taken at p_i time points for every patient. Thus, vectors T_{ij} and S_{ij} for patient

j can be seen as realizations of p_i-variate random variables $\boldsymbol{T}_i$ and $\boldsymbol{S}_i$, respectively. Denoting by $\widetilde{\boldsymbol{\varepsilon}}_{T_i}$ and $\widetilde{\boldsymbol{\varepsilon}}_{S_i}$ the residual random errors corresponding to $\boldsymbol{T}_i$ and $\boldsymbol{S}_i$, respectively, it is obvious that in trial i there will be $k = 1, \ldots, p_i$ squared canonical correlations ρ_{ki}^2 for $(\widetilde{\boldsymbol{\varepsilon}}_{T_i}, \widetilde{\boldsymbol{\varepsilon}}_{S_i})$, such that $\rho_{1i}^2 \geq \rho_{2i}^2 \geq \ldots \geq \rho_{p_i i}^2$ and ρ_{ki}^2 is the eigenvalue of

$$MCC_i = \Sigma_{TTi}^{-1/2}\Sigma_{TSi}\Sigma_{SSi}^{-1}\Sigma_{TSi}^{T}\Sigma_{TTi}^{-1/2}. \tag{14.8}$$

If we further define $\rho_{vi}^2 = (\rho_{1i}^2, \rho_{2i}^2, \ldots, \rho_{p_i i}^2)$ to be the vector of the squared canonical correlations for trial i, then it can be seen very easily that

1. ρ_{vi}^2 ranges between zero and one for all i in the sense that each of its components does;
2. $\rho_{vi}^2 = 0$ for all i if and only if the error terms for the true and surrogate endpoints are independent within each trial;
3. $\rho_{vi}^2 = 1$ for all i if and only if there exists a deterministic relationship between the error terms for the true and surrogate endpoints within each trial;
4. ρ_{vi}^2 are all equal and reduce to R_{indiv}^2 when both endpoints are measured only once.

Even though all of these properties would support the idea of using ρ_{vi}^2 as a summary measure to evaluate surrogacy at the individual level, a closer look reveals some problems. For instance, for N clinical trials we would have to analyze a set of N canonical correlation vectors $\rho_{v1}^2, \rho_{v2}^2, \ldots, \rho_{vN}^2$ to study surrogacy at the individual level. It is not evident how such an analysis should be carried out and it seems clear that a practical interpretation could be difficult in the absence of a single measure. An extra problem could come from the fact that in general all ρ_{vi}^2 could have a different dimension.

As a possible way out of these problems, we could use a function of ρ_{vi}^2 which, while preserving the properties mentioned before, would summarize the information in just a single, yet meaningful, measure. In general, such a function $\theta = g(x_1, x_2, \ldots, x_p)$, should satisfy

1. $\theta : [0,1]^p \rightarrow [0,1]$;
2. $\theta = g(x_1, x_2, \ldots, x_p) = 0 \Leftrightarrow (x_1, x_2, \ldots, x_p) = 0$;
3. $\theta = g(x_1, x_2, \ldots, x_p) = 1 \Leftrightarrow (x_1, x_2, \ldots, x_p) = 1$;
4. $\theta = g(x, x, \ldots, x) = x$.

If we restrict ourselves to the narrower subclass of linear functions

$$\theta = g(x_1, x_2, \ldots, x_p) = \sum a_i x_i,$$

then it is not difficult to prove that points the four properties above are equivalent to $a_i > 0$ for all i and $\sum a_i = 1$.

Assuming that we dispose of data from several trials, we can now define the following family of parameters to study surrogacy at the individual level

$$\Theta = \left\{ \theta : \theta = \sum_i \sum_k \alpha_{ik} \rho_{ki}^2, \quad \alpha_{ik} > 0 \quad \forall (i,k), \quad \sum_i \sum_k \alpha_{ik} = 1 \right\},$$

where $i = 1, \ldots, N$ denotes the trial and $k = 1, \ldots, p_i$ denotes the designed time points for the trial.

This definition opens some new important questions. A whole family of parameters can now be used to evaluate surrogacy at the individual level. However, it is not clear at this point if there is any relationship between this family and the concepts introduced previously, like the VRF_{indiv} and the R^2_{indiv}. This issue will be investigated in the next section.

14.4.1 Relationship Between VRF, θ, and R^2_{indiv}

At the beginning of this chapter, the VRF was introduced by formula (14.4) to summarize the relationship between both endpoints at the individual level in a multivariate framework. Upon rewriting the matrix MCC_i, given by (14.8), as $MCC_i = P_i^T \Lambda_{\rho i} P_i$, where P_i is an orthogonal matrix and $\Lambda_{\rho i}$ is the diagonal matrix of the squared canonical correlations, it can be shown that

$$\text{VRF}_{\text{indiv}} = \sum_i \sum_k \alpha_{ik}^* \rho_{ki}^2, \tag{14.9}$$

where

$$\alpha_{ik}^* = \frac{(P_i^T \Sigma_{TTi} P_i)_{kk}}{\sum_i \text{tr}(\Sigma_{TTi})}.$$

Here, $(P_i^T \Sigma_{TTi} P_i)_{kk}$ denotes the kth element of the diagonal of matrix $P_i^T \Sigma_{TTi} P_i$. It appears that all coefficients α_{ik}^* are positive and sum to 1. Therefore, VRF is an element of Θ.

This new formulation of VRF, using coefficients α_{ik}^*, is difficult to interpret. In order to obtain a better insight into these coefficients let us denote the canonical variable associated with $\widetilde{\varepsilon}_{T_i}$ as $\widetilde{U}_i$. From canonical correlation analysis it is known that $\widetilde{U}_i = A_i^T \widetilde{\varepsilon}_{T_i}$, where $A_i = \Sigma_{TTi}^{-1/2} P_i$, and that variance-covariance matrix for the canonical variable and the original one is given by $\text{Cov}(\widetilde{\boldsymbol{\varepsilon}}_{T_i}, \widetilde{U}_i) = (A_i^T)^{-1}$. It follows that

$$P_i^T \Sigma_{TTi} P_i = \text{Cov}(\widetilde{\boldsymbol{\varepsilon}}_{T_i}, \widetilde{U}_i)^T \text{cov}(\widetilde{\boldsymbol{\varepsilon}}_{T_i}, \widetilde{U}_i)$$

and, finally,

$$\alpha_{ik}^* = \frac{\sum_l \text{Cov}(\widetilde{\boldsymbol{\varepsilon}}_{T_il}, u_{ik})^2}{\sum_i \text{tr}(\Sigma_{TTi})}.$$

Taking into account that $\text{tr}(\Sigma_{TTi}) = \sum_k \sum_l \text{Cov}(\widetilde{\boldsymbol{\varepsilon}}_{T_il}, u_{ik})^2$, then $\sum_l \text{Cov}(\widetilde{\boldsymbol{\varepsilon}}_{T_il}, u_{ik})^2$ can be interpreted as the part of the total variance of $\widetilde{\boldsymbol{\varepsilon}}_{T_i}$ that is accounted for by the kth canonical variable in the ith trial. Summing over all trials we get

$$\sum_i \text{tr}(\Sigma_{TTi}) = \sum_i \sum_k \sum_l \text{Cov}(\widetilde{\boldsymbol{\varepsilon}}_{T_ik}, u_{il})^2,$$

what can be seen as the total variability of the true endpoint over all trials. Thus, α_{ik}^* can be interpreted as the proportion of the total variability that can be explained by the kth canonical variable for the true endpoint in the ith trial.

Upon noting that ρ_{ki}^2 can also be obtained as the eigenvalue of

$$\Sigma_{TTi}^{-1} \Sigma_{TSi} \Sigma_{SSi}^{-1} \Sigma_{TSi}^T,$$

under model (14.1) we have that

$$\Sigma_{TTi}^{-1} \Sigma_{TSi} \Sigma_{SSi}^{-1} \Sigma_{TSi}^T = \rho_{TSi}^2 I,$$

where I denotes the identity matrix. Thus, the eigenvalues are equal to ρ_{TSi}^2 and the family Θ can be rewritten as

$$\Theta_g = \left\{ \theta : \theta = \sum_i \alpha_i \rho_{TSi}^2, \quad \alpha_i > 0 \quad \forall i, \quad \sum_i \alpha_i = 1 \right\}.$$

Formula (14.5) shows that the VRF for the covariance structure (14.2) is a special member of this family with $\alpha_i = p_i \sigma_{TTi} / \sum_i p_i \sigma_{TTi}$. Thus, the results developed above prove that (14.9) is a generalization of formula (14.5) obtained for the special case in which the covariance structure of the error terms can be modeled by (14.2).

In addition, one easily sees that not only the VRF, as explained before, but in fact all members of Θ, reduce to R_{indiv}^2 in the cross-sectional setting. This result, together with the four property-preserving requirements mentioned previously, ensures that the members of Θ can be used to assess individual-level surrogacy.

Given that Θ can be seen as a *family* of measures to study individual-level surrogacy, Alonso *et al.* (2004b), using either theoretical arguments or appropriate simulation studies, evaluated the operational characteristics of some of members of the family that one might want to consider in practice, including VRF. As a result, they suggested that a very plausible choice in practical situations could be θ_p defined as

$$\theta_p = \sum_i \frac{1}{Np_i} \text{tr}\left[\left(\Sigma_{TTi} - \Sigma_{(T|S)i}\right) \Sigma_{TTi}^{-1}\right]. \tag{14.10}$$

Note that, structurally, both VRF and θ_p are similar, the difference being the reversal of the order of summing the trace and calculating the ratio. Moreover, θ_p has the appealing property of coinciding with Pillai's trace statistic, well-known from classical multivariate analysis. In spite of this strong structural similarity, these parameters have fundamental differences. First, the VRF is not symmetric in S and T. Second, it is only invariant with respect to linear orthogonal transformations. In contrast, θ_p is both symmetric and invariant with respect to the broader class of linear bijective transformations. Based on all of these considerations, Alonso *et al.* (2004b) suggested that θ_p seems to be the preferable choice in the analysis of real problems.

14.5 R^2_Λ and the Likelihood Reduction Factor: A Unifying Approach Based on Prentice's Criteria

One serious drawback of the measures introduced in the previous sections is that they strongly rely on the normality assumption. Their extension to non-normal settings seems to be difficult. In the current section, we will consider an alternative methodology that offers some practical and conceptual advantages and allows a straightforward extension to non-normal settings.

14.5.1 The Measure R^2_Λ

We propose a new parameter, called R^2_Λ, to evaluate surrogacy at the individual level when both responses are measured over time, or when, in general, multivariate or repeated measures are available:

$$R^2_\Lambda = \frac{1}{N}\sum_i (1-\Lambda_i), \tag{14.11}$$

where

$$\Lambda_i = \frac{|\Sigma_i|}{|\Sigma_{TTi}|\cdot|\Sigma_{SSi}|}. \tag{14.12}$$

First, let us note that R^2_Λ is defined, based on Wilks' Lambda statistic used in multivariate analysis. It involves the determinants of the variance-covariance matrices. Therefore, all the elements of the covariance structure are used when calculating (14.11). This is in contrast to (14.4) and (14.10), which only use the information in the diagonal of the matrices describing the association between both endpoints, what makes them likely less informative.

It is possible to show that

1. R^2_Λ is symmetric and invariant with respect to linear bijective transformations;
2. R^2_Λ ranges between zero and one;
3. $R^2_\Lambda = 0$ if and only if $(\widetilde{\boldsymbol{\varepsilon}}_{T_i}, \widetilde{\boldsymbol{\varepsilon}}_{S_i})$ are independent for all i;
4. $R^2_\Lambda = 1$ if and only if for all i there exist a_i, b_i such that $a_i^T\widetilde{\boldsymbol{\varepsilon}}_{T_i} = b_i^T\widetilde{\boldsymbol{\varepsilon}}_{S_i}$ with probability one;
5. $R^2_\Lambda = R^2_{ind}$ in the cross-sectional case.

These properties are essentially the same as those satisfied by VRF, θ_p, and all of the members of the Θ family. However, the fourth property makes an important difference between the new proposal and the previous ones. Whereas the elements of Θ take the value 1 only when there is a deterministic relationship between both endpoints, $R^2_\Lambda = 1$ whenever there is a deterministic relationship between two linear combinations of both endpoints. This allows us to detect strong associations in situations where VRF or θ_p would fail to do so.

Here again, using canonical correlation ideas, it is possible to define an entire family of parameters to study surrogacy at the individual level, so that R^2_Λ is just a special member of this family:

$$\Theta_\Lambda = \left\{\theta_\Lambda : \theta_\Lambda = 1 - \sum_{i=1}^{N}\alpha_i\prod_{k=1}^{p_i}(1-\rho^2_{ik}), \quad \alpha_i > 0 \quad \forall i, \quad \sum_i \alpha_i = 1\right\}.$$

14.5.2 Relationship Between R^2_Λ and θ_P

It might be worthwhile to make a connection between the parameters defined previously ($\text{VRF}_{\text{indiv}}$, θ_p) and R^2_Λ.

Let us first consider the special case defined by model (14.2). Under this model, the variance-covariance matrix of the error vectors is "decomposed" into two basic components, describing the association between sequences of repeated measurements (Σ_i) and within the sequences (R_i). These two components are then put together using the Kronecker product. It is easy to show that under this assumption (separability for the covariance structure)

$$\begin{aligned} \theta_P &= \frac{1}{N}\sum_i \rho^2_{TSi}, \\ R^2_\Lambda &= 1 - \frac{1}{N}\sum_i (1-\rho^2_{TSi})^{p_i}, \end{aligned}$$

where $\rho^2_{TSi} = \sigma_{TSi}/\sigma_{TTi}\sigma_{SSi}$.

Taking into account that

$$(1-\rho^2_{TSi})^{p_i} = (1-\rho^2_{TSi}) + (1-\rho^2_{TSi})\{(1-\rho^2_{TSi})^{p_i-1} - 1\},$$

we obtain

$$R^2_\Lambda = \theta_P + \frac{1}{N}\sum_i (1-\rho^2_{TSi})\{1-(1-\rho^2_{TSi})^{p_i-1}\}. \qquad (14.13)$$

Formula (14.13) clearly shows that θ_P can be seen as an approximation to R^2_Λ when the second part of the sum on the right-hand side of the equation is negligible.

Moreover, as

$$\frac{1}{N}\sum_i (1-\rho^2_{TSi})\{1-(1-\rho^2_{TSi})^{p_i-1}\} \geq 0,$$

we have

$$\theta_P \leq R^2_\Lambda. \qquad (14.14)$$

The equality in (14.14) is obtained for the following, special cases:

1. $p_i = 1$ for all i, which is just the cross-sectional setting, when both proposals reduce to R^2_{ind};
2. $\rho^2_{TSi} = 0$ for all i, in which case $(\widetilde{\varepsilon}_{T_i}, \widetilde{\varepsilon}_{S_i})$ are independent and $R^2_\Lambda = \theta_p = 0$;

3. $\rho^2_{TSi} = 1$ for all i, what implies a deterministic relationship between $\widetilde{\boldsymbol{\varepsilon}}_{T_i}$ and $\widetilde{\boldsymbol{\varepsilon}}_{S_i}$ and, as a consequence, $R^2_\Lambda = \theta_p = 1$.

If we now consider a completely general framework, where the separability assumption does not necessarily hold, then it is easy to see that for all θ_Λ in Θ_Λ we have

$$\begin{aligned}\theta_\Lambda &= \sum_{i=1}^{N}\sum_{h=1}^{p_i}\frac{\alpha_i}{p_i}\rho^2_{ih} + \sum_{i=1}^{N}\sum_{k=1}^{p_i}\frac{\alpha_i}{p_i}(1-\rho^2_{ik})\left(1-\prod_{h\neq k}(1-\rho^2_{ih})\right)\\ &= \theta + \sum_{i=1}^{N}\sum_{k=1}^{p_i}\frac{\alpha_i}{p_i}(1-\rho^2_{ik})\left(1-\prod_{h\neq k}(1-\rho^2_{ih})\right). \qquad (14.15)\end{aligned}$$

Expression (14.15) allows to conclude that any θ_Λ in Θ_Λ can be approximated by a θ in Θ, as long as the last term in the sum at the right-hand side of (14.15) is negligible.

It can be noted that, as

$$\sum_{i=1}^{N}\sum_{k=1}^{p_i}\frac{\alpha_i}{p_i}(1-\rho^2_{ik})\left(1-\prod_{h\neq k}(1-\rho^2_{ih})\right) \geq 0,$$

(14.15) indicates that for all θ_Λ in Θ_Λ there exists θ in Θ such, that

$$\theta \leq \theta_\Lambda. \qquad (14.16)$$

Thus, we can conclude that (14.14) holds in general, and not only under the separability assumption implied by (14.2).

14.5.3 The Likelihood Reduction Factor

Buyse *et al.* (2000a) considered the case of normally distributed surrogate and true endpoints and proposed assessing the validity of the surrogate at the individual level using the coefficient of determination R^2_{indiv}, which is the square of the correlation between the surrogate and the true endpoints after adjusting for treatment and trial effects (see Chapter 7). In earlier work, different measures of the association between the surrogate and the true endpoint were used in different settings. For instance, when both endpoints of a failure time type, Burzykowski *et al.* (2001) use Kendall's τ (see also Chapter 11). On the other hand, when the true endpoint is a failure time and the surrogate is a longitudinal sequence, Renard *et al.* (2002) propose to use $R^2_{\text{indiv}}(t) = \text{Corr}[W_1(t), W_2(t)]^2$, where $[W_1(t), W_2(t)]$ is a latent bivariate Gaussian process (see Chapter 13). Note that, in the latter case, the value of the coefficient depends on time. Other proposals have been suggested in other settings.

All of these examples clearly show one of the main limitations of the meta-analytic approach so far: different settings require different definitions for the surrogacy measures. In some of these settings, it has even been proposed to estimate the association between both endpoints at a latent level, which could be clinically less relevant or, at least, difficult to interpret.

It is possible, however, to develop a more general procedure, which allows to evaluate surrogacy at the individual level in very general settings. By way of illustration, let us consider the two following two generalized linear models for trial i:

$$g_T\{E(T_{ij})\} = \mu_{T_i} + \beta_i Z_{ij}, \tag{14.17}$$

$$g_{T|S}\{E(T_{ij}|S_{ij})\} = \gamma_{0i} + \gamma_{1i} Z_{ij} + \gamma_{2i} S_{ij}, \tag{14.18}$$

where g_T and $g_{T|S}$ are two link functions, linking the expected values $E(T_{ij})$ and $E(T_{ij}|S_{ij})$, respectively, to the linear predictors. In general, other more complex settings could be analyzed in a very similar way using the methodology that will be described below. It is also possible to consider models that assume non-linear relationships between S and $E(T|S)$, such as, for instance,

$$g_{T|S}\{E(T_{ij}|S_{ij})\} = \gamma_{0i} + \gamma_{1i} Z_{ij} + f(S_{ij}).$$

If we further consider the log-likelihood ratio test statistic, G_i^2 say, to compare (14.17) and (14.18) for trial i, then one could quantify the association between both endpoints at the individual level using the *Likelihood Reduction Factor* (LRF) defined as

$$LRF = 1 - \frac{1}{N}\sum_i \exp\left(-\frac{G_i^2}{n_i}\right). \tag{14.19}$$

Following ideas in Kent *et al.* (1983), one can think of (14.19) as a sample estimate of a general measure of association between both endpoints based on the information gain about the true endpoint, by using the surrogate. It is also possible to show that

1. LRF is always between 0 and 1;

2. $LRF = 0$ if the surrogate and the true endpoints are independent in each trial;

3. if, for continuous outcomes, $LRF \to 1$, then there is degeneracy present in the true joint distribution of S and T in each trial, which often implies a deterministic relationship between both variables;

4. when both endpoints are longitudinal, LRF becomes R^2_Λ defined in (14.11);

5. for two univariate normally distributed endpoints, LRF reduces to R^2_{indiv}.

It is worth noting that (14.18) is the model corresponding to the fourth criterion (5.10), proposed by Prentice (1989). The criterion thus comes back to play a key role in the unifying procedure quantifying the individual-level surrogacy using LRF. One of the most appealing characteristics of this procedure is that we can avoid the fitting of complicated joint models for the surrogate and the true endpoints. Models like (14.17) and (14.18) can usually be fitted using standard commercial software. This formulation also allows to generalize both the Prentice (1989) and Buyse *et al.* (2000a) methodologies, bridging the gap between both paradigms.

14.6 Analysis of Case Studies

In this section, we apply the proposed definitions to two case studies. The first one is the meta-analysis of five double-blind randomized clinical trials, comparing the effects of risperidone to conventional antipsychotic agents for the treatment of chronic schizophrenia (Section 4.2.6). The second one is the clinical trial for patients with age-related macular degeneration (Section 4.2.1).

14.6.1 Study in Schizophrenia

The meta-analysis contains five trials. This is insufficient to apply the meta-analytic methods described in previous chapters, in line with findings reported in Buyse *et al.* (2000a), where it is shown that a sufficient amount of replication at all levels is necessary to identify all of the variance components, preferably with a decent amount of precision (see also Chapter 8). Fortunately, in all the trials information is also available on the countries where patients were treated. Hence, we can use country within trial as a unit of analysis. A total of 20 units are thus available for analysis, with the number of patients ranging from 9 to 128. The number of patients per country is tabulated in Table 14.1. We consider Clinician's Global Impres-

TABLE 14.1. *Meta-analysis in schizophrenia. Number of patients and measurements per country-unit.*

Country Id	1	2	3	4	5	6	7	8	9	10
No. patients	31	29	26	44	44	9	37	32	68	49
Country Id	11	12	13	14	15	16	17	18	19	20
No. patients	43	21	25	39	36	17	33	69	30	128

sion scale (CGI) as our primary measure (true endpoint), while we treat PANSS as a surrogate (see Section 4.2.6 for a short description of these scales). Admittedly, this is not a standard situation for surrogate validation due to the lack of a clear "gold standard." Our analysis does allow us to address some very important issues. At the trial level, it will allow a flexible assessment of a common question among practitioners, i.e., how a treatment effect on PANSS can be translated into a treatment effect on CGI, which is easier to interpret clinically. On the other hand, at the individual level it will allow us to estimate the accuracy with which CGI could be estimated or predicted from PANSS.

For most patients, measurements of CGI and PANSS at six different occasions were available. In units 9 and 10, only five measurements were collected.

In our analysis, rather than using the original observations, we use linearly transformed outcomes with a non-linear transformation of time (ξ) to stabilize the variances:

$$\begin{aligned} T &= -3.63495 + 0.8538 \times \text{CGI}, \\ S &= -3.5675 + 0.04484 \times \text{PANSS}, \\ \xi_{new} &= e^{-\xi/4}. \end{aligned}$$

From graphical inspection (not shown), it follows that the transformed data have approximately a stable variance and normal distribution.

We applied the two-stage approach, introduced in Chapter 7, to these data. Model (14.1), with a linear trend over time, $g_{T_{ij}}(\xi) = \gamma_{T_{ij}}\xi$ and $g_{S_{ij}}(\xi) = \gamma_{S_{ij}}\xi$, turned out to be the best choice after a model selection procedure where the most complex model considered was a random spline approach (Verbyla *et al.* 1999, Alonso *et al.* 2004c). Figure 14.1 shows the estimated variances of T ($\hat{\sigma}_{TTi}$) and S ($\hat{\sigma}_{SSi}$), correlation coefficients for the T–S correlation, as well as the correlation parameter ρ_i, corresponding to the correlation matrix (14.3), separately for each unit. The figure shows that the assumption of a constant covariance structure over all trials is not plausible, justifying the use of a more general paradigm.

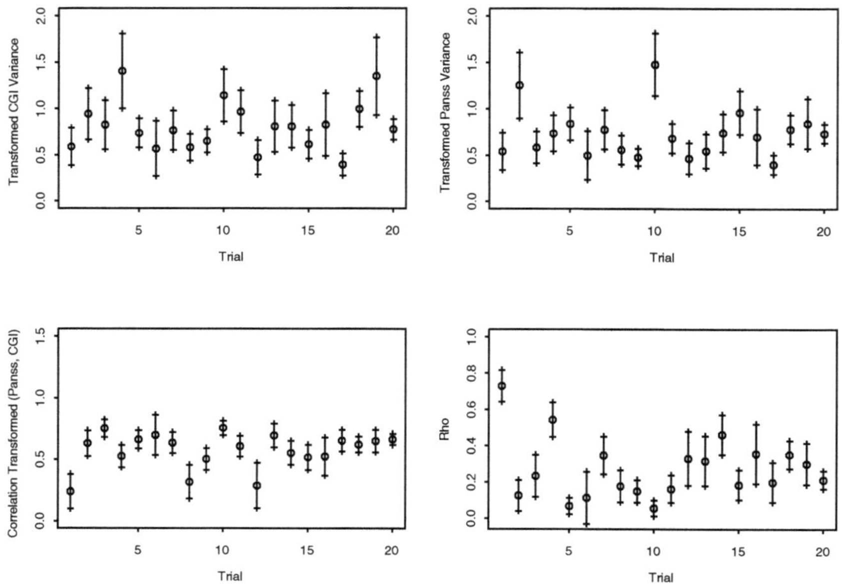

FIGURE 14.1. *Meta-analysis in schizophrenia. Variance-covariance parameters per trial.*

If we want to study the relationship between T and S, it is clear that R^2_{indiv} measure proposed by Buyse *et al.* (2000a) is no longer applicable due to the longitudinal nature of the data, while the corresponding measure at the trial level still is. The results are reported in Table 14.2.

Clearly, the association at the trial level is very strong. At the individual level, several observations can be made. First, the association at the individual level is much weaker than at the trial level: both VRF and θ_p suggest that about 35–36% of the variability in one outcome is explained by the other. However, a much stronger association is indicated by the estimated value of $R^2_\Lambda = 0.85$, in agreement with inequalities (14.14)–(14.16). This discrepancy might point to the potential of a nearly deterministic relationship between two linear combinations of both endpoints, which could not be captured by neither VRF nor θ_p. It is worth stressing the importance of this possibility: the low values of VRF and θ_p suggest that an accurate prediction of CGI given PANSS at each time point is not possible, but the large value of R^2_Λ implies that it might be possible to construct linear summary statistics of the measurements for the two endpoints that could be highly correlated. On the scale defined by these linear transformations, PANSS might have a high predictive value for CGI. Second, a less desirable side effect of the VRF definition is its asymmetry. As indicated earlier, while the difference between $VRF(S,T)$ and $VRF(T,S)$ is not dramatic in this case, it cannot be excluded that more worrying differences might

TABLE 14.2. *Meta-analysis in schizophrenia. Trial-level and individual-level validation measures.*

Parameter	Estimate	95% C.I.
Trial-level measures		
$R^2_{\text{trial}}(T,S)$	0.866	[0.668, 0.942]
$R^2_{\text{trial}}(S,T)$	0.820	[0.611, 0.920]
Individual-level measures		
$VRF(T,S)$	0.363	[0.335, 0.391]
$VRF(S,T)$	0.365	[0.336, 0.394]
θ_p	0.349	[0.324, 0.375]
$LRF = R^2_\Lambda$	0.85	[0.81, 0.88]

be seen in different sets of data. In contrast, θ_p and R^2_Λ are symmetric and therefore more appealing in a situation like the current one, where one could argue that both endpoints are actually in a symmetric relationship to one other. Indeed, there is no consensus as to whether either CGI or PANSS should be considered the gold standard. Thus, in this setting, the use of a symmetric measure to assess the individual-level surrogacy would be recommended (see also Chapter 16).

Figure 14.2 displays a graphical summary of the previous analysis. The upper-left panel shows the association between estimates of treatment effects $\gamma_{T_{ij}}$ and $\gamma_{S_{ij}}$ at the trial level, with the different sizes of the points accounting for the different sample sizes of the units. It is clear from this picture that a reliable prediction of the treatment effect on CGI, given the treatment effect on PANSS, seems to be possible. The other panels show the behavior of VRF, θ_p and R^2_Λ per unit, as well as their overall values. The similarities between VRF and θ_p panels are noticeable, but this is not surprising, since they are both special members of the same family Θ.

14.6.2 Age-related Macular Degeneration Trial

We now illustrate the use of the LRF in the analysis of the ARMD data set (Section 4.2.1). In this study, the true endpoint (visual acuity at 1 year, T), as well as the surrogate (visual acuity at 6 months, S) are binary outcomes. To obtain an estimate for LRF, the following three models need to be fitted separately to the data:

$$\text{logit}(\pi^T_{ij}) = \mu_{T_i} + \beta_i Z_{ij}, \tag{14.20}$$

$$\text{logit}(\pi^{T|S}_{ij}) = \mu^S_{T_i} + \beta^S_i Z_{ij} + \gamma_{ij}\text{vis6}_{ij}, \tag{14.21}$$

$$\text{logit}(\pi^S_{ij}) = \mu_{S_i} + \alpha_i Z_{ij}. \tag{14.22}$$

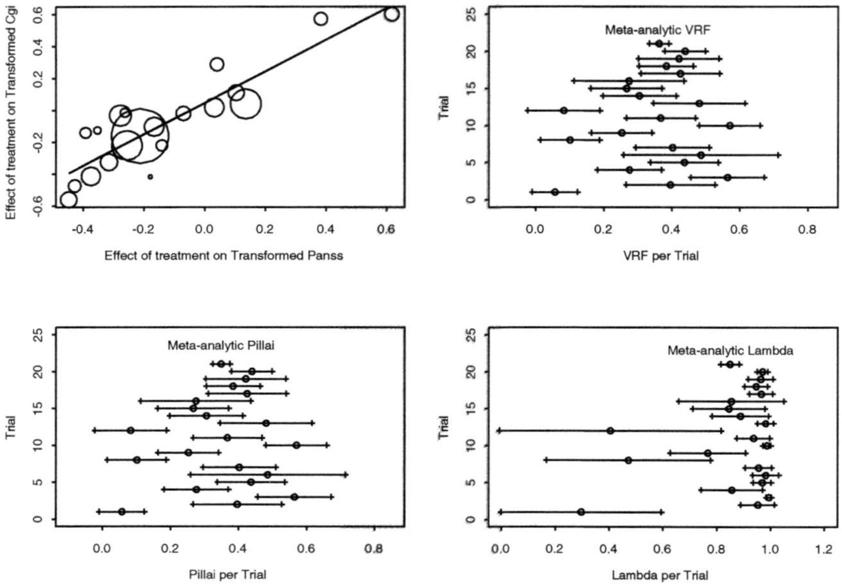

FIGURE 14.2. *Meta-analysis in schizophrenia. Summary of the meta-analytic approach.*

In (14.20)–(14.22), we use the notation $\pi_{ij}^T = \mathrm{E}(T_{ij})$, $\pi_{ij}^{T|S} = \mathrm{E}(T_{ij}|S_{ij})$, and $\pi_{ij}^S = \mathrm{E}(S_{ij})$.

At the trial level, surrogacy can be evaluated by computing the coefficient of determination R^2_{trial} using the estimated values of $(\mu_{S_i}, \alpha_i, \beta_i)$, obtained from models (14.20)–(14.22). At the individual level, however, R^2_{indiv} can no longer be used but fortunately LRF can be used instead. Assuming that the association between both variables is constant across trials, (14.20)–(14.21) can be used to compute LRF as

$$LRF = 1 - \exp\left(-\frac{G^2}{n}\right),$$

where G^2 is the log-likelihood ratio statistic to compare models (14.20) and (14.21), and $n = \sum n_i$ is the total number of patients.

Note that, as pointed out by Kent *et al.* (1983), if the true endpoint has a fixed discrete distribution and if the conditional distribution of the true endpoint given the surrogate is modeled by a family of discrete distributions, then the conditional information gain and hence LRF is bounded above by a number strictly less than one. This motivates reporting the value of $LRF_{\text{adj}} = LRF/\max(LRF)$, which can always reach one and hence is more meaningful. Table 14.3 shows the results of the analysis for both the trial and individual levels.

TABLE 14.3. *Age-related macular degeneration trial. Validation measures for the binary-binary case.*

Parameter	Estimate	95% C.I.
R^2_{Trial}	0.384	[0.149, 0.614]
LRF	0.265	[0.221, 0.370]
LRF_{adj}	0.495	[0.325, 0.604]

All of the estimated values are too low to make visual acuity at 6 months a reliable surrogate for visual acuity at 12 months. At the trial level, $R^2_{\text{trial}} = 0.38$ clearly showing that an accurate prediction of treatment effect at one year based on the treatment effect observed at 6 months does not seem to be possible. At the individual level, LRF_{adj} also provides evidence of a weak association. These results are similar to those reported by Molenberghs, Geys, and Buyse (2001) and presented in Chapter 6, who used a joint bivariate probit model based on latent variables. They reported a lower association at the trial level ($R^2_{\text{trial}} = 0.22$) and a stronger relationship at the individual level ($R^2_{\text{indiv}} = 0.64$). Nevertheless, these coefficients describe the association at an unobservable latent scale, rendering their interpretation more awkward than in the proposal made in this chapter.

14.7 Discussion

In this chapter, we have approached the problem of surrogate endpoint validation using repeated measurements. This is a setting frequently occurring in practice; a setting also where the R^2 measures originally proposed by Buyse *et al.* (2000a) are no longer applicable. We have proposed several alternative measures, from which R^2_{trial} and R^2_{indiv} result as special cases. Moreover, we have introduced a new measure, the likelihood reduction factor, which, unlike R^2_{indiv}, applies to a wide variety of settings (normal, binary, categorical, survival, and longitudinal outcomes) and reduces to R^2_{indiv} for normally distributed endpoints. It can also be linked to both the Prentice (1989) and Buyse *et al.* (2000a) validation methods, bridging the gap between the two approaches. It is also worth noting that R^2_{Λ}, which corresponds to LRF in the longitudinal setting, has the ability to detect stronger associations between both endpoints, which might go unnoticed when other, more conventional, methods are applied.

Finally, and in spite of the appeal of these methodological developments, we would like to emphasize that surrogate endpoint validation should never be done purely on statistical grounds, as important clinical and biological considerations should be factored into the decision.

15

Bayesian Evaluation of Surrogate Endpoints

Ziv Shkedy and Franz Torres Barbosa

15.1 Introduction

In randomized clinical trials, the main interest lies in assessing the effect of treatment (Z) on the primary ("true") endpoint (T). However, as outlined in Chapters 2 and 5, there are cases where the use of the endpoint may be difficult due to, for example, high measurement costs or a long observation time. This happens, for example, when the primary endpoint is time to event. In these cases, one might benefit from using a "surrogate" endpoint (S) that would allow to determine the treatment effect quicker or in a less expensive way.

In his landmark paper, Prentice (1989) proposed a formal definition of a surrogate endpoint and suggested operational criteria for its validation in the case of a single trial and single surrogate. (See also Chapters 5 and 19.) According to the definition, a surrogate endpoint is a random variable for which a test for the null hypothesis of no treatment effect is also a valid test for the corresponding null hypothesis for the true endpoint. In view of some limitations of Prentice's criteria, Freedman, Graubard, and Schatzkin (1992) proposed to use the proportion of treatment effect explained by the surrogate endpoint as a measure of the validity of a potential surrogate. Several authors have pointed towards drawbacks of the measure. For instance, De Gruttola *et al.* (1997) and Buyse and Molenberghs (1998) have shown that the proportion of treatment effect explained by the surrogate is not truly a proportion, as it is not restricted to the $[0, 1]$ interval. As an alternative, Buyse and Molenberghs (1998) proposed to replace the proportion of treatment effect explained by the surrogate by two measures closely related to it: the relative effect and the adjusted association. The first one, defined at the population level, is the ratio of the overall treatment effect on the true endpoint over that on the surrogate endpoint. The second one is the individual-level association between both endpoints, after accounting for the effect of treatment.

In this chapter, we focus on the meta-analytic approach, that is, the situation when a potential surrogate is evaluated using data from multiple, say N, trials. We further assume that the distribution of the true and surrogate endpoint come from the exponential family and that true treatment effects on the endpoints are given by

$$\begin{aligned} g[E(S_{ij}|Z_{ij}=1)] - g[E(S_{ij}|Z_{ij}=0)] &= \alpha_i, \\ g[E(T_{ij}|Z_{ij}=1)] - g[E(T_{ij}|Z_{ij}=0)] &= \beta_i, \end{aligned} \tag{15.1}$$

where $g(\cdot)$ denotes an appropriate link function, i indexes trials, and j indexes patients within trials. Within the meta-analytic or hierarchical approach, the first goal is to establish the association between β_i and α_i, to assess the quality of the surrogate at the trial level. To this aim, the precision of the prediction of the treatment effect on the true endpoint β_i from the effect on the surrogate α_i should be assessed. This can be achieved by formulating a model for the joint distribution of treatment effects $[\alpha_i, \beta_i]$ (where $[\cdot]$ is shorthand for the corresponding distribution), or a model of the conditional distribution $[\beta_i|\alpha_i]$. Note that a joint model $[\alpha_i, \beta_i]$ imposes a conditional model for $[\beta_i|\alpha_i]$. The second goal is to assess the quality of the surrogate at the individual level, i.e., the precision of the prediction of the true endpoint from the surrogate for an individual patient. This can be evaluated from the strength of the association between the two endpoints in the joint distribution of S_{ij} and T_{ij} given Z_{ij}, $[T_{ij}, S_{ij}|Z_{ij}]$.

The evaluation of a surrogate endpoint within the meta-analytic setting has been discussed, among others, by Daniels and Hughes (1997), Buyse *et al.* (2000a), and Gail *et al.* (2000). (See also Chapters 7 and 9.) All of these authors considered a multiple-trial setting with normally distributed true and surrogate endpoints and proposed a two-stage model for the evaluation of the potential surrogate. Daniels and Hughes (1997) only used summary data from the trials. They formulated a hierarchical Bayesian model for the estimated treatment effects $(\hat{\alpha}_i, \hat{\beta}_i)$, in which the joint distribution of the estimated effects was specified at the first stage and the conditional distribution of $[\beta_i|\alpha_i]$ was specified at the second stage. Buyse *et al.* (2000a) assumed the availability of individual patient data and formulated a two-stage model, with the joint distribution $[T_{ij}, S_{ij}|Z_{ij}]$ specified at the first stage and the joint distribution of the treatment effects $[\beta_i, \alpha_i]$ specified at the second stage. A simplified version of the two-stage model was proposed by Tibaldi *et al.* (2003), who used a bivariate approach within the meta-analytic framework to evaluate surrogacy from the conditional distribution $[\hat{\beta}_i|\hat{\alpha}_i]$. Simplified strategies are discussed in Section 7.4.2 and, for survival type endpoints, in Section 11.7. The advantage of the model proposed by Daniels and Hughes (1997) is that one does not need to specify the joint distribution of T_{ij} and S_{ij}. However, the price for this advantage is that the quality of the individual-level surrogacy cannot be assessed, a possibility retained in the approach developed by Buyse *et al.* (2000a).

In this chapter, we consider the Bayesian approach under the assumption that individual data are available. In Section 15.2, we discuss two bivariate approaches for meta-analytic data proposed by McIntosh (1996) and van Houwelingen, Arends, and Stijnen (2002). We then make a link (Section 15.3) between these and the model proposed by Daniels and Hughes (1997, see also Chapter 17) for the evaluation of surrogate endpoints. Moreover, we review the two-stage model proposed by Buyse *et al.* (2000a). In Section 15.4, we formulate a fully Bayesian hierarchical model for the surrogate endpoints validation corresponding to the model of Buyse *et al.* (2000a). Results of an application of the model to two case studies are presented in Section 15.5. Section 15.6 is devoted to a simulation study, in which the performance of the hierarchical Bayesian model is evaluated (see also Shkedy *et al.* 2003).

15.2 Bivariate Models for Meta-analytic Data

Consider a clinical trial in which treatment effects were estimated for the surrogate and the true endpoints. Let S_{ij} be the surrogate measurement of the jth subject, $j = 1, \ldots, n_i$, in trial i, $i = 1, \ldots, N$. We denote the measurement for the true endpoint by T_{ij}. For simplicity, we assume that subjects were randomized into two treatment groups. Let Z_{ij} be an indicator variable which takes the value of 1 if the subject was randomized to the treatment group and 0 otherwise. Finally, we denote by $\hat{\alpha}_i$ and $\hat{\beta}_i$ the maximum likelihood (ML) estimates of the treatment effects for the surrogate and the true endpoints, respectively, in trial i.

In this section, we review a two-stage bivariate model for the treatment effects proposed by McIntosh (1996). As a special case of McIntosh's modeling strategy, we also discuss the bivariate approach to the analysis of meta-analytic data proposed by van Houwelingen, Arends, and Stijnen (2002). The latter was developed for the case where individual data are not available.

15.2.1 The Two-stage Model of McIntosh (1996)

In the context of the multivariate approach within the meta-analytic framework, McIntosh (1996) discusses a bivariate model for the measurement error of a bivariate vector of maximum-likelihood estimates of the trial-specific treatment effects. Specifically, he assumes that the estimated treatment effects follow a bivariate normal distribution, i.e., that the measurement error model is given by

$$\begin{pmatrix} \hat{\alpha}_i \\ \hat{\beta}_i \end{pmatrix} \sim N\left[\begin{pmatrix} a_i \\ b_i \end{pmatrix}, \Omega_i\right], \qquad i = 1, \ldots N, \tag{15.2}$$

where

$$\Omega_i = \begin{pmatrix} \sigma^2_{a_i} & \rho_i \sigma^2_{a_i} \sigma^2_{b_i} \\ \rho_i \sigma_{a_i^2} \sigma^2_{b_i} & \sigma^2_{b_i} \end{pmatrix}.$$

Here, a_i and b_i are the true trial-specific treatment effects and Ω_i is the variance-covariance matrix of the maximum likelihood estimates. This matrix accounts for the within-trial variability and the possible correlation between $\hat{\alpha}_i$ and $\hat{\beta}_i$. McIntosh (1996) further assumes a structural model for the true treatment effects in which b_i linearly depends on a_i,

$$\begin{cases} b_i \sim N[b + \beta_b(a_i - a), \tau_b^2], \\ a_i \sim N(a, \tau_a^2). \end{cases} \tag{15.3}$$

Note that (15.3) implies a bivariate distribution for a_i and b_i and that the structural model can be rewritten as

$$\begin{pmatrix} a_i \\ b_i \end{pmatrix} \sim N\left[\begin{pmatrix} a \\ b \end{pmatrix}, D\right], \tag{15.4}$$

with variance-covariance matrix given by

$$D = \begin{pmatrix} \tau_a^2 & \beta_b \tau_a^2 \\ \beta_b \tau_a^2 & \tau_b^2 + \beta_b^2 \tau_a^2 \end{pmatrix}.$$

Combining the measurement error model (15.2) with the structural model (15.4), results in the marginal distribution of $\hat{\alpha}_i$ and $\hat{\beta}_i$

$$\begin{pmatrix} \hat{\alpha}_i \\ \hat{\beta}_i \end{pmatrix} \sim N\left[\begin{pmatrix} a \\ b \end{pmatrix}, D + \Omega_i\right]. \tag{15.5}$$

15.2.2 The Model of van Houwelingen, Arends, and Stijnen (2002)

A modification of (15.2) was given in van Houwelingen, Arends, and Stijnen (2002), who assumed the same measurement error model but with a diagonal variance-covariance matrix Ω_i. It was further assumed that the true trial-specific treatment effects, (a_i, b_i), were normally distributed with unstructured variance-covariance matrix. Hence, the structural model is

$$\begin{pmatrix} a_i \\ b_i \end{pmatrix} \sim N\left[\begin{pmatrix} a \\ b \end{pmatrix}, D\right], \qquad \text{with} \qquad D = \begin{pmatrix} d_{aa} & d_{ab} \\ d_{ab} & d_{bb} \end{pmatrix}. \tag{15.6}$$

The two variance-covariance matrices D and Ω_i cannot be estimated separately. In practice, van Houwelingen, Arends, and Stijnen (2002) assumed Ω_i to be known, replaced it by an estimate $\hat{\Omega}_i$, and kept it fixed during the estimation process. The primary interest is placed on the covariance matrix D since, as discussed in van Houwelingen, Arends, and Stijnen (2002, p. 601), it determines the bivariate relationship between the true treatment effects a_i and b_i. Note that, in contrast to the variance-covariance matrix in (15.2), the matrix in the structural model (15.6) is kept unstructured. That is because the conditional distribution of $[b_i|a_i]$ is not formulated in advance. But the distribution can easily be derived from (15.6). For example, the slope of the regression line of b_i on a_i is equal to d_{ab}/d_{aa}, while the residual variance equals $d_{bb} - d_{ab}^2/d_{aa}$. The residual variance is minimized when $d_{bb} = d_{ab}^2/d_{aa}$, i.e., when $R^2 = d_{ab}^2/d_{aa}d_{bb}$ is equal to 1.

15.3 Models for the Validation of Surrogate Endpoints Using Meta-analytic Data

In this section, we describe two models proposed for the validation of surrogate endpoints using data from multiple randomized trials. The first is the hierarchical Bayesian model of Daniels and Hughes (1997). The second is the two-stage model of Buyse *et al.* (2000a). The model of Daniels and Hughes (1997) was developed for the case where individual data are not available. Therefore, it focuses on the joint distribution of the maximum likelihood estimates for the treatment effects $\hat{\alpha}_i$ and $\hat{\beta}_i$. The model formulated by Buyse *et al.* (2000a) assumes that individual data are available and focuses on the joint distributions of $[T_{ij}, S_{ij}|Z_{ij}]$ and $[\alpha_i, \beta_i]$.

15.3.1 The Hierarchical Bayesian Model of Daniels and Hughes (1997)

Daniels and Hughes (1997) developed a meta-analytic approach for the evaluation of surrogate endpoints. They focus on the distribution of the maximum likelihood estimates for the trial-specific treatment effects for the surrogate and true endpoints. The estimates are assumed to be correlated, and the same measurement error model as in (15.2) is postulated. A simple linear association between the true treatment effects is assumed and modeled by means of the conditional distribution of $[b_i|a_i]$:

$$b_i \sim \mathrm{N}(\theta + \gamma a_i, \tau_b^2) \qquad i = 1, 2, \ldots, N. \qquad (15.7)$$

In contrast with MacIntosh (1996), the true treatment effect on the surrogate a_i is assumed to be a fixed effect. Under this assumption, the marginal model in (15.5) can be rewritten as

$$\begin{pmatrix} \hat{\alpha}_i \\ \hat{\beta}_i \end{pmatrix} \sim N\left[\begin{pmatrix} a_i \\ \theta + \gamma a_i \end{pmatrix}, \begin{pmatrix} \sigma^2_{a_i} & \rho_i \sigma^2_{a_i} \sigma^2_{b_i} \\ \rho_i \sigma^2_{a_i} \sigma^2_{b_i} & \sigma^2_{b_i} + \tau^2_b \end{pmatrix}\right]. \tag{15.8}$$

Note that the above model, with the additional assumption that a_i is a normally distributed random, rather than fixed, effect is identical to the model of McIntosh (1996).

It is also worth noting here that Daniels and Hughes (1997) and van Houwelingen, Arends, and Stijnen (2002) approach the same problem from opposite directions. van Houwelingen, Arends, and Stijnen (2002) specify the joint distribution of $[a_i, b_i]$, and hence the marginal distribution of $[\hat{\alpha}_i, \hat{\beta}_i]$), and derive the conditional distribution $[b_i|a_i]$ from it. Daniels and Hughes (1997), on the other hand, explicitly specify the conditional distribution $[b_i|a_i]$ and derive from it the marginal distribution of $[\hat{\alpha}_i, \hat{\beta}_i]$. The two approaches treat the variance-covariance matrix Ω_i, which represents the within-trial variablity, in a similar way. Because neither approach uses individual data for the estimation of D (van Houwelingen, Arends, and Stijnen 2002) or τ_b (Daniels and Hughes 1997), the matrix Ω_i is kept fixed during the estimation procedure.

In the approach of Daniels and Hughes (1997), the trial-level surrogacy is evaluated using the posterior means of the parameters in (15.7). In the hierarchical model discussed above, γ measures the association between the surrogate and the true endpoints. Indeed, $\gamma = 0$ implies that S cannot be surrogate to T. Furthermore, the case that $\gamma \neq 0$ and $\tau^2_b = 0$ implies a deterministic relationship between the treatment effects, i.e., given a_i, γ, and θ, we can predict b_i in a perfect fashion. In this case, one can call S a "perfect surrogate" for T at the trial level. Moreover, if $\theta = 0$, $\gamma \neq 0$, and $\tau^2_b = 0$, the surrogate endpoint fulfills the definition of Prentice (1992): no treatment effect on the surrogate endpoint implies no treatment effect on the true endpoint.

15.3.2 The Two-stage Model of Buyse et al. *(2000a)*

The Full Model

Buyse *et al.* (2000a) proposed a two-stage model in which the linear predictors of the true and the surrogate endpoints are given by

$$\begin{cases} E(S_{ij}|Z_{ij}) = \mu_{Si} + \alpha_i Z_{ij}, \\ E(T_{ij}|Z_{ij}) = \mu_{Ti} + \beta_i Z_{ij}. \end{cases} \tag{15.9}$$

Here, α_i and β_i are trial-specific fixed treatment effects, μ_{S_i} and μ_{Ti} are trial-specific fixed intercepts. Model (15.9) is termed a "full fixed-effects" model. It is further assumed that the two endpoints are normally distributed,

$$\begin{pmatrix} S_{ij} \\ T_{ij} \end{pmatrix} \sim N\left[\begin{pmatrix} \mu_{S_i} + \alpha_i Z_{ij} \\ \mu_{T_i} + \beta_i Z_{ij} \end{pmatrix}, \Sigma\right], \tag{15.10}$$

where Σ is given by

$$\Sigma = \begin{pmatrix} \sigma_{SS} & \sigma_{ST} \\ \sigma_{ST} & \sigma_{TT} \end{pmatrix}. \tag{15.11}$$

At the second stage of the model, it is assumed that

$$\begin{cases} \mu_{Si} = \mu_S + m_{S_i}, \\ \mu_{Ti} = \mu_T + m_{T_i}, \\ \alpha_i = \alpha + a_i, \\ \beta_i = \beta + b_i, \end{cases} \tag{15.12}$$

where $(m_{S_i}, m_{T_i}, a_i, b_i)$ is a normally distributed random vector with mean zero and variance-covariance matrix D given by

$$D = \left(\begin{array}{cc|cc} d_{SS} & d_{ST} & d_{Sa} & d_{Sb} \\ d_{ST} & d_{TT} & d_{Ta} & d_{Tb} \\ \hline d_{Sa} & d_{Ta} & d_{aa} & d_{ab} \\ d_{Sb} & d_{Tb} & d_{ab} & d_{bb} \end{array}\right). \tag{15.13}$$

Combining (15.10) and (15.13) leads to a linear mixed-effects model

$$\begin{pmatrix} S_{ij} \\ T_{ij} \end{pmatrix} \sim N\left[\begin{pmatrix} \mu_S + m_{Si} + (\alpha + a_i) Z_{ij} \\ \mu_T + m_{Ti} + (\beta + b_i) Z_{ij} \end{pmatrix}, \Sigma\right]. \tag{15.14}$$

Let us present the key elements of surrogate marker validation, based on this model, in agreement with the meta-analytic developments for normally distributed endpoints, as detailed in Section 7.2. In order to assess the trial level surrogacy, Buyse *et al.* (2000a) proposed to use the coefficient of determination defined as:

$$R^2_{\text{trial(f)}} = \frac{\begin{pmatrix} d_{Sb} \\ d_{ab} \end{pmatrix}^T \begin{pmatrix} d_{SS} & d_{Sa} \\ d_{Sa} & d_{aa} \end{pmatrix}^{-1} \begin{pmatrix} d_{Sb} \\ d_{ab} \end{pmatrix}}{d_{bb}}. \tag{15.15}$$

Similarly, to measure the individual level surrogacy, they proposed to use the coefficient of determination given by

$$R^2_{\text{indiv}} = \frac{\sigma^2_{ST}}{\sigma_{SS}\sigma_{TT}}. \tag{15.16}$$

Indeed, $R^2_{\text{trial(f)}} = 1$ and $R^2_{\text{indiv}} = 1$ indicate perfect surrogacy at trial and individual level, respectively, in the sense that perfect prediction is possible at both levels. In practical setting, one should adopt a more pragmatic attitude and merely look for R^2 values that are sufficiently high.

The Reduced Model

Buyse *et al.* (2000a) also proposed a reduced model in which the linear predictors for the expected values of S_{ij} and T_{ij} do not include trial-specific intercepts (see also Section 7.2). In the hierarchical model, the likelihood at the first stage of the model can be specified by omitting the trial specific random intercepts from (15.10). This leads to

$$\begin{pmatrix} S_{ij} \\ T_{ij} \end{pmatrix} \sim N\left[\begin{pmatrix} \mu_S + (\alpha + a_i)Z_{ij} \\ \mu_T + (\beta + b_i)Z_{ij} \end{pmatrix}, \Sigma\right]. \tag{15.17}$$

At the second stage of the model, the distribution of the trial-specific random treatment effects (a_i, b_i) is assumed to be bivariate normal with mean zero and variance-covariance matrix D

$$\begin{pmatrix} a_i \\ b_i \end{pmatrix} \sim N\left[\begin{pmatrix} 0 \\ 0 \end{pmatrix}, D\right], \qquad D = \begin{pmatrix} d_{aa} & d_{ab} \\ d_{ab} & d_{bb} \end{pmatrix}. \tag{15.18}$$

Note that model (15.18) is identical to the second-stage model (15.6), with $a = b = 0$, presented by van Houwelingen, Arends, and Stijnen (2002).

For the reduced model, the coefficient of determination (15.15), measuring the trial level surrogacy, reduces to

$$R^2_{\text{trial(r)}} = \frac{d_{ab}^2}{d_{aa}d_{bb}}. \tag{15.19}$$

Note that if the full model is used and D is a block diagonal matrix, i.e., the random intercepts are uncorrelated with the random treatment effects,

$$D = \left(\begin{array}{cc|cc} d_{SS} & d_{ST} & 0 & 0 \\ d_{ST} & d_{TT} & 0 & 0 \\ \hline 0 & 0 & d_{aa} & d_{ab} \\ 0 & 0 & d_{ab} & d_{bb} \end{array}\right).$$

In this case, one can also use (15.19) to evaluate trial-level surrogacy, as the bivariate relationship between a_i and b_i is not influenced by the trial-specific random intercepts. Of course, this is under the assumption that the simplified model is deemed plausible.

15.4 A Hierarchical Bayesian Model for the Validation of Surrogate Endpoints

We now define a hierarchical Bayesian model for the validation of surrogate endpoints using individual data from multiple randomized trials. First, we will consider a construction based on the full model presented in Section 15.3.2. At the first level of the hierarchical Bayesian model, we specify the likelihood as in (15.14). At the second level of the hierarchical model, the priors for the "fixed" effects are specified:

$$\begin{aligned} \mu_S &\sim N(0, \theta^2_{\mu_S}), \\ \mu_T &\sim N(0, \theta^2_{\mu_T}), \\ \alpha &\sim N(0, \tau^2_\alpha), \\ \beta &\sim N(0, \tau^2_\beta). \end{aligned} \tag{15.20}$$

For the precision parameters in (15.20) (flat) hyperprior models are specified using Gamma distributions (e.g., $\theta^{-2}_{\mu_S} \sim \text{gamma}(0.001, 0.001)$, etc.). Similar to the model proposed by Daniels and Hughes (1997), we need to specify a prior distribution to model the association between the treatment effects of the two endpoints. Note that, while Daniels and Hughes (1997) based their model on $[b_i|a_i]$, Buyse *et al.* (2000a) used the joint distribution of the random effects $(m_{Si}, m_{Ti}, a_i, b_i)$ in order to evaluate the trial-level surrogacy. This is done by using (15.13) as a prior distribution for the random effects. As the hyperprior distribution for the variance-covariance matrices in (15.13) and (15.10), a Wishart distribution is assumed:

$$D^{-1} \sim \text{Wishart}(R_D) \qquad \text{and} \qquad \Sigma^{-1} \sim \text{Wishart}(R_\Sigma). \tag{15.21}$$

The trial-level and individual-level surrogacy are assessed using the posterior means for the coefficients of determination (15.15) and (15.16), respectively.

The construction of the hierarchical model corresponding to the reduced model presented in Section 15.3.2 is similar to the one presented above. At the first level of the hierarchical Bayesian model, we specify the likelihood as in (15.17). At the second level of the model, the priors for the "fixed" effects are specified in the same way as in (15.20) and (15.21). The trial-level and individual-level surrogacy is assessed using the posterior means for the coefficients of determination (15.19) and (15.16), respectively.

TABLE 15.1. *Age-related macular degeneration trial. Posterior means (standard errors) for components of D. For the full model, only the variance components needed for the calculation of R^2_{trial} are reported.*

	Full model	Reduced model
d_{aa}	46.18 (24.05)	38.03 (20.96)
d_{ab}	55.67 (30.71)	45.27 (27.30)
d_{bb}	94.29 (46.96)	76.10 (41.62)
d_{SS}	18.79 (10.84)	–
d_{Sa}	-17.32 (13.31)	–
d_{Sb}	-19.70 (17.41)	–

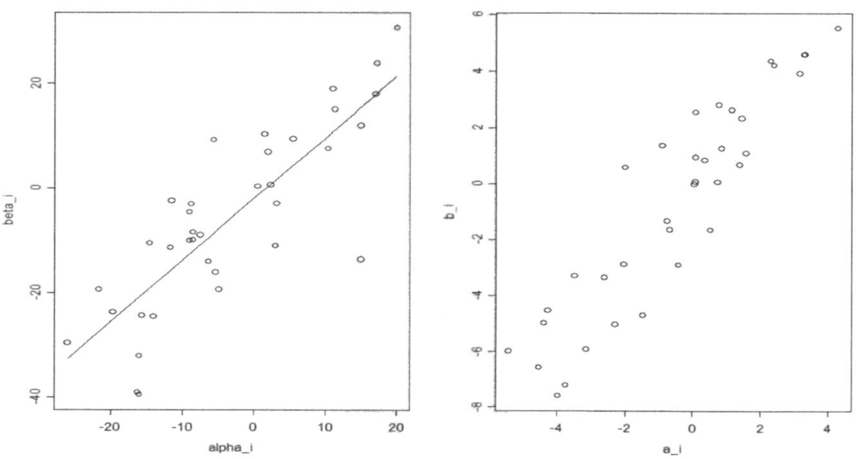

FIGURE 15.1. *Age-related macular degeneration trial. Maximum likelihood estimates for the center-specific treatment effects from the full fixed-effects model (left panel) and posterior means for the random treatment effects (right panel).*

15.5 Analysis of Case Studies

In this section, we use the full Bayesian hierarchical model described in the previous section to re-analyze the data discussed in Buyse *et al.* (2000a) and analyzed in various previous chapters. Precisely, we consider the age-related macular degeneration study (Section 4.2.1) and a meta-analysis of trials in advanced ovarian cancer (Section 4.2.2). All models were fitted using Markov Chain Monte Carlo (MCMC) methods implemented in WINBUGS 1.3 (Gilks *et al.* 1996, Gelman *et al.* 1996).

TABLE 15.2. *Age-related macular degeneration trial.* R^2_{trial} *and* R^2_{indiv} *(standard errors). The full fixed-effects model corresponds to (15.9), whereas the reduced fixed-effects model corresponds to (15.17) without trial-specific intercepts. The results for the fixed-effects models were obtained by Buyse* et al. *(2000a).*

Model	Trial level R^2_{trial}	Individual level R^2_{indiv}
Full (Fixed)	0.692 (0.085)	0.483 (0.053)
Full (Bayesian)	0.739 (0.154)	0.521 (0.054)
Reduced (Fixed)	0.776 (0.066)	0.508 (0.052)
Reduced (Bayesian)	0.771 (0.138)	0.536 (0.051)

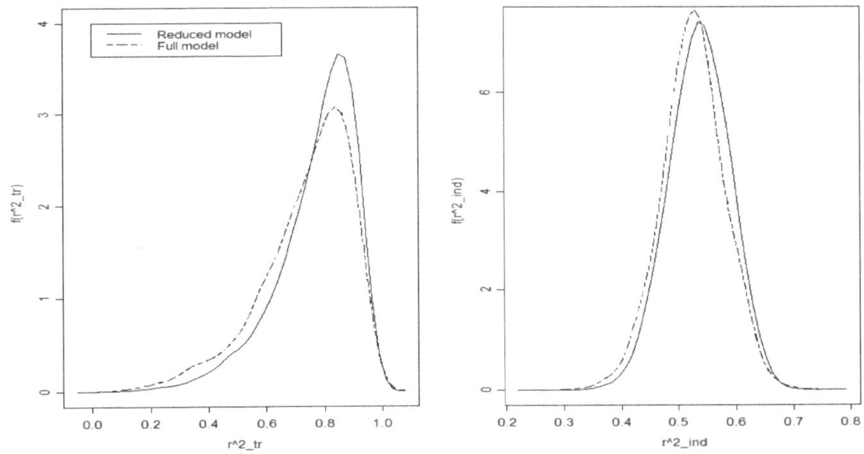

FIGURE 15.2. *Age-related macular degeneration trial. Density estimate for the posterior distribution of* R^2_{trial} *(left panel) and* R^2_{indiv} *(right panel).*

15.5.1 Age-related Macular Degeneration (ARMD) Trial

The data are described in Section 4.2.1. They come from a multicenter trial in which patients were randomized into two treatment groups: placebo and interferon α. The surrogate endpoint is the visual acuity at 6 months and the true endpoint is the visual acuity at 12 months. Patients were treated in 36 centers, which are considered the units of the analysis, with sample sizes ranging between 2 to 18 patients. Figure 15.1 (left-hand panel) shows the ML estimates for the trial specific treatment effects obtained from the full fixed-effects model in (15.9). The straight line is obtained by regressing $\hat{\beta}_i$ on $\hat{\alpha}_i$. The observed variance-covariance matrix for $\hat{\alpha}_i$ and $\hat{\beta}_i$ is

$$\begin{pmatrix} 149.63 & 175.53 \\ 175.53 & 300.77 \end{pmatrix}.$$

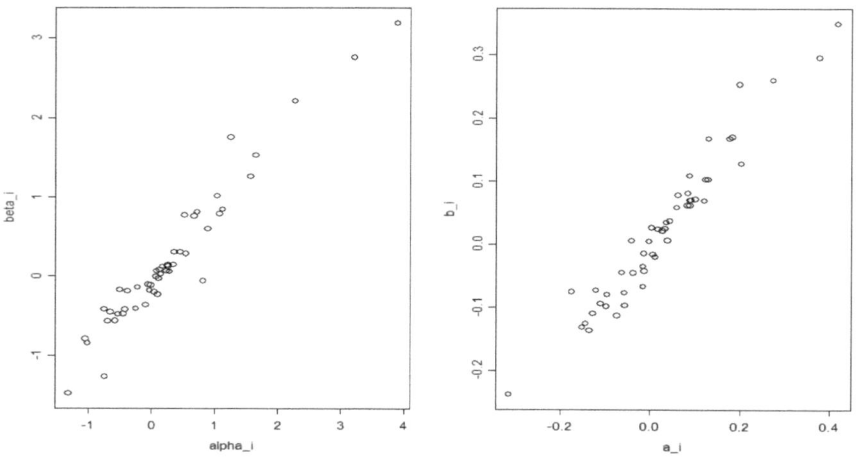

FIGURE 15.3. *Advanced ovarian cancer. Maximum likelihood estimates for the center-specific treatment effects (left panel) and posterior means for the center-specific random treatment effects (right panel).*

Although this variance-covariance matrix reflects the two sources of variability in (15.5), we use it as the mean of the prior distribution of D. We apply model (15.10)–(15.21) to analyze the data. All reported posterior means and credible intervals are based on 10,000 MCMC iterations following a burn-in period of 1000 iterations.

The right-hand panel in Figure 15.1 shows the posterior means for the trial specific (random) treatment effects. The correlation between a_i and b_i is modeled with the variance-covariance matrix of the prior distribution specified in (15.10). Note that the variability of the posterior mean is smaller than the variablity among the maximum likelihood estimates. This is reflected in the posterior mean for D obtained from the reduced model:

$$\bar{D} = \begin{pmatrix} 38.03 & 45.27 \\ 45.27 & 76.10 \end{pmatrix}.$$

Posterior means (and standard error) for the elements of the matrix D in the full model are reported in Table 15.1.

Buyse *et al.* (2000a) used the two-stage full fixed-effects model to obtain $R^2_{\text{trial}} = 0.692$ (standard error, s.e., 0.087) and $R^2_{\text{indiv}} = 0.483$ (s.e. 0.053). The posterior means and credible intervals for both individual- and trial-level surrogacy measures, resulting from the hierarchical Bayesian models, are reported in Table 15.2. For the full model, the posterior mean for $R^2_{\text{trial}} =$ 0.739 (s.e. 0.154), whereas the mean for $R^2_{\text{indiv}} = 0.521$ (s.e. 0.054). Both values are comparable to those obtained by Buyse *et al.* (2000a) using the full fixed-effects model. Figure 15.2 shows the density estimate of the

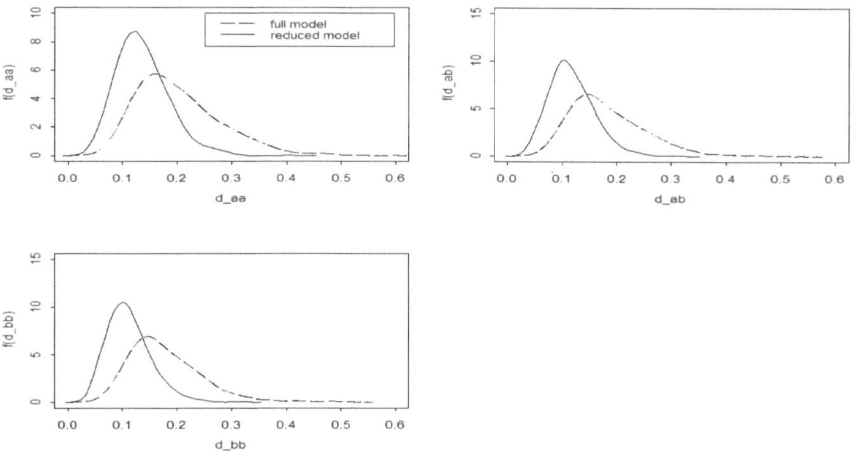

FIGURE 15.4. *Advanced ovarian cancer. Density estimate for the posterior distribution of* d_{aa}, d_{ab} *and* d_{bb}. *Reduced model: long dashed line, full model: solid line.*

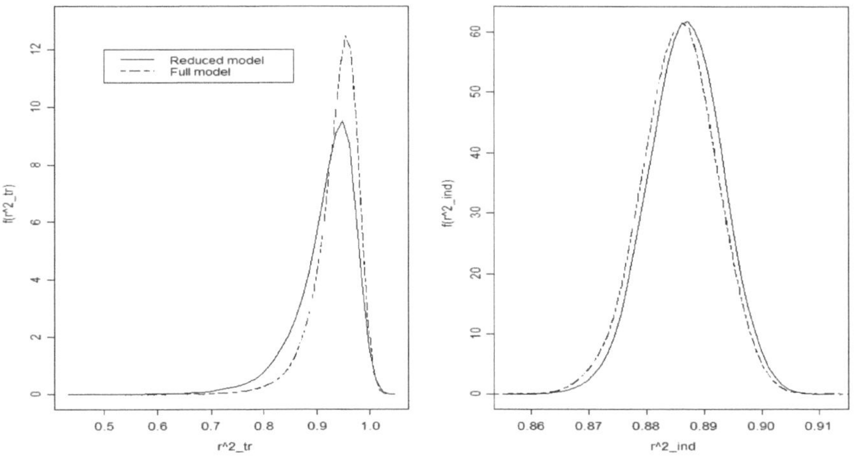

FIGURE 15.5. *Advanced ovarian cancer. Density estimate for the posterior distribution of* $R^2_{trial(f)}$ *(left panel) and* R^2_{indiv} *(right panel).*

posterior distribution for both R^2_{trial} (left-hand panel) and R^2_{indiv} (right-hand panel). Both surrogacy measures increase when the reduced model (15.17) is used in order to evaluate surrogacy. This is reflected in the right shift of the posterior distributions for R^2_{trial} and R^2_{indiv} (solid lines) in Figure 15.2.

TABLE 15.3. *Advanced ovarian cancer.* R^2_{trial} *and* R^2_{indiv} *(standard errors). The full fixed-effects model corresponds to (15.9), whereas the reduced fixed-effects model corresponds to (15.17) without trial-specific intercepts. The results for the fixed-effects model were obtained by Buyse* et al. *(2000a).*

Model	Trial level R^2_{trial}	Individual level R^2_{indiv}
Full (Fixed)	0.940 (0.017)	0.886 (0.0006)
Full (Bayesian)	0.937 (0.039)	0.885 (0.0006)
Reduced (Fixed)	0.928 (0.020)	0.888 (0.0006)
Reduced (Bayesian)	0.917 (0.054)	0.885 (0.0006)

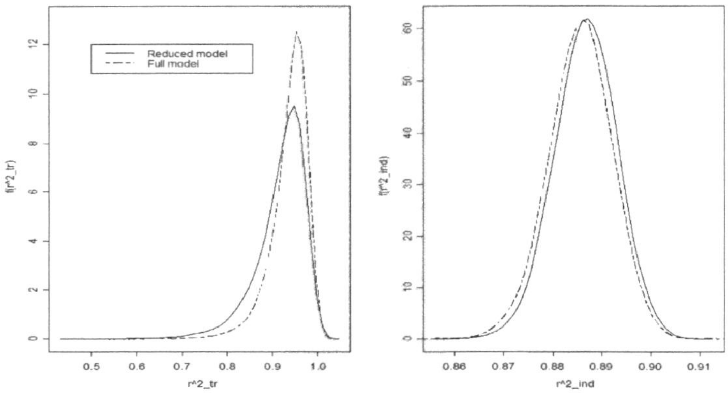

FIGURE 15.6. 95% *confidence and credible intervals for* R^2_{trial} *and* R^2_{indiv}. *F denotes the full model and R denotes the reduced model. (a) Advanced ovarian cancer; (b) age-related macular degeneration trial.*

15.5.2 Advanced Ovarian Cancer

We consider the data from four randomized multicenter trials in advanced ovarian cancer, described in Section 4.2.2. The data have previously been analyzed by Buyse *et al.* (2000a) and in various earlier chapters of this book. The true endpoint is defined as the logarithm of survival time in years, and the surrogate endpoint is taken as the logarithm of progression-free survival time in years. We use center as the unit of analysis given that the number of trials is insufficient to apply meta-analytic methods. A total of 50 centers are available for the analysis, with the number of patients varying from 2 to 274 per center.

Figure 15.3 (left-hand panel) shows the maximum likelihood estimates for the center-specific treatment effects. Analogous to the previous example,

TABLE 15.4. *Simulation results. Mean estimates for the trial- and individual-level validity of a surrogate.*

		$R^2_{\text{trial(r)}}$					
		0.65	0.7	0.75	0.80	0.85	0.9
$\bar{R}^2_{\text{trial}}$	Mean	0.726	0.757	0.787	0.808	0.837	0.866
	Lower quartile	0.515	0.543	0.674	0.619	0.674	0.699
	Upper quartile	0.871	0.904	0.946	0.932	0.946	0.962
	Relative bias (%)	11.78	8.08	4.93	1.09	-1.50	-3.69
$\bar{R}^2_{\text{indiv}}$	Mean	0.764	0.765	0.763	0.770	0.766	0.770
	Lower quartile	0.652	0.652	0.628	0.656	0.658	0.656
	Upper quartile	0.849	0.849	0.857	0.849	0.854	0.849
	Relative bias (%)	-4.45	-4.62	-4.62	-3.78	-4.21	-3.78

the observed variance-covariance matrix between $\hat{\alpha}_i$ and $\hat{\beta}_i$,

$$\begin{pmatrix} 0.98 & 0.86 \\ 0.86 & 0.81 \end{pmatrix},$$

is used as the mean of the prior distribution for (a_i, b_i). The right-hand panel in Figure 15.3 shows the posterior means of a_i and b_i and reveals, similar to the previous example, a reduction in variability of the posterior mean compared to the variability among the maximum likelihood estimates. Figure 15.4 shows the density estimate for the posterior distribution of d_{aa}, d_{ab}, and d_{bb}.

Table 15.3 presents the posterior means and the maximum likelihood estimates for R^2_{trial} and R^2_{indiv} obtained from the hierarchical Bayesian models and from the two-stage fixed-effects models. Figure 15.5 shows the density estimate for the posterior distributions. For the full model, the posterior mean for $R^2_{\text{trial}} = 0.937$ (s.e. 0.039) and for $R^2_{\text{indiv}} = 0.885$ (s.e. 0.0006). The results from the full fixed-effects model are comparable, $R^2_{\text{trial}} = 0.940$ (s.e. 0.017) and $R^2_{\text{indiv}} = 0.885$ (s.e. 0.0006). For the reduced hierarchical model, the posterior mean for $R^2_{\text{trial}} = 0.917$ (s.e. 0.054) can be compared to $R^2_{\text{trial}} = 0.928$ (s.e. 0.020) obtained from the fixed-effects model. At the individual level, the standard error associated with R^2_{indiv} is the same for the Bayesian and fixed-effects models. However, at the trial level, the variability of R^2_{trial} is higher in the Bayesian models. This is reflected in the width of the confidence intervals (for the fixed-effects models) and the credible intervals (for the Bayesian models) as shown in Figure 15.6.

15.6 Simulation Study

We studied the performance of the hierarchical Bayesian model, in terms of estimation (point and interval) of both R^2_{indiv} and $R^2_{\text{trial(r)}}$. Data were generated according to (15.14) with $\mu_S = 10$, $\mu_T = 20$, $\alpha_i = 10$, and $\beta_i = 5$. For the joint distribution of the trial-specific random effects it was assumed that $(m_{S_i}, m_{T_i}, a_i, b_i) \sim N(0, D)$,

$$D = \sigma^2 \begin{pmatrix} 1 & 0.8 & 0 & 0 \\ 0.8 & 1 & 0 & 0 \\ 0 & 0 & 1 & \rho \\ 0 & 0 & \rho & 1 \end{pmatrix}, \tag{15.22}$$

with $R^2_{\text{trial(r)}} = \rho^2$ equal to either 0.65, 0.7, 0.75, 0.8, 0.85, or 0.9. It was further assumed that $(\varepsilon_{S_{ij}}, \varepsilon_{T_{ij}}) \sim N(0, \Sigma)$ with

$$\Sigma = \begin{pmatrix} 1 & 0.8 \\ 0.8 & 1 \end{pmatrix}.$$

The parameter σ^2 was chosen to equal 15. Each simulated dataset consisted of 50 trials with 50 patients within each trial. One hundred datasets were generated for each setting, and the hierarchical Bayesian model was fitted using WINBUGS 1.4. The MCMC simulation for each one of the simulated datsets consisted of 100,000 iterations. The first 10,000 iterations were considered "burn-in" and discarded. Hence, posterior means for both R^2_{indiv} and $R^2_{\text{trial(r)}}$ were calculated based on the last 90,000 iteration of each MCMC run. For each simulation setting, the mean of the posterior means was calculated by $\bar{R}^2 = \sum_{i=1}^{100} \bar{R}_i^2$, where $\bar{R}_i^2$ is the posterior mean in the ith simulation. The relative bias was calculated by

$$\left(\frac{\bar{R}^2}{R^2} - 1\right) \times 100.$$

Results are presented in Table 15.4. For R^2_{indiv}, regardless of the value of $R^2_{\text{trial(r)}}$, the model underestimated the true value with relative bias ranging between -3.33% and -4.45%. For $R^2_{\text{trial(r)}}$, the model overestimated the true value for lower values of $R^2_{\text{trial(r)}}$ and underestimated it for higher values of $R^2_{\text{trial(r)}}$. Figure 15.7 (panel (a)) shows that the relative bias decreased from 11.77% for $R^2_{\text{trial(r)}} = 0.65$ to -3.69% for $R^2_{\text{trial(r)}} = 0.9$. Note that the relative bias changed in almost a linear fashion as $R^2_{\text{trial(r)}}$ increased. The absolute relative bias (panel (b) in Figure 15.7) was minimized for $R^2_{\text{trial(r)}} = 0.8$, which was also the true value of R^2_{indiv}.

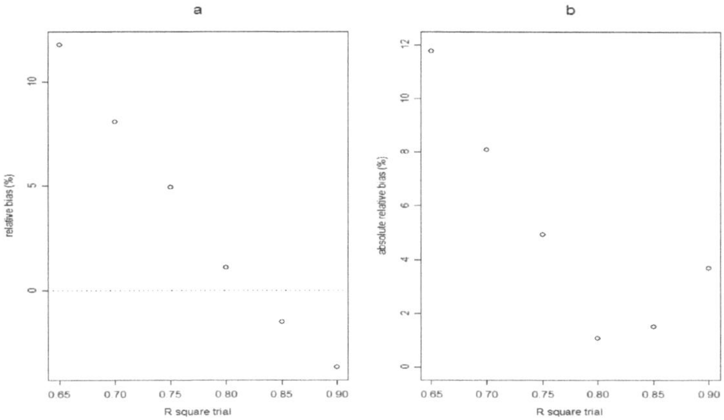

FIGURE 15.7. *Simulations Results. (a) Relative bias; (b) absolute bias.*

15.7 Discussion

The meta-analytic approach in surrogate marker validation built upon the initial concepts of Prentice (1989), Freedman, Graubard, and Schatzkin (1992), and Buyse and Molenberghs (1998). Within the meta-analytic framework, the evaluation of the trial-level validity of a surrogate requires specification of the joint or the conditional distribution for the true treatment effects. All models discussed in this chapter used the bivariate relationships between the latent true (random) treatment effects to evaluate the trial-level validity. The advantage of the approach proposed by Daniels and Hughes (1997) is that it does not require specification of the joint distribution of S and T. The trial-level validity of a surrogate is assessed using the variance of the conditional distribution. However, in the case of two normally distributed endpoints, one can specify a two-stage model in which the joint distribution of S and T is assumed at the first stage and the joint distribution of the true trial-specific treatment effects is specified at the second stage of the model. We have shown that the individual-level validity of a surrogate can be evaluated using the posterior distribution of the variance-covariance matrix specified at the first stage of the model. Similar to Daniels and Hughes (1997), the trial-level validity can be evaluated using the bivariate relation of the true trial-specific treatment effects, i.e., from the posterior distribution of variance-covariance matrix D specified at the second stage of the model. By using the two-stage model we can avoid the need for fixing the variance-covariance matrix Σ, which represents the within trial variablity.

In the cases studies analyzed, the density estimate for the posterior distribution of $R^2_{\text{trial(r)}}$ was skewed to the left, whereas the density estimate for R^2_{indiv} revealed a symmetric distribution. We have shown that, for both examples, the posterior means for both R^2_{indiv} and $R^2_{\text{trial(r)}}$ were comparable with the maximum likelihood estimates reported in Buyse *et al.* (2000a). However, for the trial-level validity, the 95% credible intervals were wider from the 95% confidence intervals. This pattern was observed for both the advanced ovarian cancer and the ARMD trials, though the trials differ in the number of observations per unit.

The simulation study in Section 15.6 reveals a clear pattern of over and under estimation of $R^2_{\text{trial(r)}}$. The fact that the estimation bias of $R^2_{\text{trial(r)}}$ changed in a linear fashion as the value of R^2_{trial} got away form R^2_{indiv} suggests that a bias correction factor should be added to the posterior mean of $R^2_{\text{trial(r)}}$. This is a topic for future investigation.

16

Surrogate Marker Validation in Mental Health

Tony Vangeneugden, Ariel Alonso Abad, Helena Geys, and Annouschka Laenen

16.1 Introduction

In this chapter, we describe how the framework for surrogate marker validation in clinical trials can easily be adapted and used to assess the so-called *criterion validity* of psychiatric symptom scales. This concept will be described further in this cahpter (see also Laenen *et al.* 2004).

One feature of the psychiatric health sciences literature, devoted to measuring subjective states, is the daunting area of available scales (Steiner and Norman 1995). The development of scales to assess subjective attributes is not easy and subject to many controversial debates. One particular drawback, of course, lies in the fact that the filling-in of a scale may vary from one person to another. Because of the subjective nature of many of these scales, one may encounter scales that are not adequate to assess a particular concept. Therefore, whenever a mental health measurement scale is developed, translated, or used in a new population, its psychometric properties have to be assessed. Two important properties are *reliability* and *validity*.

Reliability consists in determining the extent to which the measurement is free from random error. This can be performed through analyzing *internal consistency* and *reproducibility* of the questionnaire. Internal consistency is the extent to which individual items are consistent with each other and reflect a single underlying construct. Essentially, internal consistency represents the average of the correlations among all the items in the instrument. Several measures that are often used to provide proof of internal consistency are: Cronbach's alpha coefficient (Cronbach 1951), Kuder and Richardson (1953), and factor analysis. Intra-observer or test-retest reliability is the degree to which a measure yields stable scores at different points in time for patients who are assumed not to have changed clinical status on the domains being assessed. The calculation of intraclass correlation coefficients

(Fleiss and Cohen 1973, Deyo, Dierh, and Patrick 1991) is one of the most commonly used methods. For interviewer-administered questionnaires, the inter-observer reliability is the degree to which a measurement yields stable scores when administered by different interviewers, rating the same patients. The calculation of interclass correlation coefficients is also one of the most commonly used methods. In classical test theory, the outcome of a test is frequently modeled as

$$X = \tau + \varepsilon, \tag{16.1}$$

where X represents an observation or measurement, τ is the true score, and ε the corresponding measurement error. It is further assumed that the measurement errors are mutually uncorrelated as well as with the true scores, and under this assumption they obtain

$$\text{Var}(X) = \text{Var}(\tau) + \text{Var}(\varepsilon). \tag{16.2}$$

The reliability of a measuring instrument is defined as the ratio of the true score variance to the observed score variance, i.e.,

$$R = \frac{\text{Var}(\tau)}{\text{Var}(\tau) + \text{Var}(\varepsilon)}. \tag{16.3}$$

For interviewer-administered questionnaires, the inter-observer reliability is the degree to which a measurement yields stable scores when administered by different interviewers, rating the same patients. Also here the interclass correlation coefficient is commonly used.

The validity of a questionnaire is defined as the degree to which the questionnaire measures what it purports to measure. This can be performed through the analysis of *content*, *construct*, and *criterion* validity. Content validity can be defined as the extent to which the instrument assesses all the relevant or important content or domains. Also the term *face validity* is used to indicate whether the instrument appears to be assessing the desired qualities at face. This form of validity consists of a judgment by experts in the field. Construct validity refers to a wide range of approaches which are used when what we are trying to measure is a "hypothetical construct" (e.g., anxiety, irritable bowel syndrome, ...) rather than something that can readily be observed. The most commonly used methods to explore construct validity are extreme groups (apply instrument for example to cases and non-cases), convergent and discriminant validity testing (correlate with other measures of this construct and not correlate with dissimilar or unrelated constructs), and multitrait-multimethod matrix (Campbell and Fisk 1959). Criterion validity can be divided into two types: *concurrent validity* and *predictive validity*. With concurrent validity we correlate the measurement with a criterion measure (gold standard), both of which are given at the same time. In predictive validity, similar as with surrogate markers, the criterion will not be available until some time in the future. The most commonly used method to assess the validity is by calculation of the Pearson correlation coefficient.

In spite of the utmost importance of these psychometric concepts, the statistical methods used to study them have mainly been based on elementary tools. The most commonly used method to assess validity is by calculation of the Pearson correlation coefficient. On the other hand, even though very frequently psychiatric patients are followed for a long period of time, the traditional approach to validity is often limited to the simpler cross-sectional case.

The idea is to provide a new way of investigating criterion validity of psychiatric symptom scales, using the theme of the book: criteria applied in surrogate marker validation for clinical trials, not only for the cross-sectional setting, but also making use of the longitudinal developments in Chapter 14. In particular, we will show how the meta-analytic approach of Buyse *et al.* (2000a), presented in Chapter 7, can be used to investigate the concurrent validity of two psychiatric rating scales. In cases where a gold standard scale can be assigned, we can almost directly apply their methodology for the validation of surrogate markers with the standard scale playing the role of true endpoint. In many mental health studies and psychiatric trials, however, a more "symmetric" situation is encountered where different scales are measured in conjunction without knowing their relationships. In such cases, one will need to "symmetrize" the validation techniques. Although our data setting does not allow us to investigate the predictive validity, the methods proposed here could be applied to "validate" one scale *versus* another in that sense as well using clinical trial data.

The case studies will, obviously, be the equivalence trial in schizophrenic patients (Section 4.2.7 and the meta-analysis of clinical trials comparing antipsychotic agents for the treatment of chronic schizophrenia (Section 4.2.6). A brief overview of the mental health area, in particular schizophrenia, is given in Section 16.2. Section 16.3 gives a brief discussion of how the different criteria to validate surrogate endpoints in randomized clinical trials (described in Chapters 5 and 7) could be adapted and used to investigate the criterion validity of psychiatric measurement scales. The drawbacks of some of these approaches will be pointed out. In Section 16.4, we apply the different methods to the data. We will show how some of these methods can usefully be applied to investigate the criterion validity of two rating scales, whereas others may lead to misleading or inconclusive results. The multi-trial approach of Buyse *et al.* (2000a) will turn out to be really superior.

16.2 Mental Health

When compared with all other diseases (such as cancer, HIV, or heart disease), mental illness ranks first in terms of causing disability in the United States, Canada, and Western Europe, according to a study by the World Health Organization (WHO 2001). This groundbreaking study found that mental illness (including depression, bipolar disorder, and schizophrenia) accounts for 25% of all disability across major industrialized countries (`http://www.who.int`).

However, actions from governments are not always proportional to the magnitude of the problem. Forty percent of countries have no mental health policies, and 25% have no legislation in the field of mental health. Many large countries, including China, Iran, Nigeria, Thailand, and Turkey, have no specific legislation for mental health, though some are in the process of developing legislation. Of the countries reporting, about one-third spend less than 1% of their federal health budget on mental health-related activities. Community care facilities have yet to be developed in about half of the countries in the African, Eastern Mediterranean, and Southeast Asia regions. In other regions, these facilities are absent in at least one-third of the countries. Of the total number of psychiatric beds in the world, about 65% are still in mental hospitals.

Among all the psychiatric disorders, schizophrenia is one of the most disabling and emotionally devastating illnesses. In a recent 14-country study on disability associated with physical and mental conditions, active psychosis was ranked the third most disabling condition, higher than paraplegia and blindness, by the general population. The economic cost of schizophrenia to society is also high. It has been estimated that, in 1991, the cost of schizophrenia to the United States was US$ 19 billion in direct expenditure and US$ 46 billion in lost productivity (`http://www.who.int`).

A substantial number of individuals with schizophrenia attempt suicide at some time during the course of their illness. Recent studies showed that 30% of patients diagnosed with this disorder had attempted suicide at least once during their lifetime. About 10% of persons with schizophrenia die by suicide. Globally, schizophrenic illness reduces an affected individual's lifespan by an average of 10 years. Frequently, schizophrenic patients show lack of interest and initiative in daily activities and work, social incompetence, and inability to take interest in pleasurable activities. These can cause continued disability and poor quality of life (`http://www.who.int`).

The study and evaluation of these symptoms play a key role in the diagnosis and treatment of schizophrenic patients and, as a result, several measures have been developed to assess a patient's global condition. When psychiatric health measurements are either developed or used in a new population, of course, their reliability and validity must be investigated.

16.2.1 Mental Health and Schizophrenia

The impact of psychiatric disorders on public health is not fully known, but as early as the 1980s studies began to show that it was greater than first believed. Lee Robins, a psychiatric epidemiologist at Columbia University, first reported the following findings in 1984: At any given time, 15 to 23 percent of the U.S. population has a diagnosable mental disorder. At some point in their lives, between 28 and 38 percent of people will develop a mental disorder. Ten to 20 percent of people will have an episode of clinical depression, and 10 to 15 percent will experience unmanageable anxiety. Severe personality disorders will affect 5 to 10 percent and each year at least 30,000 people will commit suicide. An additional 3,000 to 15,000 deaths per year can be attributed to other causes stemming from suicide attempts. The economic impact of these diseases is huge: the United States loses more than US $185 billion each year due to invalidity or temporary disability related to mental illnesses, and the annual cost of mental health treatments ranges between US $20 billion and US $50 billion (`http://biosun1.harvard.edu/ lobrien/psych.html`).

More recent investigations carried out by the World Health Organization confirm these preliminary findings (`http://www.who.int`). These studies show that mental and behavioral disorders are common, affecting more than 25% of all people at some time during their lives. They are also universal, affecting people of all countries and societies, individuals at all ages, women and men, the rich and the poor, from urban and rural environments. They have an economic impact on societies and on the quality of life of individuals and families. Mental and behavioral disorders are present at any point in time in about 10% of the adult population. Around 20% of all patients seen by primary health care professionals have one or more mental disorders. One in four families is likely to have at least one member with a behavioral or mental disorder. These families not only provide physical and emotional support, but also bear the negative impact of stigma and discrimination. It was estimated that, in 1990, mental and neurological disorders accounted for 10% of the total DALYs (disability-adjusted life years) lost due to all diseases and injuries. This was 12% in 2000. By 2020, it is projected that the burden of these disorders will have increased to 15%. Factors associated with the prevalence, onset, and course of mental and behavioral disorders include poverty, sex, age, conflicts and disasters, major physical diseases, and the family and social environment.

A few studies in Europe have estimated expenditure on mental disorders as a proportion of all health service costs. In The Netherlands, this was 23.2% and in the United Kingdom, for in-patient expenditure only, the proportion equaled 22%. Though scientific estimates are not available for other regions of the world, it is likely that the costs of mental disorders as a proportion of the overall economy are generally high. Although estimates of direct costs may be low in countries where there is low availability and coverage of mental health care, these estimates are spurious. Indirect costs arising from productivity loss account for a larger proportion of overall costs than direct costs. Furthermore, low treatment costs (because of lack of treatment) may actually increase the indirect costs by increasing the duration of untreated disorders and associated disability. All of these estimates of economic evaluations are most likely underestimates, since lost opportunity costs to individuals and families are not taken into account (`http://www.who.int`).

Mental diseases have also affected relevant figures of our history, sciences, and arts. Abraham Lincoln, the revered 16th president of the United States, suffered from severe, incapacitating, and occasionally suicidal depressions. Lincoln's major depressions are well-documented in his own writings and in reports from contemporaries. Virginia Woolf, the British novelist who wrote *To The Lighthouse* and *Orlando*, experienced manic depressive disorder as did the German musician Ludwig von Beethoven and the Dutch painter Vincent Van Gogh. Leo Tolstoy, author of *War and Peace*, revealed the extent of his own mental illness in *My Confession* and a recent Nobel Laureate in Economics, the mathematician John Forbes Nash Jr., has a lifetime history of schizophrenia.

Schizophrenia, a disease of the brain, is one of the most disabling and emotionally devastating illnesses known to man. But because it has been misunderstood for so long, it has received relatively little attention, and its victims have been undeservingly stigmatized. In 1911, Eugen Bleuler first used the word "schizophrenia." The term schizophrenia comes from the Greek words "schizo" (=split) and "phrenia" (=mind) and therefore

$$\text{schizophrenia} = \text{split} + \text{mind}.$$

However, schizophrenia is not seen nowadays as a split personality, a rare and very different disorder. Like cancer and diabetes, schizophrenia has a biological basis; it is not caused by bad parenting or personal weakness. Schizophrenia is, in fact, a relatively common disease: it affects 1 in 100 people worldwide, irrespective of races, culture, and social class. Although there is no known cure for schizophrenia, it is a very treatable disease. Most of those afflicted by schizophrenia respond to drug therapy, and many are able to lead productive and fulfilling lives.

Schizophrenia is characterized by a constellation of distinctive and predictable symptoms. The symptoms that are most commonly associated with the disease are called positive symptoms, denoting the presence of grossly abnormal behavior. These include thought disorder, delusions, and hallucinations. Thought disorder is the diminished ability to think clearly and logically. Often it is manifested by disconnected and nonsensical language that renders the person with schizophrenia incapable of participating in conversation, contributing to his alienation from his family, friends, and society. Delusions are common among individuals with schizophrenia. An affected person may believe that he or she is being conspired against (called "paranoid delusion"). "Broadcasting" describes a type of delusion in which the individual with this illness believes that his thoughts can be heard by others. Hallucinations can be heard, seen, or even felt; most often they take the form of voices heard only by the afflicted person. Such voices may describe the person's actions, warn him of danger, or tell him what to do. At times the individual may hear several voices carrying on a conversation. Less obvious than the "positive symptoms" but equally serious are the deficit or "negative symptoms" that represent the absence of normal behavior. These include flat or blunted affect (i.e., lack of emotional expression), apathy, and social withdrawal.

Although schizophrenia can affect anyone at any point in life, the disease has a very strong genetic component. The probability of developing schizophrenia as the offspring of two parents, neither of whom has the disease, is 1 percent. The probability of developing schizophrenia being the offspring of one parent with the disease is approximately 13 percent. The probability of developing schizophrenia as the offspring of both parents with the disease is approximately 35 percent. Three-quarters of persons with schizophrenia develop the disease between 16 and 25 years of age. Onset is uncommon after age 30, and rare after age 40. In the 16–25 year old age group, schizophrenia affects more men than women. In the 25–30 year old group, the incidence is higher in women than in men.

16.3 Surrogate Endpoint Validation Criteria

Chapter 5 gave a general overview of the history of surrogate marker validation measures, and Chapter 7 sketched the meta-analytic framework of Buyse *et al.* (2000a). In this section, we summarize the main arguments, but now focusing on the assessment of concurrent validity for mental health symptom scales. A key difference is that the natural asymmetry that exists between the surrogate (S) and true endpoints (T) will often have to be replaced by a more symmetric treatment of two endpoints (scales), i.e., S_1 and

S_2. Let us first introduce notation particular to this chapter. Throughout, we assume that S_1 and S_2 are random variables that represent two scales for which we want to assess the criterion validity. Traditional approaches investigate the concurrent validity by correlating one measurement scale (S_2) with the other assumed to be a gold standard (S_1). In many cases, an ordinary Pearson's correlation coefficient is used. Here, we propose to assess the criterion validity based on criteria similar to the ones used in surrogate marker validation in randomized clinical trials. Although the criteria could equally well be applied to investigate the predictive validity (where one of the two criteria will not be available until some time in the future), this is beyond the scope of the data analyses presented in this chapter. Further, we assume that Z is an indicator variable for treatment. We restrict attention to a binary treatment indicator ($Z = 0$ or 1).

16.3.1 Prentice's Criteria

Prentice's criteria (Prentice 1989) have been presented in Section 5.2.2. They can be applied to our setting, treating the gold standard scale S_1 as the true endpoint. Consequently, criteria (5.2) and (5.3) measure departures from the null hypothesis of no treatment effect on S_2 and S_1, respectively, implicit in Prentice's definition of a surrogate endpoint. Criterion (5.4) implies that S_2 has prognostic value for the gold standard. Criterion (5.5) requires S_2 to capture fully the effect of treatment on S_1, that is: there is no effect of treatment on one scale after correction for the other scale. Of course, this last condition is so restrictive that it rarely holds in practice and it is hard to verify since it would formally require equivalence testing.

Although in many practical applications one of the symptom scales may be regarded as "the standard," this is not always evident with psychiatric diagnostic tools. In that case, we may have to add two extra criteria:

$$f(S_2|S_1) \neq f(S_2), \tag{16.4}$$

$$f(S_2|S_1) = f(S_2|S_1, Z). \tag{16.5}$$

Further, in an equivalence trial designed to demonstrate the equivalence of a new treatment with a standard therapy, the first two Prentice criteria are bound not to be fulfilled. Yet, from a clinical perspective there is no reason why the symptom scales used as responses in such a trial cannot be validated. This will be illustrated further in this chapter.

16.3.2 Freedman's Proportion Explained

Freedman, Graubard, and Schatzkin (1992) supplemented Prentice's criteria with their *proportion explained*, given by (5.19). In the current context, it can be interpreted as the proportion of the treatment effect on one scale that is explained by the other. Let $PE(S_1, S_2, Z)$ stand for the proportion of the effect of Z on S_1, which can be explained by S_2. An estimate of $PE(S_1, S_2, Z)$ can be obtained from (5.19). Note that this quantity is subject to the same asymmetry as criteria (5.4)–(5.5) and (16.4)–(16.5). Therefore, one might also have to look at $PE(S_2, S_1, Z)$ whenever there is no clear standard among the two instruments considered. Prentice's criterion (5.5) requires that S_2 fully captures the effect of treatment on S_1, what leads to $PE(S_1, S_2, Z) = 1$.

It was believed that an instrument for which $PE < 1$ explains only part of the treatment effect on the other instrument. Hence, following the ideas of Freedman, Graubard, and Schatzkin (1992), one could suggest that the criterion validity of two instruments is assessed when the PE is close to unity. In cases where it is not clear which scale can serve as "the standard," both $PE(S_1, S_2, Z)$ and $PE(S_2, S_1, Z)$ should be close to unity. However, this reasoning is not valid. Several conceptual difficulties surrounding the PE have been outlined in the literature (Lin, Fleming, and De Gruttola 1997, Buyse and Molenberghs 1998, Flandre and Saidi 1999, Buyse *et al.* 2000a, 2000b, Molenberghs *et al.* 2002) and presented in Sections 5.3.2 and 5.4.2. In particular, a fundamental problem with PE is that it is not a proportion: it can be estimated to be anywhere on the real line, which makes its interpretation problematic.

16.3.3 Relative Effect and Adjusted Association

Buyse and Molenberghs (1998) suggested to replace the PE by two related quantities: the relative effect (RE), which is the ratio of the treatment effects upon the two instruments, and the treatment-adjusted association, ρ_Z, which is the subject-specific association, adjusted for treatment (Section 5.4). From (5.22), one can see that in our setting two versions of RE can be formally written: $RE(S_1, S_2)$ and $RE(S_2, S_1)$, depending on which scale is treated as the "true" endpoint. Note that RE is anti-symmetric in the sense that $RE(S_1, S_2) = 1/RE(S_2, S_1)$, whereas the adjusted association (5.23) is fully symmetric.

16.3.4 Hierarchical Approach

Buyse *et al.* (2000a) adopted an alternative approach to the validation of surrogate endpoints based on a meta-analysis of several trials (Chapter 7). We will show that this setting is very much fit for the validation of psychiatric symptom scales.

The approach of Buyse *et al.* (2000a) is based on the two-stage model (7.1)–(7.5) or its random-effects representation (7.6)–(7.7). The models can be naturally applied to the case of two measurement scales considered in this chapter. In particular, the first-stage model (7.1)–(7.2) can be re-written as

$$S_{1ij} = \mu_{S_{1i}} + \beta_i Z_{ij} + \varepsilon_{S_{1ij}}, \qquad (16.6)$$

$$S_{2ij} = \mu_{S_{2i}} + \alpha_i Z_{ij} + \varepsilon_{S_{2ij}}, \qquad (16.7)$$

where α_i and β_i are trial-specific effects of treatment Z on the endpoints in a trial, $\mu_{S_{1i}}$ and $\mu_{S_{2i}}$ are trial-specific intercepts, and $\varepsilon_{S_{1i}}$ and $\varepsilon_{S_{2i}}$ are correlated error terms, assumed to be mean-zero normally distributed with covariance matrix

$$\Sigma = \begin{pmatrix} \sigma_{S_1S_1} & \sigma_{S_1S_2} \\ \sigma_{S_1S_2} & \sigma_{S_2S_2} \end{pmatrix}.$$

At the second stage, it can be assumed that

$$\begin{pmatrix} \mu_{S_{1i}} \\ \mu_{S_{2i}} \\ \beta_i \\ \alpha_i \end{pmatrix} = \begin{pmatrix} \mu_{S_1} \\ \mu_{S_2} \\ \beta \\ \alpha \end{pmatrix} + \begin{pmatrix} m_{S_{1i}} \\ m_{S_{2i}} \\ b_i \\ a_i \end{pmatrix}, \qquad (16.8)$$

where the second term on the right-hand side of (16.8) follows a zero-mean normal distribution with dispersion matrix

$$D = \begin{pmatrix} d_{S_1S_1} & d_{S_1S_2} & d_{S_1b} & d_{S_1a} \\ d_{S_2S_1} & d_{S_2S_2} & d_{S_2b} & d_{S_2a} \\ d_{bS_1} & d_{bS_2} & d_{bb} & d_{ba} \\ d_{aS_1} & d_{aS_2} & d_{ab} & d_{aa} \end{pmatrix}.$$

The setting described above naturally lends itself to the validation of two scales at both the trial level as well as the individual level.

To investigate the trial-level concurrent and/or predictive validity of two psychiatric scales, it is of interest to investigate how a change in treatment effect on one measurement scale can be translated into the other psychiatric measurement instrument. Therefore, it is essential to explore the quality of the prediction of the treatment effect on S_1 in trial i by (a) information obtained in the validation process based on trials $i = 1, \ldots, N$, and (b) the estimate of the effect of Z on S_2 in a new trial $i = 0$. Whenever there is no clear standard but simply relations are studied, as is often the case with psychometric instruments, the reverse prediction (on S_2 based on the effect on S_1) is also important.

To this end, the developments presented in Section 7.2.1 can be used. It follows that, to assess the validity of S_2 with respect to S_1, the following coefficient of determination can be used:

$$\begin{aligned} R^2_{\text{trial(f)}} &= R^2_{b_i|m_{S_2i},a_i} \\ &= \frac{1}{d_{bb}} \begin{pmatrix} d_{S_2b} \\ d_{ab} \end{pmatrix}^T \begin{pmatrix} d_{S_2S_2} & d_{S_2a} \\ d_{S_2a} & d_{aa} \end{pmatrix}^{-1} \begin{pmatrix} d_{S_2b} \\ d_{ab} \end{pmatrix}. \end{aligned} \quad (16.9)$$

Again, when none of the two scales can be assumed to be a standard, we may also have to look at the second coefficient of determination:

$$\begin{aligned} R^2_{\text{trial(f)}} &= R^2_{a_i|m_{S_1i},b_i} \\ &= \frac{1}{d_{aa}} \begin{pmatrix} d_{S_1a} \\ d_{ab} \end{pmatrix}^T \begin{pmatrix} d_{S_1S_1} & d_{S_1b} \\ d_{S_1b} & d_{bb} \end{pmatrix}^{-1} \begin{pmatrix} d_{S_1a} \\ d_{ab} \end{pmatrix}. \end{aligned} \quad (16.10)$$

These coefficients are unitless and range in the unit interval, two desirable features for interpretation. Whenever these quantities are sufficiently close to 1, we can say that one scale is a good surrogate for the other at trial level.

An attractive special case of (16.9) applies when the prediction of the treatment effect can be done independently of the trial-specific random intercept m_{S0}. In this case, in agreement with (7.12), the following, simplified coefficient of determination results:

$$R^2_{\text{trial(r)}} = R^2_{b_i|a_i} = \frac{d^2_{ab}}{d_{aa}d_{bb}}, \quad (16.11)$$

which is now symmetric in the two scales. Clearly, this is a very attractive property when validating two psychometric scales for which in many cases no gold standard can be assigned. In contrast to previous approaches, only one quantity suffices to assess the validity.

To validate two scales at the individual level, following the developments by Buyse *et al.* (2000a), one can consider using the squared correlation between the two instruments after adjustment for both the trial effects as well as the treatment effect:

$$R^2_{\text{indiv}} = R^2_{\varepsilon_{S_1i}|\varepsilon_{S_2i}} = \frac{\sigma^2_{S_1S_2}}{\sigma_{S_1S_1}\sigma_{S_2S_2}}. \quad (16.12)$$

16.3.5 Variance Reduction Factor and Likelihood Reduction Factor

Just as we discussed symmetries and asymmetries in the single-trial measures case as well as for the original meta-analytic framework sketched, one may want to investigate the longitudinal setting, too, as, in mental health studies and psychiatric trials, data are often collected repeatedly over time.

In Chapter 14, several particular measures were introduced, members of a wide family of validation measures. Specific instances were the variance reduction factor (VRF), the canonical correlation based measure θ_p, and the likelihood reduction factor (LRF). On page 241, it is stated that the variance reduction factor is not symmetric in S_1 and S_2 and hence it differs depending on the "directionality" chosen. In contrast, θ_p is symmetric. This issue is discussed in some detail on page 248. In addition, the measure R^2_Λ, introduced in Section 14.5.1, is symmetric in both endpoints. A nice overview of the symmetries and asymmetries in both the traditional meta-analytic coefficient of determination based measures,, supplemented with those in the newly proposed measures of Chapter 14, is given in Table 14.2.

16.4 Analysis of Case Studies

In the analysis of the case studies, our interest will focus on the extent to which the Positive and Negative Syndrome Scale (PANSS) and the Brief Psychiatric Rating Scale (BPRS) scales are related with each other and with Clinician's Global Impression (CGI). We will show that for this purpose, we can use analogous techniques as when validating a surrogate endpoint from meta-analytic data.

16.4.1 A Meta-analysis of Trials in Schizophrenic Subjects

In this section, we will apply the methods of Section 16.3 to the data from a meta-analysis of five clinical trials in schizophrenic patients, described in Section 4.2.6. Evidently, there is no natural "true endpoint" associated with such data. Nevertheless, we will show how these methods can be used to investigate the criterion validity between the three scales of interest: PANSS, BPRS, and CGI. We will successively consider the relationships between (i) PANSS and BPRS, (ii) PANSS and CGI, and (iii) BPRS and CGI. Within each of these comparisons, missing values (if any) were deleted first. The

TABLE 16.1. *Meta-analysis in schizophrenia. Prentice's criteria for the comparison of PANSS* versus *BPRS.*

Effect tested	Criterion	Estimate (standard error)	p-value
Z on S_1	(5.2)	−4.63 (1.65)	0.005
Z on S_2	(5.3)	−2.43 (0.95)	0.011
S_2 on S_1	(5.4)	1.66 (0.01)	0.000
Z on S_1 adjusted for S_2	(5.5)	−0.57 (0.46)	0.217
S_1 on S_2	(16.4)	0.55 (0.01)	0.000
Z on S_2 adjusted for S_2	(16.5)	0.13 (0.27)	0.641

binary indicator for treatment (Z_{ij}) will be set to 0 for the conventional antipsychotic agents and to 1 for risperidone.

The meta-analysis contains only five trials. This is insufficient to apply the meta-analytic methods of Buyse *et al.* (2000a). Fortunately, in all of the trials information is also available on the investigators that treated the patients. Hence, we can also use investigator as the unit of analysis. A total of 138 units are thus available for analysis, with the number of patients per unit ranging from 2 to 30.

Relationship Between PANSS and BPRS

The relationship between PANSS and BPRS was studied first. Because the BPRS is essentially constructed from the PANSS by selecting 18 of its 30 items, there is a natural link between these two scales, but it remains difficult to assign one of the two endpoints as the "true endpoint." With our notation we assume that PANSS plays the role of S_1 and BPRS plays the role of S_2. Figure 16.1(a) shows a scatterplot of BPRS *versus* PANSS. Clearly, both scales are highly correlated. The Pearson's correlation coefficient equals $\rho = 0.96$.

Let us now apply the different validation methods, described in Section 16.3. Starting with the Prentice criteria, all of them are fulfilled: the treatment is prognostic for both PANSS and BPRS, BPRS is prognostic for PANSS and vice-versa, and there is no effect of treatment on either scale after correction for the other scale. A summary of these results is shown in Table 16.1. However, one has to keep the conceptual difficulties with this formalism in mind. In addition, the lack of symmetry of this approach is a further drawback. Next, we calculated Freedman's proportion explained as $PE(S_1, S_2) = 0.875$ with 95% confidence interval, C.I., [0.65, 1.05]. Because of the symmetry in the endpoints, we also needed to calculate

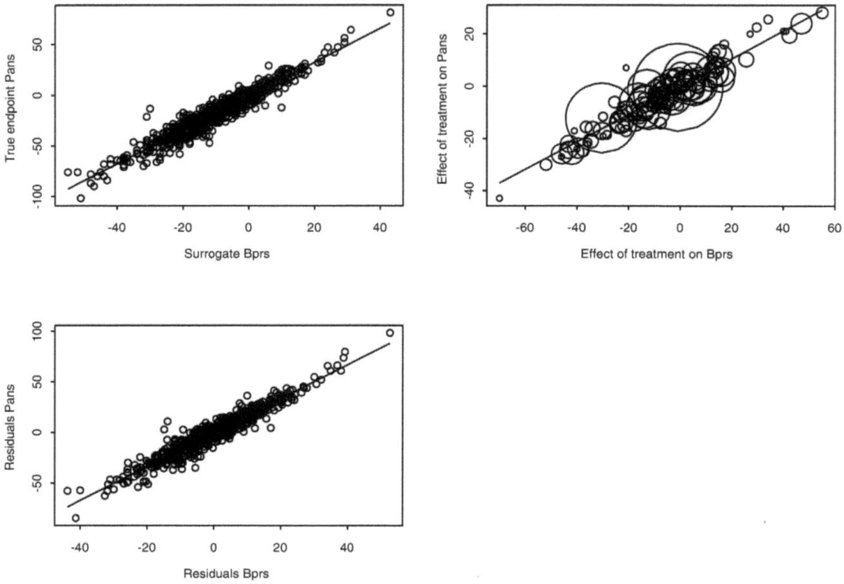

FIGURE 16.1. *Meta-analysis in schizophrenia. (a) Scatter plot of PANSS* versus *BPRS (top left); (b) treatment effects on PANSS by treatment effects on BPRS (top right). The size of each point is proportional to the number of patients examined by the corresponding investigator. (c) Plot of the residuals of PANSS* versus *BPRS (bottom left).*

$PE(S_2, S_1) = 1.052$ (95% C.I. [0.87, 1.41]). Note that, with this approach we might not only find a value of PE that is larger than 1, but in addition the confidence intervals tend to be rather wide. The relative effect and adjusted association were respectively calculated as $RE(S_1, S_2) = 1.90$ (95% C.I. [0.70, 5.77]), $RE(S_2, S_1) = 1/RE(S_1, S_2) = 0.53$ (95% C.I. [0.17, 1.43]), and $\rho_Z = 0.96$ (95% C.I. [0.95, 0.97]). The confidence intervals around the REs may be too large to convey any useful information. In contrast, the adjusted association is very close to one and estimated with high precision. This implies that, after accounting for treatment, a very large part of the variability of BPRS can be explained by PANSS (and vice versa) at the individual level. In addition, one can observe the closeness with the Pearson's correlation coefficient ρ, which is traditionally calculated to investigate the concurrent validity between two psychometric rating scales.

Let us now consider the multi-trial approach of Buyse *et al.* (2000a). Throughout, the sample sizes of the units were used to weight the observations in the calculation of the R^2 values. Figure 16.1(b) shows a plot of the treatment effects on the PANSS *versus* the treatment effects on BPRS for the different units. These seem to be highly correlated. Indeed, using the multi-trial method, we found high conclusive values for the coefficients

TABLE 16.2. *Meta-analysis in schizophrenia. Prentice's criteria for the comparison of PANSS* versus *CGI.*

Effect tested	Criterion	Estimate (standard error)	p-value
Z on S_1	(5.2)	−0.24 (0.103)	0.016
Z on S_2	(5.3)	−4.46 (1.656)	0.007
S_2 on S_1	(5.4)	0.04 (0.001)	0.000
Z on S_1 adjusted for S_2	(5.5)	-0.04 (0.071)	0.513
S_1 on S_2	(16.4)	11.66 (0.402)	0.000
Z on S_2 adjusted for S_2	(16.5)	−1.59 (1.152)	0.167

of determination at the trial *and* individual level. Becuase no clear "true endpoint" could be assigned, we calculated both $R^2_{b_i|a_i,m_{S_2}} = 0.91$ (95% C.I. [0.86, 0.94]) and $R^2_{a_i|b_i,m_{S_1}} = 0.91$ (95% C.I. [0.86, 0.94]). However, calculating the estimate (16.11) based on the reduced model, we found $R^2_{b_i|a_i} = 0.92$ (95% C.I. [0.91, 0.93]), which is very close to the previous values but has the advantage of being symmetric in both scales. Its value indicates that not much would be gained in the precision of the prediction if instead of the full model the reduced model were used to predict the treatment effect. The individual coefficient of determination was calculated as $R^2_{\text{indiv}} = 0.92$ (95% C.I. [0.91, 0.93]). Note that this quantity is symmetric in both scales. Graphically this correlation is represented by the residual plot shown in Figure 16.1(c).

Relationship Between PANSS and CGI

As pointed out before, there is no natural true endpoint associated with this kind of data. Therefore, we will study the symmetric relationship between PANSS (S_2) and CGI (S_1), i.e., we will let each of the endpoints play the role of "true" endpoint. This way, we will be able to study the impact of changing the role of surrogate and true endpoints on the scales.

Again, the Prentice criteria were fulfilled as can be seen from the summary presented in Table 16.2: the treatment is prognostic for both PANSS and CGI, PANSS is prognostic for CGI (and vice versa), and there is no effect of treatment on either scale after correcting for the other scale.

However, as pointed out by Buyse and Molenberghs (1998) and Buyse *et al.* (2000a), one has to be very careful in interpreting these results, as Prentice's criteria are surrounded with a number of conceptual difficulties, possibly leading to wrong conclusions. The point estimates for Freedman's

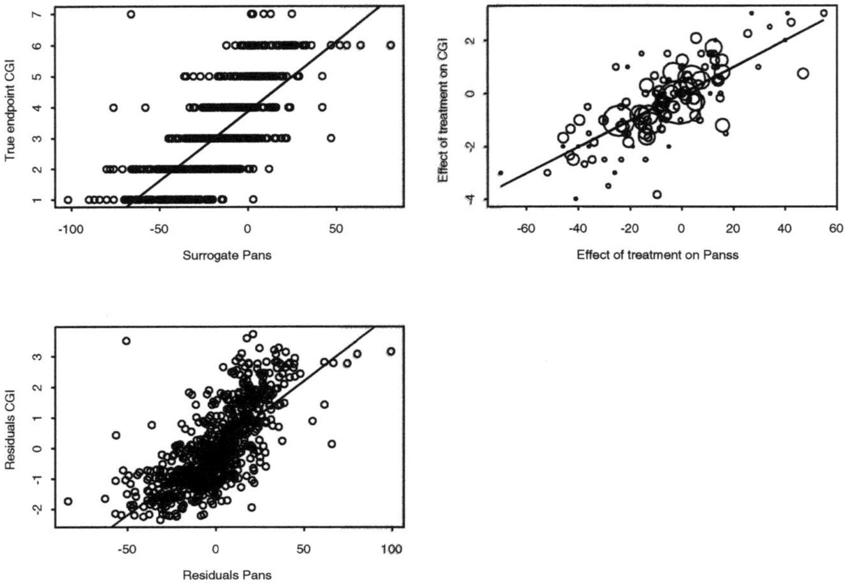

FIGURE 16.2. *Meta-analysis in schizophrenia. (a) Scatter plot of CGI* versus *PANSS (top left); (b) treatment effects on CGI by treatment effects on PANSS (top right). The size of each point is proportional to the number of patients examined by the corresponding investigator. (c) Plot of the residuals of CGI* versus *PANSS (bottom left).*

proportions explained were estimated as $PE(S_1, S_2) = 0.81$ (95% C.I. [0.46, 1.67] and $PE(S_2, S_1) = 0.64$ (95% C.I. [0.31, 1.12]). Clearly the confidence intervals are too wide to be informative. In addition, the upper bounds again exceed 1, which is hard to justify for a proportion. The estimated values for the relative effect were $RE(S_1, S_2) = 0.055$ (95% C.I. [0.01, 0.16]) and $RE(S_2, S_1) = 18.07$ (95% C.I. [6.24, 61.93]).

The treatment-adjusted association had an estimated value of $\rho_Z = 0.72$ (95% C.I. [0.69, 0.75]). Although the point estimate for ρ_Z is smaller than in the previous case, which is not so surprising given the nature of the data, it is still estimated with high precision (in contrast to the RE measures). The meta-analytic approach yielded $R^2_{b_i|m_{S_i},a_i} = 0.56$ (95% C.I. [0.43, 0.68]), $R^2_{a_i|m_{T_i},b_i} = 0.56$ (95% C.I. [0.43, 0.68]) at the trial level and $R^2_{\text{indiv}} = 0.51$ (95% C.I. [0.47, 0.55]) at the individual level. Clearly, these quantities were estimated with sufficient precision, at the same time indicating that the agreement between PANSS and CGI, is smaller than would have been anticipated from the classical validation approaches such as the Prentice criteria and the proportion explained. The individual level correlation between the two endpoints is relatively strong with a value of 0.71 (95%

TABLE 16.3. *Meta-analysis in schizophrenia. Frequency table of the number of units with a given number of patients.*

No. patients per unit n	No. units with n patients	No. patients per unit n	No. units with n patients
2	29	10	2
3	18	11	4
4	23	12	2
5	16	13	3
6	9	15	1
7	12	18	1
8	10	21	1
9	6	30	1

C.I. [0.68, 0.74]). This agrees closely with the treatment-adjusted association parameter ρ_Z and even the Pearson's correlation coefficient $\rho = 0.73$.

Figures 16.2(a) and (b) show a scatterplot of CGI *versus* PANSS and a plot of the treatment effects on CGI by the treatment effects on PANSS, the latter being a graphical representation of R_{trial}. The R_{indiv} is graphically represented by the residual plot in Figure 16.2(c). Clearly, these effects are less correlated than in the previous section. In addition we calculated the R^2 measure at the trial level for the "reduced" model. This yielded $R^2_{b_i|a_i} = R^2_{a_i|b_i} = 0.56$ (95% C.I. [0.43, 0.67]) which coincides with the trial-level values obtained from the "full" model. Apart from the attractive feature that this quantity is symmetric in both scales, the result again indicates that not much would be gained in the precision of the treatment prediction if instead of the full model, the reduced model were used.

In the above meta-analytic analyses, we used the investigator as the unit of analysis. As pointed out at the beginning of Section 16.4.1, this leads to a total of 138 units with the number of patients per unit ranging from 2 to 30. Table 16.3 shows the frequency table of the number of units with a given number of patients. Clearly, the majority of units consists of less than 5 patients.

Alternatively, one could also consider the main investigator as unit of analysis. For 4 out of the 5 trials, only one main investigator was used, leading to extremely large investigator sites. This led to a total number of 29 units with the number of patients per unit ranging from 4 to 450, 4 of which represent trials. When redoing the meta-analytic approach for this setting, we found similar results as before (we now consider the reduced model only); the trial-level and individual-level association measures are respectively given by $R^2_{\text{trial(r)}} = 0.58$ (95% C.I. [0.45, 0.71]) and $R^2_{\text{indiv(r)}} = 0.52$

TABLE 16.4. *Meta-analysis in schizophrenia. Predictions for the treatment effects on CGI based on the observed treatment effects on PANSS. Estimates (standard errors) are shown.*

Unit	No. patients	$\hat{\alpha}_0$	$E(\beta + b_0 \| a_0)$	$\widehat{\beta + b_0}$
1	8	14.00 (16.35)	0.53 (0.63)	0.50 (1.26)
2	6	−43.33 (29.02)	−1.99 (0.63)	−2.33 (1.25)
3	9	−13.50 (12.75)	−0.75 (0.60)	0.30 (1.18)
4	4	7.50 (35.28)	0.08 (0.58)	1.50 (1.80)
5	9	−7.60 (7.65)	−0.45 (0.63)	−0.40 (0.99)
6	8	−42.00 (18.93)	−1.88 (0.63)	−2.50 (1.04)
7	7	−39.58 (18.71)	−2.07 (0.61)	−1.00 (1.18)
8	6	−13.33 (13.79)	−0.69 (0.62)	−1.33 (1.56)
9	6	−7.33 (23.35)	−0.44 (0.63)	−0.33 (1.33)
10	4	−2.00 (18.06)	−0.18 (0.63)	−0.50 (1.80)
11	68	−4.84 (4.46)	−0.32 (0.63)	−0.47 (0.36)
12	8	−14.25 (30.53)	−0.72 (0.62)	−1.50 (0.89
13	7	−6.33 (11.24)	−0.37 (0.63)	−0.83 (0.95)
14	4	−36.5 (14.77)	−1.96 (0.58)	−0.50 (0.50)
15	5	−13.00 (26.93)	−0.66 (0.61)	−1.66 (1.72)
16	8	−22.75 (10.45)	−1.13 (0.63)	−1.25 (0.63)
17	8	−9.00 (10.93)	−0.52 (0.63)	−0.50 (0.65)
18	450	−3.57 (2.13)	−0.28 (0.63)	−0.15 (0.13)
19	7	−23.5 (12.02)	−1.16 (0.63)	−1.25 (0.74)
20	5	−5.33 (13.52)	−0.33 (0.63)	−0.83 (0.57)
21	70	2.75 (5.79)	−0.00 (0.63)	0.21 (0.38)
22	7	−7.50 (16.13)	−0.46 (0.63)	−0.25 (1.40)
23	7	−20.66 (15.39)	−1.00 (0.62)	−1.83 (1.06)
24	9	−4.00 (11.06)	−0.31 (0.63)	0.05 (0.93)
25	5	−7.83 (11.16)	−0.43 (0.61)	−1.33 (0.86)
26	45	−20.15 (9.68)	−1.01 (0.63)	−1.18 (0.50)
27	9	1.14 (19.19)	−0.06 (0.63)	0.00 (0.95)
28	5	−10.50 (10.96)	−0.63 (0.59)	0.66 (0.86)
29	8	−3.25 (10.71)	−0.24 (0.63)	−0.49 (0.79)

(95% C.I. [0.48, 0.56]). Although the point estimates of these R^2 values are similar to the ones found in the previous setting, the confidence interval for R^2_{trial} is much wider, probably due to the smaller number of trials.

Based on the results of the above meta-analytic method, we are able to predict for example the treatment effect on the CGI response based on the observed treatment effect on PANSS (or vice versa). The details hereof have been described in Section 7.2.1. Table 16.4 reports prediction intervals for the 29 units together with the number of patients per unit. In this table, $\hat{\alpha_0}$ and $\widehat{\beta + b_0}$ are values estimated from the data; $E(\beta + b_0)$ is the predicted treatment effect on CGI, given its effect on PANSS. Clearly, in all cases, the

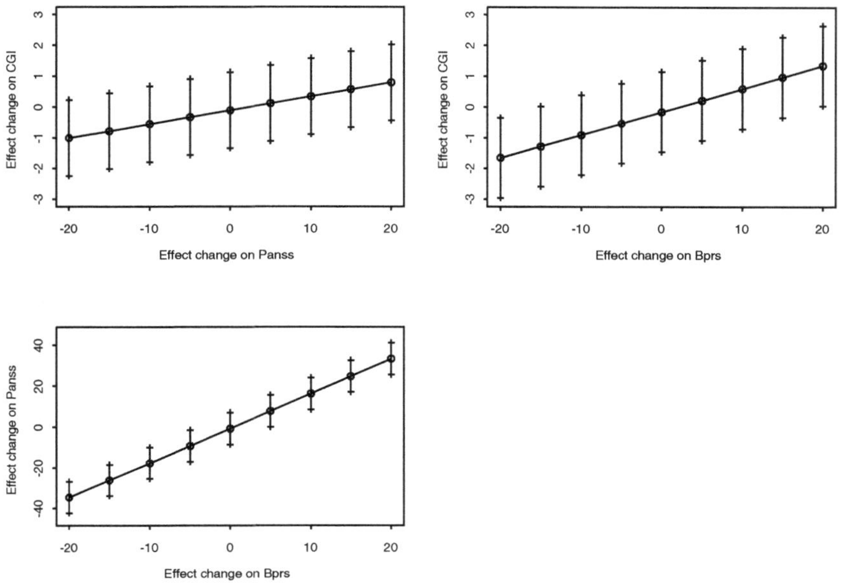

FIGURE 16.3. *Meta-analysis in schizophrenia. Effect changes on one outcome by the effect changes on another outcome.*

predicted values for $\beta + b_0$ agree reasonably well with the effects estimated from the data.

Figure 16.3 indicates how effect changes on one outcome can be translated into effect changes on another outcome. Translating effect changes of PANSS or BPRS to the CGI scale is more or less similar. But, as expected, the translation of an effect change on BPRS to PANSS is much more precise.

Relationship Between BPRS and CGI

When studying the relationship between CGI (S_1) and BPRS (S_2), we found similar results to the ones obtained above for PANSS and CGI. This is not so surprising given the strong relationship found between BPRS and PANSS. Because results for the full and reduced models almost coincide, we only present the values for the reduced model here.

Again, the Prentice criteria were fulfilled as can be seen from the summary presented in Table 16.5: Freedman's proportion explained was estimated as $PE(S_1, S_2) = 0.72$ with a wide 95% confidence interval of [0.37, 1.49] and $PE(S_2, S_1) = 0.09$ (95% C.I. [0.33, 1.34]). The estimated value for the relative effect $RE(S_1, S_2)$ was 0.10 (95% C.I. [0.03, 0.34]) and the

TABLE 16.5. *Meta-analysis in schizophrenia. Prentice's criteria for the comparison of BPRS* versus *CGI.*

Effect tested	Criterion	Estimate (standard error)	p-value
Z on S_1	(5.2)	−0.24 (0.103)	0.016
Z on S_2	(5.3)	−2.35 (0.954)	0.013
S_2 on S_1	(5.4)	0.07 (0.002)	0.000
Z on S_1 adjusted for S_2	(5.5)	−0.06 (0.072)	0.363
S_1 on S_2	(16.4)	6.62 (0.235)	0.000
Z on S_2 adjusted for S_2	(16.5)	−0.73 (0.673)	0.279

TABLE 16.6. *Equivalence trial in schizophrenia. Prentice's criteria for the comparison of PANSS* versus *BPRS.*

Effect tested	Criterion	Estimate (standard error)	p-value
Z on S_1	(5.2)	1.06 (4.050)	0.792
Z on S_2	(5.3)	−0.33 (2.398)	0.887
S_2 on S_1	(5.4)	1.65 (0.024)	0.000
Z on S_1 adjusted for S_2	(5.5)	1.62 (0.834)	0.052

treatment-adjusted association had an estimated value of $\rho_Z = 0.71$ (95% C.I. [0.68, 0.73]). Using the meta-analytic approach we find a value of 0.59 for R^2_{trial} (95% C.I. [0.46, 0.73]) and $R^2_{\text{indiv}} = 0.49$ (95% C.I. [0.44, 0.53]). Figure 16.4(a)–(c), as before, shows the scatterplot of CGI *versus* BPRS, the treatment effects on CGI by the treatment effects on BPRS and a residual plot, respectively.

16.4.2 An Equivalence Trial in Schizophrenic Patients

The data have been described in Section 4.2.7. They come from an international equivalence trial (INT-10) on schizophrenic patients, described by Nair (1998) and the Risperidone Study Group. Like in the previous study, interest lies in determining the extent to which CGI, PANSS, and BPRS are related with each other. Because we only had information available on a single trial with one main investigator, we chose to use investigator as the unit of analysis in the multi-trial approach. A total of 34 units were thus available for analysis with the number of patients per unit ranging from 2 to 15.

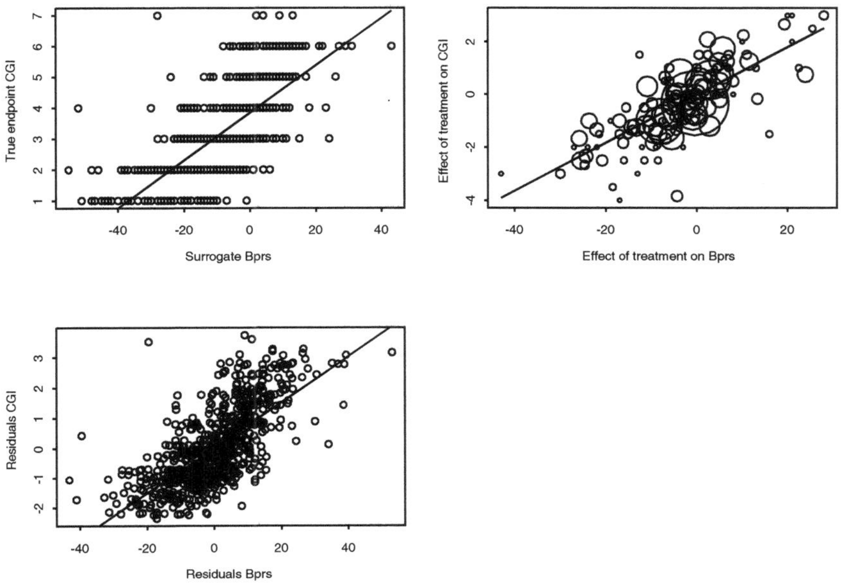

FIGURE 16.4. *Meta-analysis in schizophrenia. (a) Scatter plot of CGI* versus *BPRS (top left); (b) treatment effects on CGI by treatment effects on BPRS (top right). The size of each point is proportional to the number of patients examined by the corresponding investigator. (c) Plot of the residuals of CGI* versus *BPRS (bottom left).*

In the current section, we illustrate on the basis of these data how the classical approaches can hide the possible "agreement" of variables in an equivalence study and how they can produce misleading or even wrong results. Like in the previous section, we will subsequently consider the relationships between (i) PANSS and BPRS and (ii) PANSS and CGI. Results about the BPRS *versus* CGI agreement are not shown, as they are very similar to the results obtained for PANSS and CGI.

PANSS *versus* BPRS

For the sake of illustration, we let PANSS play the role of "true" endpoint. The Prentice criteria now utterly failed to show the high agreement between both scales. Results are summarized in Table 16.6. By definition of an equivalence trial, the first two criteria are bound to be unfulfilled.

As usual, Freedman's proportion explained cannot give a conclusive answer, being estimated at $PE = -0.525$ with an infinite 95% confidence interval. Apart from the confidence interval, which is too wide to be of any practical use, the PE is even negative, which can hardly be justified for a proportion and makes it hard to interpret. The relative effect was estimated at $RE = -3.14$ with an unbounded confidence interval as well, which makes it inconclusive. However, the adjusted association equals $\rho_Z = 0.97$ with 95% confidence interval [0.97, 0.98], giving evidence of a high individual level association corrected for treatment. The meta-analytic approach produced values, $R^2_{\text{trial(r)}} = 0.96$ (95% C.I. [0.82, 1.09]) at the trial level, and $R^2_{\text{indiv(r)}} = 0.94$ (95% C.I. [0.92, 0.95]) at the individual level. Both give conclusive results, which are in agreement with the ones found for PANSS and BPRS in Section 16.4.1. This "robust" behavior clearly confirms the superiority of the meta-analytic approach. Thus, we have illustrated the meta-analytic approach is the only that is able to use data from equivalence trials for validation. All other approaches give inconclusive results, with the Prentice criteria being even utterly useless by definition.

PANSS *versus* CGI

Let us now investigate the agreement between PANSS and CGI with CGI playing the role of "true" or "standard" endpoint. A summary of the Prentice criteria is found in Table 16.7. As could have been anticipated, the first two criteria are again not fulfilled. Freedman's proportion explained takes a negative value of $PE = -0.94$ with an infinite confidence interval. The relative effect estimate was estimated at $RE = -0.03$ with also an infinite confidence interval. The adjusted association was estimated as $\rho_Z = 0.74$ (95% C.I. [0.69, 0.79]), which closely corresponds to the value obtained for PANSS and CGI in Section 16.4.1. The meta-analytic approach yielded values, $R^2_{\text{trial(r)}} = 0.70$ (95% C.I. [0.44, 0.96]) at the trial level, and $R^2_{\text{indiv(r)}} = 0.55$ (95% C.I. [0.47, 0.62]) at the individual level. This illustrates again that the multi-trial approach is the only one that seems to give conclusive results, which are consistent with the ones found in Section 16.4.1.

16.5 Discussion

In this chapter, we have shown how a well-known psychometric property such as the criterion validity can be assessed using surrogate marker validation methodology. Although psychiatric studies, such as the ones presented here, differ from clinical trials by the fact that no true endpoint can be assigned, we show that the developed methodology can equally well be applied on softer endpoints.

Traditional psychometric techniques that try to assess the criterion validity are often limited to the calculation of a simple Pearson's correlation coeffi-

TABLE 16.7. *Equivalence trial in schizophrenia. Prentice's criteria for the comparison of PANSS* versus *CGI.*

Effect tested	Criterion	Estimate (standard error)	p-value
Z on S_1	(5.2)	−0.03 (1.186)	0.835
Z on S_2	(5.3)	1.06 (4.050)	0.792
S_2 on S_1	(5.4)	0.03 (0.002)	0.000
Z on S_1 adjusted for S_2	(5.5)	−0.07 (0.124)	0.544

cient. In contrast, the multi-trial approach described in this paper allows us to relate or predict a treatment effect on one scale with a treatment effect on the other scale. Further, one is able to distinguish between trial-level and individual-level agreement, which the classical techniques do not. In addition, treatment effects on aggregate scores can be translated to effects on more understandable measures.

17

The Evaluation of Surrogate Endpoints in Practice: Experience in HIV

Michael D. Hughes

17.1 Introduction and Background

As for many life-threatening diseases, there has been intense interest in evaluating rapidly the effects of new treatments on the progression of human immunodeficiency virus (HIV) infection. In this chapter, we describe some of the work that was undertaken to evaluate potential surrogate endpoints for use in HIV clinical trials and which contributed to policies for anti-HIV drug approval, for example the United States Food and Drug Administration's (FDA's) "Guidance for Industry: Antiretroviral Drugs Using Plasma HIV RNA Measurements—Clinical Considerations for Accelerated and Traditional Approval" (2002). (See also Chapter 3.)

Early clinical trials of anti-HIV treatments focused on the effects on progression to the acquired immunodeficiency syndrome (AIDS) or to death. However, the progression of HIV infection is typically characterized by a period of asymptomatic infection that may last many years, followed by the development of more minor symptoms of immunodeficiency prior to the onset of AIDS or death. Early in the epidemic, it became clear that this course of clinical disease progression was associated with a decline in the count of $CD4^+$ T-lymphocytes (referred to as CD4 cells forthwith) from levels that are typically greater than 1000 cells/μl prior to HIV infection, with the onset of AIDS usually occurring at levels below 200 cells/μl. The CD4 cell is instrumental in the HIV life cycle because replication of the virus occurs within the cell. Early anti-HIV treatments produced, however, only modest improvements in CD4 cell count. Typically, these involved mean changes of only 50 to 100 cells/μl during the first weeks and months of treatment, followed by declines. Furthermore, there is considerable measurement error and within-subject biological variation in CD4 cell count. For example, a doubling or halving in two successive counts taken a few days apart on the same patient is not unusual. Thus, from the perspectives of both drug regulation and patient management, there was considerable debate about the value of changes in CD4 cell count as a surrogate for longer-term disease progression.

In the mid-1990s, the technology to quantify the amount of viral RNA became available. This was usually measured in an HIV-infected subject's plasma. Worldwide, the most common type of HIV is type 1, and the viral load is referred to as HIV-1 RNA, measured in copies per milliliter of plasma (copies/ml) or $\log_{10}$ copies/ml. Using plasma specimens stored in natural history studies of HIV-infected subjects, it was quickly established that the HIV-1 RNA level was strongly predictive of disease progression.

About the same time as the development of assays to measure HIV-1 RNA levels, drug development began to focus on the use of combination anti-HIV treatment, which typically included drugs from two different classes of drugs. Usually, these combinations involved two nucleoside reverse transcriptase inhibitors (NRTIs) and either a non-nucleoside reverse transcriptase inhibitor (NNRTI) or a protease inhibitor (PI), often described as highly active antiretroviral therapy (HAART). In individual patients, the magnitude of the acute suppression of HIV-1 RNA following initiation of these combination therapies was often larger than the changes that might be explainable by measurement error or within-subject biological variation. In clinical trials, it was also quickly established that these changes in HIV-1 RNA were accompanied by larger and more sustained increases in CD4 cell count and more substantial reductions in the risk of progression to AIDS or death compared with single or two-drug NRTI treatment. Hence, based on reasonable biological arguments, strong opinions developed that treatment-mediated suppression of HIV-1 RNA was associated with improved immunologic status and hence reduced risk of progression to AIDS or death. Furthermore, the sensitivity of assays to measure HIV-1 RNA levels provided physicians and patients with a readily available tool for monitoring the antiviral effects of treatments over time including both the initial suppression and any subsequent rebound (for example, due to the development of viral resistance to the drugs being taken). This also made it very difficult to conduct randomized clinical trials to evaluate the effects of a specific combination of drugs using the traditional endpoint of progression to AIDS or death because many patients changed treatments quickly after seeing poor initial HIV-1 RNA response or subsequent loss of response.

Thus in the mid-1990s, there was substantial interest in the pharmaceutical industry as well as in drug regulatory agencies and academia to evaluate formally the value of HIV-1 RNA and CD4 cell count as surrogate markers for use as endpoints in clinical trials and as a basis for patient management. This interest led to broadly based collaborations including the HIV Surrogate Marker Collaborative Group. This group was a somewhat informal collaboration primarily involving statisticians and clinicians from pharmaceutical companies and government-funded cooperative clinical trials groups. As well as undertaking a formal meta-analysis of clinical trials to evaluate treatment-mediated changes in HIV-1 RNA and CD4 cell count as surrogate endpoints, it also provided a forum for the development and discussion of other relevant research and for interactions on the surrogacy issue with regulatory agencies. Much of the work presented in this chapter benefited from this collaboration and so this chapter is in many respects a tribute to its success.

17.2 Framework for Evaluating Surrogacy

The framework for evaluating surrogacy was largely based on issues and a meta-analysis approach discussed by Hughes, DeGruttola, and Welles (1995), and built upon Temple's definition (1995): "A surrogate endpoint of a clinical trial is a laboratory measurement or physical sign used as a substitute for a clinically meaningful endpoint that measures directly how a patient feels, functions, or survives. Changes induced by a therapy on a surrogate endpoint are expected to reflect changes in a clinically meaningful endpoint." The framework can be defined in terms of the following hierarchy with three levels:

- Evaluate whether HIV-1 RNA and CD4 cell count are separately and jointly predictors of HIV-related disease progression in the absence of treatment.
- Evaluate whether changes in HIV-1 RNA and CD4 cell count following initiation of anti-HIV treatment initiation are separately and jointly predictors of HIV-related disease progression.
- Evaluate whether differences between randomized treatments in changes in HIV-1 RNA and CD4 cell count following initiation of anti-HIV treatment predict differences between the same randomized treatments in HIV-related disease progression.

The first two levels of the hierarchy concern whether marker levels and treatment-mediated changes are *prognostic markers* and should be seen as necessary but not sufficient conditions for establishing the markers as potential surrogate endpoints. In essence, the first requirement reflects the first condition of Prentice (1989; see Section 5.2). The first two levels also relate broadly to the concept of individual-level surrogacy subsequently proposed by Buyse and Molenberghs (1998; see Section 5.4) inasmuch this concept concerns the prognostic value of markers in the presence of treatment, while the third level relates to their concept of trial-level surrogacy (see Section 7.2.1).

17.3 Defining the True Endpoint

Temple defined a surrogate endpoint of a clinical trial as a laboratory measurement or physical sign used as a substitute for a clinically meaningful endpoint that measures directly how a patient feels, functions or survives (Temple 1995). Thus, a key issue that needs to be considered in any evaluation of a potential surrogate endpoint concerns the definition of the clinically meaningful endpoint. In the requirements listed in the previous section, this concerns the definition of "HIV-related disease progression." Arguably the most relevant and objectively defined endpoint of HIV-related disease is death. This is particularly so given that HIV infection is most prevalent in younger adults and so there is minimal risk of non-HIV-related competing causes of death among HIV-infected subjects. However, except in very late-stage HIV infection, HIV clinical trials tended to use a composite endpoint of progression to the first AIDS-defining event or death, whichever occurred first. The definition of AIDS typically used comprised the set of events defined in 1987 by the U.S. Centers for Disease Control and Prevention (CDC) for disease surveillance purposes (Centers for Disease Control 1987). In some ways, this endpoint was itself being used as a surrogate for death allowing trials to be smaller and shorter in duration than if death was used as the primary endpoint.

Although this set of events is reasonably well-defined, there are important issues that need recognition and that could impact the evaluation of a potential surrogate endpoint. First, the clinical significance of the events included in the definition is highly varied. For example, Neaton *et al.* (1994) ranked AIDS-defining events in terms of their prognostic value for death. Some AIDS-defining events, for example herpes simplex infection and cryptosporidiosis, showed no clear association with death, whereas other events, for example lymphoma and progressive multifocal leukoencephalopathy, showed very high relative risks (8 and 18, respectively). Second, different clinical trials used different definitions as to what constituted an endpoint, for example according to whether a subject had or had not experienced an AIDS-defining event prior to randomization. Some trials considered any event, whereas other trials only considered an event that was different from any that a patient had previously experienced. Some trials allowed recurrences of certain events (typically those such as *Pneumocytis carinii* pneumonia that could be treated), whereas other trials categorized events as severe or less severe and, for patients who had previously experienced an AIDS-defining event, only considered events as endpoints if a patient advanced from a previous less severe event to a severe event or death, or from a previous severe event to death. Third, as with most diagnoses, there are gradations of evidence ranging from presumptive diagnoses based on largely subjective evidence to reasonably definitive diagnoses based upon a combination of evidence including, for example, the ability to culture a causative organism. Related to this, it is notable that in practice patients may not be worked up for a definitive diagnosis not only when the event is considered less severe but also when it is considered more severe, for example when a patient chooses to remove himself or herself from hospital to hospice care. Fourth, over time, the availability and use of prophylaxes and treatments for AIDS-defining events may change, affecting not only the incidence of AIDS and death but also the relative importance of the various AIDS events in the AIDS/death endpoint. Fifth, it is notable that a subsequent definition of AIDS by the CDC actually incorporated a CD4 cell count below 200 cells/μl as an AIDS-defining event. Naturally, CD4 cell count will be a better surrogate for progression to AIDS if the definition of AIDS is dominated by CD4 cell count (because most AIDS-defining clinical events occur at counts below 200 cells/μl). These points serve to highlight the fact that evaluation of a potential surrogate endpoint needs careful consideration not only of the definition of the potential surrogate itself but also of the so-called "clinically meaningful endpoint." Needless to say, the quality of the surrogate may be somewhat dependent on the choice of the clinically meaningful endpoint.

17.4 Defining the Potential Surrogate Endpoints

Careful definition of the potential surrogate endpoints is also important. With laboratory measurements such as HIV-1 RNA and CD4 cell count, considerations such as standardization of specimen type, specimen handling and storage, the specific assay or technology used, and the quality control programs in place across multiple laboratories might affect the levels and precision of results (e.g., absolute values of HIV-1 RNA can differ by two-fold or more between assays though the relative changes between measurement times tend not to be different). Other factors may also be important. For example, there is considerable diurnal variation in CD4 cell count so standardizing the timing of measurements particularly within individual patients at successive visits can be important for reducing variability. Standardizing the timing of measurements across clinical trials is an important part of defining a potential surrogate endpoint.

17.5 Prognostic Value of HIV-1 RNA and CD4 Cell Count

Evaluating the prognostic value of a potential surrogate endpoint may not be straightforward if the technique for measuring the surrogate, as with the assay for measuring HIV-1 RNA levels, becomes available after treatments for delaying disease progression are available. In the HIV setting, it was possible to go back to observational studies that were initiated in the 1980s and measure levels in stored serum or plasma specimens. However, it is interesting to note that the measurement of CD4 cell counts needs to be done rapidly after obtaining a blood specimen and so the same could not have been done if it was CD4 cell count that was discovered as a potential surrogate endpoint in the 1990s. The association between depletion of CD4 cells and the development of AIDS was actually identified very soon after AIDS was originally identified in the early 1980s, and hence CD4 cell counts were measured in real time in these observational studies.

The pivotal study that established the prognostic value of HIV-1 RNA levels used data from the U.S. Multicenter AIDS Cohort Study, a prospective observational study (Mellors *et al.* 1996, Mellors *et al.* 1997). This study included 1604 homosexual men who were enrolled in the mid-1980s, and had a study visit at which they were free of AIDS, had a CD4 cell count and had a stored plasma specimen available for measurement of HIV-1 RNA. Table 17.1 shows a recent summary of results from this study showing the joint prognostic value of both HIV-1 RNA and CD4 cell count (DHHS Panel on Clinical Practices for Treatment of HIV Infection, 2004). The risk of progression to AIDS/death clearly increases with HIV-1 RNA level within each of the three categories of CD4 cell count shown. There is also a clear trend of increasing risk of progression with increasing CD4 cell count within each category of HIV-1 RNA level. For both markers, the trends are evident when considering risk over both the shorter-term (over 3 years) and the longer-term (over 9 years). Formal statistical analysis showed that both markers were jointly predictive.

Current recommendations about when to initiate anti-HIV treatment are largely based upon balancing the risks of progression to AIDS or death summarized in Table 17.1 and the potential benefits of treatment (DHHS Panel on Clinical Practices for Treatment of HIV Infection 2004). These recommendations suggest initiation of treatment for all HIV-infected subjects with symptomatic disease (AIDS or other severe symptoms) or asymp-

TABLE 17.1. *Risk for progression to AIDS/death in the multicenter AIDS Cohort Study by baseline CD4 cell count and HIV-1 RNA.*

HIV-1 RNA (copies/ml)	Percentage progressing			
	n	3 years	6 years	9 years
CD4 $\leq$ 200 cells/μl				
$\leq$500	0	-	-	-
$501 - 3,000$	3	-	-	-
$3,001 - 10,000$	7	14.3	28.6	64.3
$10,001 - 30,000$	20	50.0	75.0	90.0
>30,000	70	85.5	97.9	100.0
CD4 $201 - 350$ cells/μl				
$\leq$500	3	-	-	-
$501 - 3,000$	27	0	20.0	32.2
$3,001 - 10,000$	44	6.9	44.4	66.2
$10,001 - 30,000$	53	36.4	72.2	84.5
>30,000	104	64.4	89.3	92.9
CD4 $>$ 350 cells/μl				
$\leq$500	119	1.7	5.5	12.7
$501 - 3,000$	227	2.2	16.4	30.0
$3,001 - 10,000$	342	6.8	30.1	53.5
$10,001 - 30,000$	323	14.8	51.2	73.5
>30,000	262	39.6	71.8	85.0

NOTE: No estimates were available in categories with very small numbers of subjects. Source: DHSS Panel on Clinical Practices for Treatment of HIV Infection (2004).

tomatic subjects with a CD4 cell count of less than 200 cells/μl, with a recommendation to offer treatment when CD4 cell counts are between 200 and 350 cells/μl. However, elevated HIV-1 RNA levels only play a role in the guidelines when CD4 cell counts are greater than 350 cells/μl. Thus the treatment guidelines for initiation of therapy place a greater emphasis on CD4 cell counts than HIV-1 RNA levels, reflecting the fact that CD4 cell count is the more important predictor of imminent risk of progression to AIDS.

17.6 Prognostic Value of Changes in HIV-1 RNA and CD4 Cell Count

Establishing that the improvements in a marker that occur after initiating treatment are predictive of improvements in the true endpoint should be considered an important necessary condition for a good surrogate endpoint, though it is not sufficient. To understand the latter caveat, it is possible that a treatment would have the intended improvement in marker levels and hence also on the clinical endpoint via the intended mechanism of action yet have unintended adverse effects on the true endpoint via other mechanisms of action that would reduce or outweigh the intended benefit. Alternatively, it is possible that a treatment could alter marker levels with no or minimal effect on the clinical endpoint. In the HIV setting, the latter concern is sometimes voiced for immune based therapies. As an example, IL2 has been shown to improve substantially CD4 cell counts in HIV-infected patients, but it is still a matter of debate whether this has any effect on progression to AIDS or death. Biologically, this might reflect increases in CD4 cells that have no or limited functionality against the virus. This is currently being evaluated in two major large randomized trials, which are powered to using clinical events as the primary endpoints.

It is also possible that an association would be observed because it is the patients with a better prognosis in terms of the clinical endpoint who show the greater improvements in marker levels. This latter point was illustrated for short-term changes in CD4 cell count among HIV-infected patients receiving placebo: those showing a defined CD4 cell count response had a lower rate of progression to AIDS/death than those who did not show a CD4 cell count response (Hughes *et al.* 1995).

Two meta-analyses evaluated the prognostic value of changes in HIV-1 RNA and CD4 cell count following initiation of a new anti-HIV treatment. The treatments ranged from NRTI monotherapy through to early HAART regimens. The first meta-analysis was a pooled analysis of data from seven trials undertaken by the AIDS Clinical Trials Group including 1000 subjects who had measurements of change in HIV-1 RNA and CD4 cell count at 24 weeks after starting the new treatment and had no evidence of clinical disease progression during those 24 weeks (Marschner *et al.* 1998). Of these 1000 patients, 120 subsequently experienced clinical progression after week 24.

The major focus of this meta-analysis was on evaluating the prognostic value of changes in HIV-1 RNA following treatment initiation. The study established that each 10-fold reduction in HIV-1 RNA (i.e., each 1 $\log_{10}$ copies/ml reduction) from baseline to week 24 was associated with a 72% reduction in the risk of progression after adjusting for baseline HIV-1 RNA level. Furthermore, the association between the adjusted log relative risk of progression and the change in $\log_{10}$ HIV-1 RNA level was strikingly linear. The latter result suggested proportionately larger reductions in risk associated with greater treatment-mediated antiviral effects. This association was also shown to be very similar across categories of baseline HIV-1 RNA level.

Marschner *et al.* (1998) also evaluated the joint prognostic value of changes in HIV-1 RNA and CD4 cell count. This was complicated by a significant interaction between changes in the two markers. This interaction was characterized in different ways but the general conclusion was that patients who showed an improvement in either or both markers had similar risks of progression during up to about 3 years of follow-up, and these patients had better outcomes than patients who showed no change or a deterioration in both markers.

The second meta-analysis was undertaken by the HIV Surrogate Marker Collaborative Group (HSMCG 2000). It included data from 13,045 patients from all 16 randomized trials that compared NRTI-based therapies and which, by September 1997, (a) had completed follow-up of patients with at least one subject progressing to AIDS or death, and (b) had HIV-1 RNA data measured in some or all patients at baseline and at 24 weeks of follow-up. CD4 cell counts were measured in all patients in all of the trials. A total of 3369 subjects (26%) developed AIDS or died, and 3146 (93%) subjects had measurements of both markers at week 24. The fact that a marker may only be measured in a subset of patients may be a common issue when marker measurement involves new and hence often costly technology. In the description of results that follows, wherever possible, all available data were incorporated in analyses. Obviously, there may be concern about potential selection bias when only subsets of patients are evaluated for an outcome. However, in general, the selection of subjects was determined by factors that might not be expected to be related to outcome (including not being related to the treatment to which a patient was randomized) or involved designs such as a case-cohort design where analysis could take account of the design. However, similar results were obtained when the analysis was restricted to subjects with data on both markers and on the clinical endpoint though with the expected loss of precision.

Decreases in HIV-1 RNA and increases in CD4 count between baseline and week 24 were highly significant predictors of reduced risk of progression to AIDS or death in multivariate analysis that adjusted for baseline marker levels (which were also highly significant). As in the pooled analysis of Marschner *et al.* (1998), approximately linear associations were identified between the log relative risk of progression to AIDS or death and changes in $\log_{10}$ HIV-1 RNA and $\log_{10}$ CD4 cell count (Figure 17.1). However, in contrast to the study of Marschner *et al.* (1998), no interaction between changes in HIV-1 RNA and CD4 cell count was found: patients showing improvements from baseline in both markers experienced a lower rate of progression than patients who showed an improvement in one marker but not the other, while patients who showed deteriorations in both markers had the worst outcome (Figure 17.2).

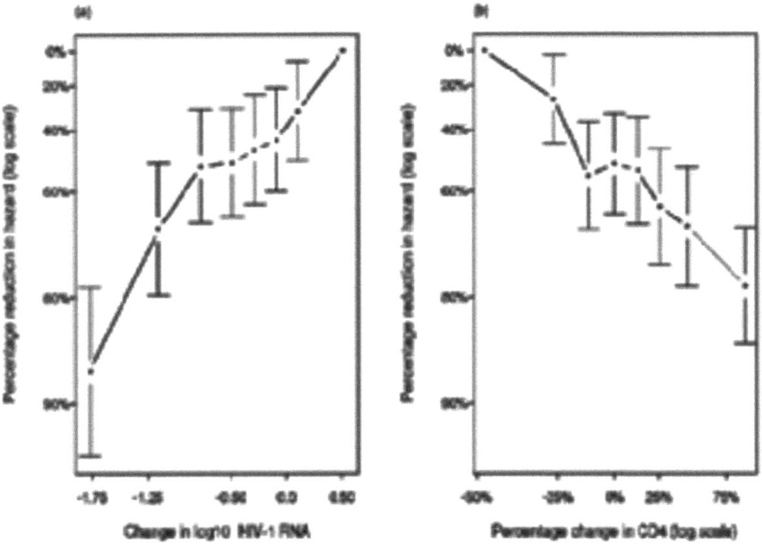

FIGURE 17.1. *Associations between the reduction in hazard of progression to AIDS or death and change in* log_{10} *HIV-1 RNA and relative change in CD4 cell count at 24 weeks after starting study treatment. [Source: HIV Surrogate Marker Collaborative Group (2000)].*

For a marker to be a good surrogate endpoint, a defined change in the marker following the initiation of treatment should be associated with similar (ideally the same) changes in the clinical endpoint irrespective of the treatment being used or the population being treated. This would then mean that the interpretation of a particular magnitude of change in a marker for patient/treatment management decision-making would be similar for all treatments and in all patient populations. Conversely, if the associations are not similar across treatments, then this would mean the marker would be less appealing as a surrogate endpoint for evaluating future treatments because there would be greater uncertainty about the likely associated effect on the clinical endpoint. This issue was evaluated in the HSMCG meta-analysis by quantifying the reduction in risk of progression to AIDS/death associated with changes in each of HIV-1 RNA and CD4 cell count for each treatment arm in the trials included in the meta-analysis (HMSCG 2000). Figure 17.3 summarizes the results including pooled estimates from standard fixed- and random-effects models. Note that the smaller confidence intervals for associations with CD4 cell count than with HIV-1 RNA primarily reflect the fact that all subjects had CD4 cell count measurements, whereas typically only subgroups of subjects had HIV-1 RNA measurements.

A key finding is that almost all of the associations reflect concordance

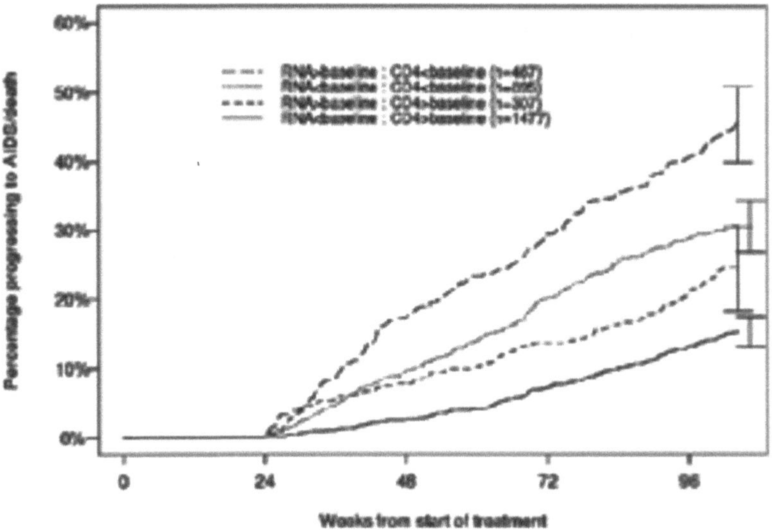

FIGURE 17.2. *Association between the risk of progression to AIDS or death by whether a patient showed improvement in both, one of, or neither HIV-1 RNA and CD4 cell count at 24 weeks after starting study treatment. [Source: HIV Surrogate Marker Collaborative Group (2000)].*

between beneficial effects on each of the markers and beneficial effects on risk of progression to AIDS/death; the two or three associations in each plot to the right of the vertical line (indicating discordance) are typically estimated with considerable imprecision and so are not incompatible with a true concordant association. In addition, with the caveat that tests of heterogeneity often lack power, there was no significant evidence that the associations varied between study populations and treatments. In addition, the average associations were very similar from both fixed- and random-effects models. Specifically, from the fixed effects model, on average, each 1 $\log_{10}$ copies/ml reduction in HIV-1 RNA was associated with a 49% reduction in risk of progression to AIDS/death, and each 33% increase in CD4 cell count was associated with a 21% reduction in risk of progression.

A third study, reported by employees of the U.S. Food and Drug Administration, focused just on the prognostic value of changes in HIV-1 RNA for progression to AIDS/death (Murray *et al.* 1999). This study presented results from selected groups of studies undertaken by different pharmaceutical companies or by the AIDS Clinical Trials Group. A potential limitation is that the analysis methods varied across the different groups of studies. However, the general conclusions from the results were similar to those obtained by Marschner *et al.* (1998) and the HSMCG (2000). A key additional result showed an association of lower risk of disease progression

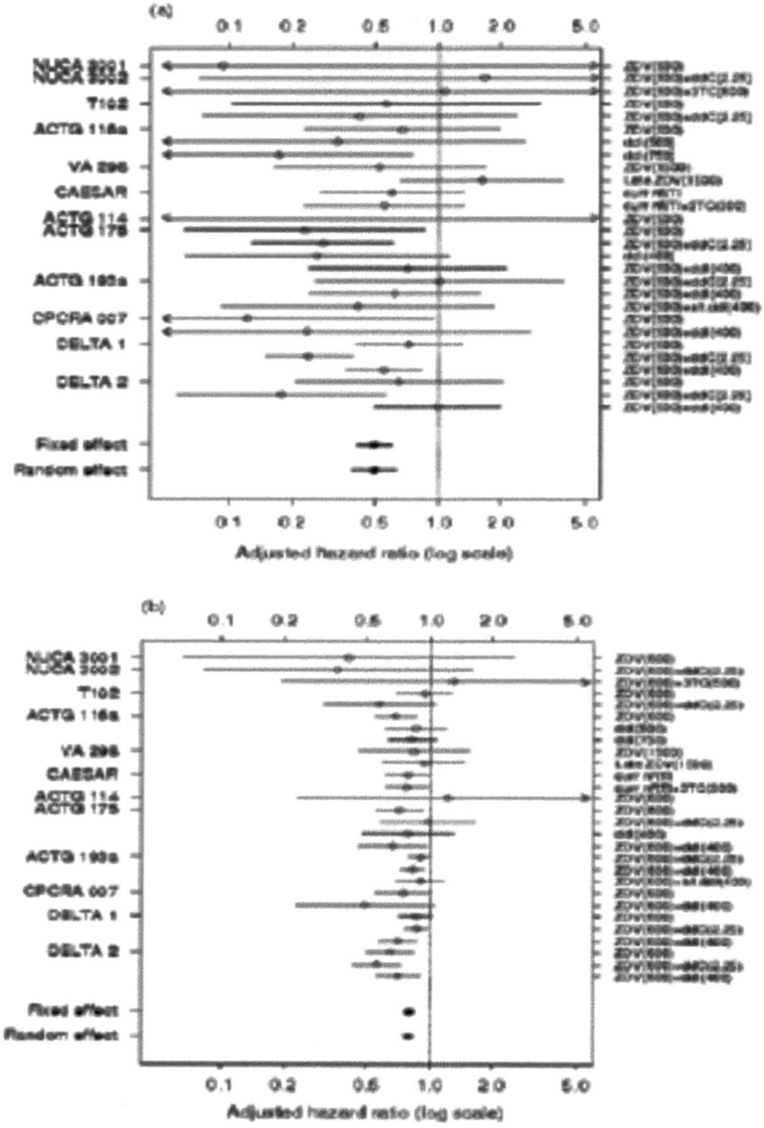

FIGURE 17.3. *Reduction in risk of progression to AIDS/death associated with (a) each 1 $\log_{10}$ copies/ml decrease in HIV-1 RNA and (b) each 33% increase in CD4 cell count at 24 weeks after starting study treatment for each treatment arm in the trials included in the meta-analysis of the HIV Surrogate Marker Collaborative Group.*

with increasing duration of virologic response (defined as the duration of suppression of HIV-1 RNA by greater than 0.5 $\log_{10}$ copies/ml below pretreatment level) during the first 24 weeks of treatment. Thus sustained virologic suppression was important for improved prognosis.

Biologically, it might be expected that short-term changes in HIV-1 RNA, and hence reductions in the amount of circulating virus in an infected person, might be associated with longer-term improvements in CD4 cell count as one measure of improved immunological status. Such an association has been found. For example, results from one clinical trial showed that each additional reduction of 1 $\log_{10}$ copies/ml in HIV-1 RNA level from baseline to week 8 after initiating a new antiretroviral treatment was significantly associated with an additional increase of 30 cells/μl in mean CD4 cell count from baseline to week 48 (Hughes *et al.* 1997). This was after adjustment for baseline HIV-1 RNA and CD4 cell count as well as the change in CD4 count from baseline to week 8. Although this observation does not directly concern the surrogacy question, it does provide supporting information for an underlying mechanistic model by which treatment-mediated suppression of HIV-1 RNA is associated with subsequent improvements in immunological status and hence also reductions in risk of progression to AIDS or death.

17.7 Association of Differences Between Randomized Treatments in Their Effects on Markers and Progression to AIDS or Death

17.7.1 Regression Approach

As part of the meta-analysis conducted by the HSMCG, the regression approach of Daniels and Hughes (1997) was used to evaluate the strength of the association of differences between a pair of randomized treatments in the rate of progression to AIDS/death and the corresponding differences between the treatments in the marker changes. The underlying model used is conceptually the same as that subsequently used by Buyse *et al.* (2000a; see also Chapter 7) to describe trial-level surrogacy. Consider trials $i = 1, \cdots, N$ which, for simplicity, each involve a randomized comparison of two treatments. Let θ_i denote the true treatment difference on the clinical endpoint (e.g., the log hazard ratio for progression to AIDS/death) and γ_i denote the true difference on the marker change (e.g., change in $\log_{10}$ HIV-1 RNA or $\log_{10}$ CD4 cell count from baseline to week 24). From each trial, estimates $\hat{\theta}_i$ and $\hat{\gamma}_i$ are obtained. It is assumed that the size of each study is sufficiently large such that, within the ith trial, the following model holds:

$$\begin{pmatrix} \hat{\theta}_i \\ \hat{\gamma}_i \end{pmatrix} \sim N\left[\begin{pmatrix} \theta_i \\ \gamma_i \end{pmatrix}, \begin{pmatrix} \sigma_i^2 & \rho_i\sigma_i\delta_i \\ \rho_i\sigma_i\delta_i & \delta_i^2 \end{pmatrix}\right], \tag{17.1}$$

where σ_i^2 and δ_i^2 are variances that reflect sampling variation, and ρ_i is the correlation between the estimated treatment differences conditional upon the true differences. This model is easily extended to handle the correlation between estimators when there are multiple treatment arms in any particular trial (see Daniels and Hughes (1997) for details). This was the case in the HSMCG meta-analysis: five, nine, and two trials randomized patients among two, three, and four treatments, respectively.

A simple linear model is assumed to describe the association between θ_i and γ_i across the N clinical trials:

$$\theta_i|\gamma_i \sim N(\alpha + \beta\gamma_i, \tau^2). \tag{17.2}$$

In this model, β measures the association between the treatment differences on the marker and on the clinical endpoint so that $\beta = 0$ corresponds to the situation in which the marker is not in fact a surrogate endpoint since knowledge about the difference in marker values between randomized treatments, γ_i, is not predictive of the corresponding difference in the clinical endpoint, θ_i. In addition, if $\beta \neq 0$, then $\tau^2 = 0$ would imply that θ_i could be predicted perfectly given γ_i. For imperfect surrogate endpoints, the closer τ^2 is to zero, the better the surrogate. It is also useful to have $\alpha = 0$. Although this is not strictly necessary in order that the difference in marker levels might provide a good prediction of the corresponding difference in the clinical endpoint, it seems desirable that a zero difference between randomized treatments for the marker should be associated with a zero difference in the clinical endpoint. This would also then be consistent with the spirit of Prentice's requirement that a test of the null hypothesis of no difference between treatments in the surrogate endpoint should be a valid test of the null hypothesis of no difference between treatments in the clinical endpoint.

Daniels and Hughes (1997) proposed an empirical Bayes approach to model fitting by proceeding as if σ_i^2, δ_i^2 and ρ_i are known and replacing them by their estimates. To avoid the need to specify a joint model within a trial for the marker and the clinical endpoint, they proposed estimating ρ_i using a bootstrap technique. This requires data from each individual patient to be available for the meta-analysis, as was the case for the HSMCG meta-analysis. This bootstrap approach has the advantage that the evaluation of trial-level surrogacy is not affected by any misspecification in a model for the prognostic value of the marker for the clinical endpoint at the within-trial patient level but has the disadvantage that some loss of efficiency may arise, though this is likely to be minimal in many practical situations (Gail *et al.* 2000). However, use of the estimates for the variances and correlation rather than the true values does mean that the precision of any trial-level association may be over-estimated particularly if the number of trials included in the meta-analysis is small. Gail *et al.* (2000) suggested a bootstrap approach to help overcome this (see Chapter 9). Alternatively a joint model for time-to-event data and marker data might be used (see Chapters 11, 12, and 13).

For the parameters α and β, Daniels and Hughes (1997) proposed using mutually independent "non-informative" prior distributions, specifically normal distributions with very large variances. If the parameters γ_i, $i = 1, \cdots, N$, are considered as fixed effects, then similar mutually independent "non-informative" prior distributions could be used for these nuisance parameters. Alternatively, they could be considered as random effects arising from, for example, a normal distribution $N(\mu, \kappa^2)$ with a "non-informative" normal prior distribution placed upon the mean, μ. This requires careful thought as there may not be a strong rationale for the choice of distribution for such random effects. For example, a normal distribution may be more plausible if all trials are comparing active treatments from the same drug class. However, if some trials compare active drugs to placebo while other trials compare active drugs from the same class, then a bimodal distribution for the random effects might be more appropriate. Empirical justification of the choice of distribution may be difficult if the meta-analysis includes only a limited number of trials.

The choice of prior distribution, $\pi(\tau^2)$, for the variance, τ^2, is less straightforward. Daniels and Hughes (1997) proposed three possibilities:

- DuMouchel prior: $\pi(\tau^2) = \frac{\sigma_c}{(\sigma_c+\tau)^2}\frac{1}{2\tau}$ where σ_c^2 is the harmonic mean of the within-study variances of the treatment difference on the clinical outcome, σ_i^2 (DuMouchel 1994).

- Shrinkage prior: $\pi(\tau^2) = \frac{\sigma_c^2}{(\sigma_c^2+\tau^2)^2}$ (Strawderman 1971).

- Flat prior: $\pi(\tau^2) = \mathrm{d}\tau^2$ (Berger 1995).

The DuMouchel and shrinkage priors permit the possibility that $\tau^2 = 0$. Provided that $\beta \neq 0$, this would indicate that the marker was a perfect surrogate endpoint. The flat prior does not allow for this possibility. In general, the DuMouchel prior tends to give a posterior distribution for τ^2 which is closer to zero compared with that for the flat prior, and the shrinkage prior is intermediate. As an alternative, a gamma prior distribution with very large variance might be used for the precision, τ^{-2} (Spiegelhalter *et al.*

1996). As noted above, the parameters γ_i, $i = 1, \cdots, N$, might also be considered as normally distributed random effects. In this case, similar types of prior distributions might be used for the variance, κ^2, or precision, κ^{-2} of that distribution.

In practice, because the number of trials in a meta-analysis might be quite small, the difficulty in defining "non-informative" prior distributions for variance parameters means that the analysis should be repeated for a range of reasonable prior distributions and the sensitivity of the conclusions to the choice of prior evaluated. In the following presentation of results from the HSMCG meta-analysis, the γ_i's were considered to be random effects from a $N(\mu, \kappa^2)$ distribution. This was confirmed to be reasonable by visual inspection of a normal plot based on the fact that $\hat{\gamma}_i \sim N(\mu, \sigma_i^2 + \kappa^2)$ and hence that $\frac{\hat{\gamma}_i - \mu}{\sqrt{(\sigma_i^2 + \kappa^2)}} \sim N(0, 1)$. The prior distributions for α, β, and μ were independent $N(0, \delta^2)$ distributions with δ^2 taken to be very large, specifically 10^8, and the prior distributions for the precisions, τ^{-2} and κ^{-2}, were taken as independent $\Gamma(0.001, 0.001)$. Although the choice of reasonable alternative prior distributions for the variances does affect the numerical values of the results presented, the conclusions that are drawn were not significantly impacted.

17.7.2 Results from the Meta-analysis

The first analysis that was conducted considered as potential surrogate endpoints the change from baseline to week 24 in either $\log_{10}$ HIV-1 RNA or $\log_{10}$ CD4 cell count. The clinical endpoint was the hazard of progression to the first AIDS-defining event or to death, whichever occurred first, within two years of randomization. The choices of week 24 and two years, respectively, were made on the basis that these time periods were typical of practice at the time for marker-based endpoints (in phase II trials) and clinical endpoints (in phase III trials).

Figure 17.4 summarizes the data for the meta-analysis. Panels A and B show the associations between differences in randomized comparisons in the rate of progression to AIDS/death (expressed as a hazard ratio on a log scale) versus the corresponding differences in the change from baseline to week 24 in $\log_{10}$ HIV-1 RNA and $\log_{10}$ CD4 cell count, respectively. Each circle in each plot represents an individual randomized comparison with the size of the circles being in proportion to the precision in estimating the log hazard of progression to AIDS/death so that larger circles indicate comparisons with greater precision. It is clear that most comparisons show, qualitatively, concordance between results for each marker and results for progression to AIDS/death. Specifically, for differences in change in $\log_{10}$

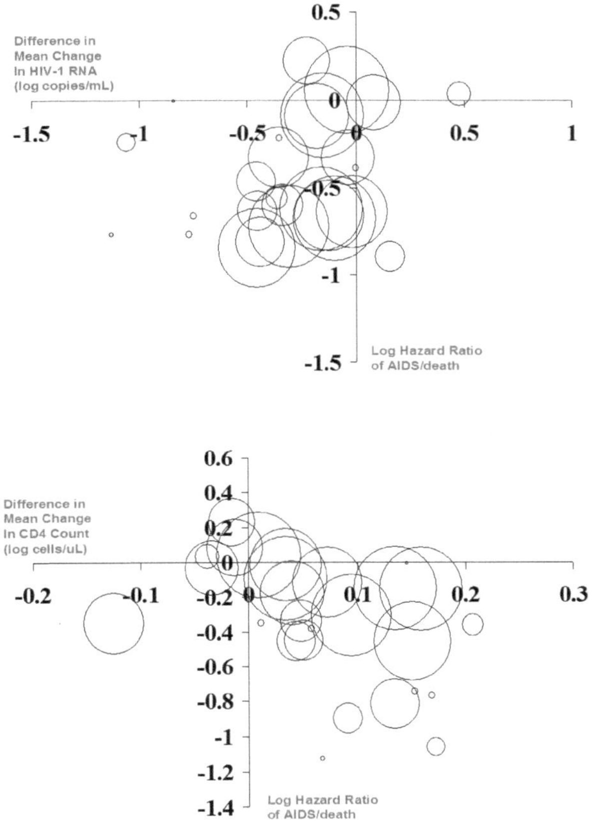

FIGURE 17.4. *Association between log hazard ratio for progression to AIDS or death for randomized comparisons of treatments and the corresponding differences in (a) change in* $\log_{10}$ *HIV-1 RNA or (b) change in* $\log_{10}$ *CD4 cell count at 24 weeks after starting study treatment, in the meta-analysis of the HIV Surrogate Marker Collaborative Group. Each circle represents a randomized comparison, and the size of the circle is in proportion to the precision in estimating the log hazard ratio.*

HIV-1 RNA, most points are in the lower left quadrant, indicating that within these randomized comparisons the treatment that showed greater suppression of HIV-1 RNA also showed greater reduction in the hazard of progression to AIDS/death. There was only one comparison in the upper right quadrant reflecting qualitative concordance but with the control treatment superior to the experimental treatment for both outcome measures. This reflects the reasonable success in HIV research in developing new treatments that are generally better than previous options.

However, five comparisons did show qualitative discordance between the estimated differences in effect for change in HIV-1 RNA and risk progression to AIDS/death. For four of these five comparisons, the discordance could reflect sampling variation because there was no significant difference between randomized treatments for either outcome measure. For the fifth comparison (a point in the lower right quadrant), however, the discordance reflects a situation in which there was a small (non-significant) difference in change in HIV-1 RNA between randomized treatments with the estimate favoring the control treatment, but a significant difference in risk of progression to AIDS/death favoring the test treatment. Hence, use of change in HIV-1 RNA in this trial would have led to a potentially incorrect conclusion versus comparing treatments based upon the clinical endpoint.

For changes in CD4 cell count, recognizing that increases in CD4 cell count are beneficial and hence qualitative concordance is reflected by points being in the upper left or lower right quadrants, there was a slightly better predominance for qualitative concordance. However, as for change in HIV-1 RNA, there was one comparison that showed discordance whereby there was a non-significant difference favoring the control treatment for change in CD4 cell count but a significant difference favoring the test treatment for risk of progression to AIDS/death. The notable discordant results for change in HIV-1 RNA and change in CD4 cell count were not, however, for the same comparison.

Focusing on the trial-level component of the regression model, $\theta_i|\gamma_i \sim N(\alpha + \beta\gamma_i, \tau^2)$, for changes in HIV-1 RNA, the median (2.5^{th}, 97.5^{th} percentile) of the posterior distribution for α and β were -0.12 (-0.34, 0.08) and 0.28 (-0.16, 0.70). Clearly, there is not strong statistical evidence for a non-zero trend. Furthermore, the median of the posterior distribution for τ was 0.16 compared with a value of 0.18 for the model with no marker effects (i.e., setting $\beta = 0$). In contrast, for changes in CD4 cell count, the medians of the posterior distributions for α and β were 0.04 (-0.16, 0.29) and -4.1 (-7.3, -1.6), showing significant evidence of a trend. The closeness of the median of the posterior distribution for α to zero suggests that a lack of a difference in a randomized comparison in mean change in $\log_{10}$ CD4 cell count was associated with a lack of a difference in the risk of progression to AIDS/death. Also, the median of the posterior distribution for τ was 0.08, which, when compared with the value of 0.18 obtained from the model with no marker effects, suggests that much more of the heterogeneity in log hazard ratios for progression to AIDS/death is explained by differences in mean change in $\log_{10}$ CD4 cell count than by differences in mean change in $\log_{10}$ HIV-1 RNA. Referring back to Figure 17.4, these results are consistent with the visual impression of a stronger trend in the association for changes in CD4 cell count than for changes in HIV-1 RNA. Furthermore, although there was only one notable qualitatively discordant comparison in both of panels A and B in Figure 17.4, the smaller median estimate for

τ for differences in change in CD4 cell count versus differences in change in HIV-1 RNA is compatible with the impression of stronger quantitative concordance in panel B than in panel A.

Biologically, it might be expected that a measure of sustained suppression of HIV-1 RNA might be a better surrogate endpoint than simply evaluating the change in HIV-1 RNA between baseline and some subsequent time. This is because sustained suppression might allow for greater improvement in the immune system and hence lower risk of progression to AIDS/death. Trials in the meta-analysis typically also measured the markers at 8 weeks after randomization. Hence it is possible to evaluate whether incorporating the 8-week measurement into the definition of a potential surrogate endpoint provides an improvement in predicting differences in the clinical endpoint versus just measuring the change from baseline to week 24. One simple metric for the two markers that was widely considered in trials was the so-called "area under the curve minus baseline" (AUCMB). In the context of having the baseline, week 8 and week 24 measurements, this is the area under the curve over time obtained by joining the baseline, week 8, and week 24 measurements and then subtracting off the baseline level. Dividing this area by the time between baseline and week 24 then gives a time-averaged AUCMB for $\log_{10}$ HIV-1 RNA over the first 24 weeks after starting study treatment. Using this time-averaged AUCMB for $\log_{10}$ HIV-1 RNA in the regression model instead of the simple changes in $\log_{10}$ HIV-1 RNA did provide a modest improvement in the model. Specifically, the median value of the posterior distribution for β was 0.28 and the 95% probability interval given by the (2.5^{th}, 97.5^{th}) percentiles was (-0.16, 0.70) and so almost excluded zero suggesting stronger statistical evidence for a trend. However, there was very little difference in heterogeneity in the log hazard ratio across trials explained by the time-averaged AUCMB versus the simple change. In contrast, there was no evidence that differences between treatments in the time-averaged AUCMB for $\log_{10}$ CD4 count was a better predictor for differences in the log hazard of progression to AIDS/death.

The regression-based approach can also be extended to a multivariate (multiple regression) model to evaluate whether differences in each of the two markers are jointly predictive of differences between randomized treatments in the log hazard of progression to AIDS/death. Table 17.2 shows the results from a univariate (simple regression) model that includes the difference in change in time-averaged AUCMB for $\log_{10}$ HIV-1 RNA from baseline to week 24 (model 1), as well as from a univariate model that includes the difference in change in $\log_{10}$ CD4 cell count (model 2), and from a multivariate model that includes differences in both time-averaged AUCMB for HIV-1 RNA and change in CD4 count (model 3) as covariates. The most notable aspect of the multivariate model is that the median of the posterior distribution for the parameter β_{RNA} is very close to zero (par-

TABLE 17.2. *Univariate and multivariate models for predicting the log hazard Ratio for progression to AIDS/death.*

	Model 1		Model 2		Model 3	
Par.	Med.	95% PI	Med.	95% PI	Med.	95% PI
α	−0.12	(−0.34, 0.08)	0.04	(−0.16, 0.29)	0.04	(−0.20, 0.31)
β_{RNA}	0.28	(−0.16, 0.70)		—	0.07	(−0.49, 0.59)
β_{CD4}		—	−4.2	(−7.3, −1.6)	−3.9	(−7.7, −0.5)
τ	0.16	(0.04, 0.31)	0.08	(0.02, 0.23)	0.08	(0.02, 0.25)

NOTE: Values presented are median (Med.) and 95% probability interval (PI) = (2.5^{th}, 97.5^{th} percentiles) of the posterior distribution.
Model 1: Difference in HIV-1 RNA AUCMB.
Model 2: Difference in change in CD4 count.
Model 3: Difference in HIV-1 RNA AUCMB & change in CD4 count.

ticularly when compared to its value in the univariate model). In contrast, the 95% probability interval for β_{CD4} excludes zero, confirming a strong association between differences in change in $\log_{10}$ CD4 count even after adjustment for differences in $\log_{10}$ HIV-1 RNA. Thus, the evidence from this meta-analysis favors change in CD4 count as a surrogate endpoint for progression to AIDS/death and suggests that differences in change in HIV-1 RNA provide little additional predictive value.

Biologically, the results of the multivariate model seem quite reasonable in that CD4 count is a measure of immunological status that is more proximal to AIDS/death than HIV-1 RNA in the sense that the clinical events that define AIDS are events that are associated with more severe immunosuppression. This general conclusion persisted in sensitivity analyses that dropped in turn either each trial or each group of randomized comparisons that included a specific treatment to evaluate whether any particular trial or treatment was overly influential in the modeling. In addition, this type of sensitivity analysis allows a comparison of what was observed for a particular dropped trial or group of comparisons with what is predicted based on a model with that trial or group of comparisons omitted (see Daniels and Hughes (1997) for details). None of these comparisons revealed any differences between the observed and predicted outcomes beyond that explainable by random variation.

The regression models can also be used to provide information about the magnitude of difference between randomized treatments in a marker that is necessary before there is reasonable evidence that there would be an associated difference in progression to AIDS/death as measured by the log hazard ratio of progression. Specifically, given a future study j with an observed marker difference $\hat{\gamma}_j$ with variance $\hat{\sigma}_j^2$, then using the past experience encapsulated in the regression model, the posterior distribution for the log hazard ratio for progression $\theta_j|\hat{\gamma}_j, \hat{\sigma}_j^2, \alpha, \beta, \tau^2$ can be obtained (see Daniels and Hughes (1997) for details). To illustrate the basic idea here, consider the situation in which the true difference, γ_j, is known. Table 17.3 shows the predictions for various values of γ_j when expressed as relative differences between treatments in CD4 cell count. The wide probability intervals show that there is considerable uncertainty in the predictions even though these are based on knowing the true relative difference in change in CD4 cell count. This reflects the variability about the regression line captured by the non-zero τ and captures the uncertainty inherent in using change in CD4 cell count as a surrogate endpoint. In a randomized comparison, the test treatment would need, in truth, to increase CD4 cell count between baseline and 24 weeks by about 15% more on average than the control treatment in order for the probability interval to exclude a hazard ratio of one and hence provide reasonable certainty of a corresponding reduction in risk of progression to AIDS/death for the test treatment versus the control treatment. This relative difference corresponds to an absolute increase of about 33 cells/μl more for a subject with the median CD4 cell count in the dataset of 220 cells/μl, and agrees well with an earlier meta-analysis which evaluated change in CD4 cell count as a surrogate endpoint (Hughes *et al.* 1998). Even then, knowing the true relative effect on CD4 cell count leaves uncertainty about whether the test treatment might have a very minimal effect on progression to AIDS/death (i.e., a hazard ratio close to 1.0) or a quite substantial effect (i.e., a hazard ratio of about 0.67 corresponding to a one-third reduction in the risk of progression). These probability intervals are, however, conservative because they are based on a meta-analysis model that was fitted using estimated variances (e.g., $\hat{\sigma}_i^2$) as if they were the true variances. Furthermore, the probability intervals would also be wider in the real situation in which the difference in change in CD4 cell count is estimated within a trial, *versus* using the true value as in Table 17.3.

A second meta-analysis of HIV randomized clinical trials further evaluated CD4 count and HIV-1 RNA level as potential surrogate endpoints (Hill *et al.* 1998). This meta-analysis included some of the same trials as in the meta-analysis described above but also included clinical trials that evaluated combination antiretroviral regimens that included two newer classes of drugs, non-nucleoside reverse transcriptase inhibitors (NNRTIs) and protease inhibitors (PIs). This meta-analysis was restricted to trials in which at least 10 patients per treatment arm showed progression to AIDS or death, over each trial's duration of follow-up, and for which data were collected on both markers. This meta-analysis focused on marker changes from baseline to 16 weeks.

One notable difference between this meta-analysis and the one conducted

TABLE 17.3. *Predicted hazard ratios for progression to AIDS/death for given true relative differences in CD4 count.*

% increase in CD4 count:	Predicted hazard ratio for AIDS/death	
Test vs. control treatment	Median	(95% PI)
0%	1.04	(0.78, 1.42)
10%	0.88	(0.69, 1.12)
20%	0.75	(0.60, 0.93)
30%	0.65	(0.49, 0.83)
40%	0.57	(0.41, 0.78)
50%	0.51	(0.34, 0.72)

NOTE: Values presented are median and 95% probability interval (PI) = (2.5^{th}, 97.5^{th} percentiles) of the posterior distribution for the hazard ratio.

by the HSMCG is that this one used summary data from publications or other public sources rather than individual patient data. In part, this reflected a desire to address the surrogacy question quickly in the face of mounting difficulties in conducting trials with clinical endpoints and difficulties in accessing individual patient data from all trials owing to issues of confidentiality. This necessitates using some approximations to provide standardized estimates of differences in treatment effect on clinical progression and each of the markers which might weaken any association.

The meta-analysis used the regression-based approach proposed by Daniels and Hughes (1997). However, model fitting was undertaken using standard methods for weighted linear regression. Each randomized comparison in the meta-analysis was weighted by the reciprocal of the sum of the variances of the estimated differences in treatment effect on HIV-1 RNA, CD4 cell count and the clinical endpoint. Conceptually, this gives greater weight to randomized comparisons that provide more precise estimates for treatment effects on all three outcomes. However, as far as we know, the validity of this system of weighting has not been evaluated and hence whether it appropriately deals with the two statistical issues in the modeling of (a) different variances for the outcome variable (i.e., for the log hazard ratio for progression to AIDS/death) for which weighted analysis is an accepted methodology and (b) imprecision in the covariates (the difference in mean changes in each of the markers) is unknown.

One other methodological issue is worth commenting on. This concerns the fact that the assays for measuring HIV-1 RNA may not be able to detect RNA at low levels, and they also have defined ranges of reliable quantification. One trial in the meta-analysis had a high proportion of subjects with HIV-1 RNA levels below the lower limit of quantification, reflecting the potency of newer drugs and combination therapies. Although statistical methods for censored data can be used to estimate treatment effects taking

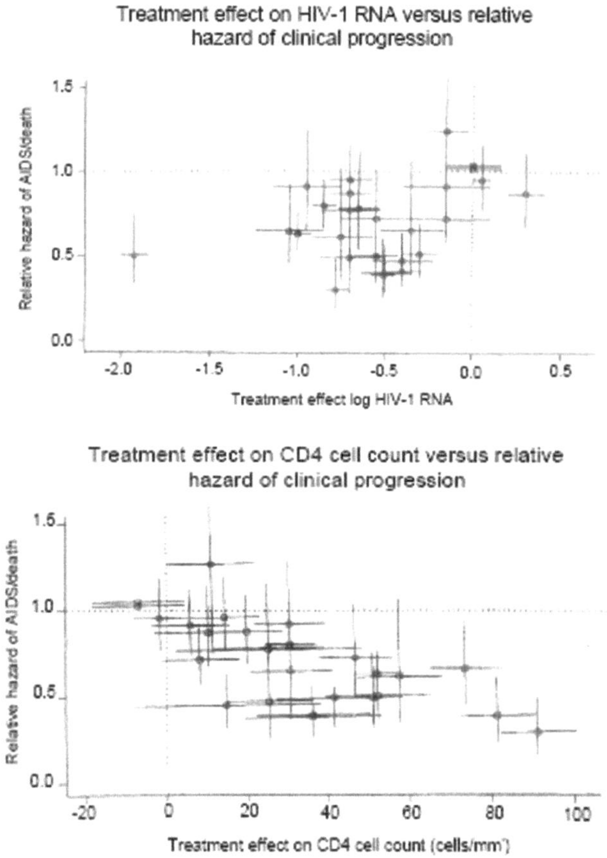

FIGURE 17.5. *Association between the hazard ratio for progression to AIDS/death and the difference in mean change in HIV-1 RNA or CD4 cell count from baseline to week 16 in the meta-analysis of Hill* et al. *(1998).*

account of the range of quantification, when a large proportion are below the lower limit (e.g., over one-half), it is difficult to validate assumptions necessary to estimate mean changes. A change in the metric of measuring a marker may circumvent the problem.

Figure 17.5 summarizes the associations between the hazard ratio for progression to AIDS/death and the difference in mean change in HIV-1 RNA or CD4 count from baseline to week 16. The general impression about possible associations in this figure is similar to that seen in Figure 17.4 for the meta-analysis of randomized comparisons only involving NRTIs. Note though that differences in change in CD4 cell count were measured on an absolute scale in this meta-analysis, whereas they were measured on a log scale or, equivalently, as relative differences in the meta-analysis described earlier. However, using the weighted regression analysis, both associations, and not just the association with the difference in change in CD4 count, were statistically significant in this meta-analysis (Hill *et al.* 1998). This might reflect greater power in this meta-analysis to detect associations because of the inclusion of trials of other drug classes and, particularly, a larger number of subjects progressing to AIDS/death. The power may also be increased by greater heterogeneity in the magnitudes of differences in effect between pairs of randomized treatments. In this respect, it is notable that one randomized comparison is a clear outlying observation in the association between the hazard ratio for clinical progression and differences in mean change in HIV-1 RNA. This comparison would obviously be influential in regression analysis. It is interesting to note that this comparison does not provide a clear outlying observation in the association with difference in mean change in CD4 cell count—suggesting some disconnect between the two markers. It is also possible that the significant association for changes in HIV-1 RNA in this analysis might reflect use of changes to week 16 rather than week 24, though Hill *et al.* (1998) state that similar results were obtained when changes to week 24 were considered. Alternatively, it is possible that there is a stronger association between effects on clinical progression and HIV-1 RNA for drugs from the NNRTI and PI classes than for drugs from the NRTI) class. This was not evaluated by Hill *et al.* (1998), though the power to show differences according to drug class is likely to be limited due to the relatively small number of trials involving NNRTIs) (three trials) or PIs (four trials).

17.8 Discussion

The validation of potential surrogate endpoints for use in HIV clinical trials highlights some of the practical problems that might be encountered as well as the need to balance empirical evaluation with an understanding of disease processes and mechanisms of action (and failure) of treatments. From a quantitative perspective, the preceding summary might suggest that change in CD4 cell count might be a more reliable surrogate endpoint than some measure of change in HIV-1 RNA, though there is undoubtedly a substantial body of evidence that treatment-mediated suppression of HIV-1 RNA is associated with increases in CD4 cell count and reductions in risk of progression to AIDS and death.

The FDA Guidance for Industry (2002) advocates use of HIV-1 RNA level in plasma as the primary basis for assessing efficacy of new antiretroviral drugs for accelerated and traditional approval. Supportive analyses for CD4 cell count and clinical endpoints are also required, particularly for traditional approval. The guidance accepts changes in HIV-1 RNA during the first 24 weeks of treatment for accelerated approval but requires longer-term effects (over 48 weeks) to be established for traditional approval. With the advent of very potent antiretroviral treatments, the proportion of subjects with HIV-1 RNA levels below the limit of quantification of an assay is the preferred endpoint though quantitative changes (including changes averaged over time along the lines of the time-averaged AUCMB) may be acceptable in certain circumstances, for example when extensive prior treatment may mean that few patients are suppressed below the limit of quantification of the assay used.

The focus on HIV-1 RNA level as the primary basis for assessing efficacy in this guidance document likely reflects a number of factors. First, for an infectious disease, it is obviously attractive to focus on effects on the specific pathogen causing the disease. A caveat here is that the level of HIV-1 RNA in plasma is only one measure of a subject's viral load and it may be that viral load in other body compartments other than in plasma, or other attributes of the virus such as its infectiousness or fitness, may also be important. Second, treatment-mediated changes in HIV-1 RNA are highly predictive of reduction in risk of progression to AIDS/death as indicated in Figures 17.1 and 17.3. Furthermore, combinations of antiretroviral drugs produce very substantial reductions in HIV-1 RNA that, if sustained, would indicate corresponding very substantial reductions in risk of progression. Such reductions were seen in randomized trials that compared, for example, PI-containing three-drug antiretroviral therapy to two-drug NRTI therapy and in disease surveillance where dramatic declines in HIV-related mortality have been seen since highly active combination antiretroviral therapy has become available. In this respect, the availability of very potent anti-HIV therapy is very important—it may be very difficult to identify a reasonable surrogate endpoint for diseases for which the effects of therapy are very limited. Third, the fact that CD4 cell counts typically increase as HIV-1 RNA levels are reduced provides a mechanism for understanding how reductions in HIV-1 RNA lead to reductions in risk of progression to AIDS/death. Of note, these improvements in CD4 cell count reflect improvements in immunological status as studies have shown that prophylaxis against AIDS-defining opportunistic infections such as *Pneumocytis carinii* pneumonia can be safely removed when increases in CD4 cell count have been achieved on antiretroviral therapy. Fourth, the meta-analyses of randomized comparisons (Figures 17.4 and 17.5) do show that there have been very few instances in which there has been a qualitative discordance between the difference between a pair of treatments in progression to AIDS/death and the corresponding difference in change in HIV-1 RNA. Fifth, there are practical issues concerning the conduct of randomized trials using other endpoints. The substantial efficacy of antiretroviral drug combinations means that clinical endpoints such as AIDS-defining events or deaths will be very rare and so randomized trials would need to be large and long. Also, the assays to quantify HIV-1 RNA are very sensitive so that treatment-mediated suppression (and subsequent loss of suppression due, for example, to the development of viral resistance to a drug) can be monitored within individual patients. Hence patients and physicians make substantial use of changes in HIV-1 RNA in deciding when to change treatments. These changes in treatment further make it almost impossible to compare reliably the rates of progression to clinical endpoints between specific drug regimens, and also complicate the interpretation of comparisons of other intermediate outcomes such as changes in CD4 cell count.

Despite these factors, the meta-analyses that evaluated the association of differences between randomized treatments in risks of progression to AIDS/death and the corresponding differences in change in HIV-1 RNA (Figures 17.4 and 17.5) do show that there is a lot of variability in this association. At a simple level, this means that a small (large) difference between treatments in short-term change in HIV-1 RNA may not necessarily indicate a small (large) difference in the rate of progression to clinical events. Thus, a ranking of treatments based upon their magnitudes of effect on HIV-1 RNA may differ somewhat from a ranking based upon their effects on progression to AIDS/death. However, both from a biological perspective and from data from observational studies, there is evidence that sustained suppression of HIV-1 RNA is important for reducing risk of progression to AIDS/death. This captures the spirit of the result from the HSMCG meta-analysis that the time-averaged AUCMB might be a better surrogate than the simple change in HIV-1 RNA albeit over an extended time frame. Furthermore, it reflects concerns that a relatively small number of mutations in the virus, sometimes just one, can appear rapidly after treatment initiation and lead to substantial resistance to a drug and hence loss of suppression of HIV-1 RNA. This is reflected in the FDA guidance through the more stringent requirements for traditional versus accelerated approval when using HIV-1 RNA level as the primary basis for evaluating antiretroviral drugs by requiring evaluation of longer-term virologic outcome and consistency of evidence from supporting immunological and clinical outcomes. Currently, applications for drug approvals often also need extensive evaluation of the development of drug resistance further reflecting understanding of how treatments fail.

Having made the step to approve antiretroviral drugs primarily on the basis of effects on HIV-1 RNA, it is useful to reflect on some of the consequences of this. Obviously, the major one is that the effects on clinical outcomes that directly affect the quality and length of lives of HIV-infected people of specific drugs or drug combinations are not likely to be well-understood. A second important consequence is that it will not be known (short of a major disaster) how well HIV-1 RNA performs as a surrogate endpoint for newer types of antiretroviral drugs. For example, some newer drugs affect HIV-1 RNA levels by inhibiting entry of the virus into the CD4 cell. This contrasts with the classes of drugs (NRTIs, NNRTIs, and PIs) that were more formally evaluated in the meta-analyses described in this chapter which inhibit replication of the virus after entry into the CD4 cell. It is important to note though that drugs that do not target the virus, for example immune-based therapies, still typically need more extensive evaluation likely including their effects on progression to AIDS/death. This requires long-term trials involving follow-up of large numbers of patients (in the thousands) over several years particularly as these therapies will almost inevitably need to be evaluated when added to potent antiretroviral therapy. A third consequence concerns the fact that the various studies that contributed to the evaluation of HIV-1 RNA as a surrogate endpoint were primarily undertaken in resource-rich countries where subtype B of the virus is prevalent. However, the HIV epidemic is predominantly in sub-Saharan Africa and other more resource-limited countries where the most prevalent viral subtypes are A, C, and D, and co-infections (e.g., tuberculosis and malaria) are common. How much these factors might affect the value of HIV-1 RNA as a surrogate endpoint is unclear.

HIV infection is now more of a chronic disease. There is considerable interest in understanding the potential benefits of treatment very close to primary infection and of the secondary effects of candidate vaccines used for the prevention of transmission of HIV on disease progression among those subjects who become infected despite being vaccinated. These interests require identification of surrogate endpoints that might be reliable early in the course of HIV infection and hence temporally distant from major morbidity and mortality. Ultimately, this is likely to require new validation techniques for use in observational studies, possibly including the linkage of follow-up in sequential shorter-term randomized trials involving the same or different cohorts of patients. This challenge is not unique to HIV but is highly relevant to many long-term chronic diseases. The validation of potential surrogate endpoints will, however, be more difficult for diseases in which these endpoints are less sensitive and for which treatments only have limited effects.

18

An Alternative Measure for Meta-analytic Surrogate Endpoint Validation

Tomasz Burzykowski and Marc Buyse

18.1 Introduction

When considering the meta-analytic approach to the validation of surrogate endpoints (Chapter 7), Gail *et al.* (2000) noted that, unless the trial-level $R^2 = 1$, the variance of the prediction of treatment effect on the true endpoint in a new trial cannot be reduced to 0, even in the absence of any estimation error in the trial. On the other hand, if the effect is estimated directly from data on the true endpoint, this estimation error can theoretically be made arbitrarily close to 0 by increasing the trial's sample size. Gail *et al.* (2000) considered this as an argument against the use of surrogate endpoints and their validation within the meta-analytic framework (see also Chapter 9). It should be noted, however, that the idea of using a surrogate endpoint is based on the assumption that the information about the surrogate can be obtained earlier than about the true endpoint. The loss of efficiency in predicting treatment effect on true endpoint, as opposed to estimating it, might be treated as the price to pay for the time gain arising from the use of the surrogate endpoint.

To study further the issue raised by Gail *et al.* (2000), it would be important to quantify this loss of efficiency and assess whether in a particular application it does not render the use of a surrogate infeasible. In this chapter, a new concept, the so-called *a surrogate threshold effect* (STE), is proposed for this purpose. One of its interesting features, apart from providing information relevant to the practical use of a surrogate endpoint, is its natural interpretation from a clinical point of view. This might facilitate communication between the statisticians and clinicians regarding results of a validation of a surrogate endpoint.

18.2 The Use of the Trial-level Validation Measures

The essential features of the meta-analytic approach to the validation of surrogate endpoints, proposed by Buyse *et al.* (2000a) for the case of normally distributed endpoints, were described in Section 7.2. Let us briefly recall that the approach is based on the linear mixed-effects model

$$S_{ij} = \mu_S + m_{Si} + \alpha Z_{ij} + a_i Z_{ij} + \varepsilon_{Sij}, \qquad (18.1)$$

$$T_{ij} = \mu_T + m_{Ti} + \beta Z_{ij} + b_i Z_{ij} + \varepsilon_{Tij}, \qquad (18.2)$$

where μ_S and μ_T are fixed intercepts, α and β are the fixed effects of treatment Z on the endpoints, m_{Si} and m_{Ti} are random intercepts, and a_i and b_i are the random effects of treatment Z on the endpoints in trial i $(i = 1, \ldots, N)$. The vector of random effects $(m_{Si}, m_{Ti}, a_i, b_i)$ is assumed to be mean-zero normally distributed with variance-covariance matrix

$$D = \begin{pmatrix} d_{SS} & d_{ST} & d_{Sa} & d_{Sb} \\ & d_{TT} & d_{Ta} & d_{Tb} \\ & & d_{aa} & d_{ab} \\ & & & d_{bb} \end{pmatrix}. \qquad (18.3)$$

The error terms ε_{Si} and ε_{Ti} are assumed to be mean-zero normally distributed with variance-covariance matrix

$$\Sigma = \begin{pmatrix} \sigma_{SS} & \sigma_{ST} \\ & \sigma_{TT} \end{pmatrix}. \qquad (18.4)$$

By considering the conditional variance of treatment effect $\beta + b_0$ on the true endpoint in a new trial, given the random intercept m_{S0} and treatment effect a_0 on the surrogate, Buyse *et al.* (2000a) proposed to measure the quality of the surrogate at the trial level by the coefficient of determination $R^2_{\mathrm{trial(f)}}$ given by (7.11). It is worth noting that $R^2_{\mathrm{trial(f)}}$ measures the relative reduction in the variability of the prediction assuming the knowledge of all the parameters of the mixed effects model (18.1)–(18.2) and of the random effects m_{S0} and a_0. In practice, these parameters and the random effects have to be estimated. By fitting the mixed-effects model (18.1)–(18.2) to data from a meta-analysis, estimates for the fixed-effects parameters and variance components are obtained. We will use

$$\vartheta \equiv (\beta, \mu_S, \alpha, d_{Sb}, d_{ab}, d_{SS}, d_{Sa}, d_{aa})^T, \qquad (18.5)$$

to denote the fixed-effects parameters and variance components, with $\widehat{\vartheta}$ denoting the corresponding estimates.

Fitting the linear model

$$S_{0j} = \mu_{S0} + \alpha_0 Z_{0j} + \varepsilon_{S0j} \qquad (18.6)$$

to data on the surrogate endpoint from the new trial provides estimates for m_{S0} and a_0:

$$\begin{aligned} \widehat{m}_{S0} &= \widehat{\mu}_{S0} - \widehat{\mu}_S, \\ \widehat{a}_0 &= \widehat{\alpha}_0 - \widehat{\alpha}. \end{aligned}$$

Formally, expressing the conditional mean $E(\beta + b_0|m_{S0}, a_0)$ as $E(\beta + b_0|\mu_{S0}, \alpha_0, \vartheta)$, we can write

$$E(\beta + b_0|\mu_{S0}, \alpha_0, \vartheta) = E[E(\beta + b_0|\widehat{\mu}_{S0}, \widehat{\alpha}_0, \widehat{\vartheta})],$$

with the outer expectation taken with respect to the conditional distribution of $(\widehat{\mu}_{S0}, \widehat{\alpha}_0, \widehat{\vartheta})$ given $(\mu_{S0}, \alpha_0, \vartheta)$. It follows that the prediction for $\beta + b_0$ can obtained by replacing the parameter involved in the conditional mean $E(\beta + b_0|m_{S0}, a_0)$ with the corresponding estimates. Moreover, using the iterated variance formula, we can write:

$$\begin{aligned} \text{Var}(\beta + b_0|\mu_{S0}, \alpha_0, \vartheta) &= \text{Var}[E(\beta + b_0|\widehat{\mu}_{S0}, \widehat{\alpha}_0, \widehat{\vartheta})] \\ &\quad + E[\text{Var}(\beta + b_0|\widehat{\mu}_{S0}, \widehat{\alpha}_0, \widehat{\vartheta})]. \end{aligned} \quad (18.7)$$

Let $f_{d,0}$ and $f_{d,1}$ be the derivatives of $E(\beta + b_0|\mu_{S0}, \alpha_0, \vartheta)$ with respect to $(\mu_{S0}, \alpha_0)^T$ and ϑ, respectively. Denoting the asymptotic variance-covariance matrices of $(\widehat{\mu}_{S0}, \widehat{\alpha}_0)^T$ and $\widehat{\vartheta}$ by V_0 and V_1, respectively, and using the delta method, it follows that

$$\text{Var}(\beta + b_0|\mu_{S0}, \alpha_0, \vartheta) \approx f_{d,0} V_0 f_{d,0}^T + f_{d,1} V_1 f_{d,1}^T + (1 - R^2_{\text{trial(f)}}) d_{bb}. \quad (18.8)$$

The third term on the right-hand side of the formula (18.8) indicates the variability of the prediction if μ_{S0}, α_0 and ϑ were known. The first two terms describe the contribution to the variability due to the use of the estimates of these parameters.

One can now consider three scenarios:

Estimation error in both the meta-analysis and the new trial.
If the parameters of models (18.1)–(18.2) and (18.6) have to be estimated, as it happens in practice, the prediction variance is given by (18.8). From the equation it is clear that in practice, the reduction of the variability of the estimation of $\beta + b_0$, related to the use of the information on m_{S0} and a_0, will always be smaller than that indicated by $R^2_{\text{trial(f)}}$. The latter coefficient can thus be thought of as measuring the "potential" validity of a surrogate endpoint at the trial-level, assuming precise knowledge (or infinite numbers of trials and sample sizes per trial available for the estimation) of the parameters of models (18.1)–(18.2) and (18.6).

Estimation error only in the meta-analysis. This scenario is possible only theoretically, as it would require an infinite sample size in the new trial. But it can provide information of practical interest since, with an infinite sample size, the parameters of the single-trial regression model (18.6) would be known. Consequently, the first term on the right hand-side of (18.8), $f_{d,0}V_0 f_{d,0}^T$, would vanish and (18.8) would reduce to

$$\mathrm{Var}(\beta + b_0|\mu_{S0}, \alpha_0, \vartheta) \approx f_{d,1}V_1 f_{d,1}^T + (1 - R^2_{\mathrm{trial(f)}})d_{bb}. \qquad (18.9)$$

Expression (18.9) can thus be interpreted as indicating the minimum variance of the predicton of $\beta + b_0$, achieveable in the actual application of the surrogate endpoint. In applications, the size of the meta-analytic data providing an estimate of ϑ will necessarily be finite and fixed. Consequently, the first term on the right-hand side of (18.9) will always be present. Note that based on this observation Gail *et al.* (2000) conclude that the use of surrogates validated through the meta-analytic approach will always be less efficient than the direct use of the true endpoint.

No estimation error. If the parameters of the mixed-effects model (18.1)–(18.2) and the single-trial regression model (18.6) were known, the prediction variance for $\beta + b_0$ would contain only the last term on the right hand side of (18.8). Thus, the variance would be reduced to

$$\mathrm{Var}(\beta + b_0|\mu_{S0}, \alpha_0, \vartheta) = (1 - R^2_{\mathrm{trial(f)}})d_{bb}, \qquad (18.10)$$

which is equivalent to (7.10). This situation is, of course, only of theoretical relevance, as it would require infinite numbers of trials and sample sizes per trial available for the estimation in the meta-analysis and in the new trial.

Based on the scenarios considered above, one can argue that in a particular application the size of the minimum variance (18.9) is of importance. The reason is that (18.9) is associated with the minimum width of the prediction interval for $\beta + b_0$ that might be approached in a particular application by letting the sample size for the new trial increase toward infinity. This minimum width will be responsible for the loss of efficiency related to the use of the surrogate, pointed out by Gail *et al.* (2000). (See also Chapter 9.) It would thus be important to quantify the loss of efficiency, as it may be counter-balanced by a shortening of trial duration. To this aim, one might consider, for example, using the ratio of (18.9) to d_{bb}, the unconditional variance of $\beta + b_0$. However, in what follows we will consider another way of expressing this information, which should be more meaningful clinically.

18.3 Surrogate Threshold Effect

18.3.1 Normally Distributed Endpoints

We will first focus on the case where the surrogate and true endpoints are jointly normally distributed.

Assume that the prediction of $\beta + b_0$ can be made independently of μ_{S0}. Under this assumption, the conditional mean and variance of $\beta + b_0$ can be respectively written as

$$E(\beta + b_0|\alpha_0, \vartheta) = \beta + \frac{d_{ab}}{d_{aa}}(\alpha_0 - \alpha), \tag{18.11}$$

$$\text{Var}(\beta + b_0|\alpha_0, \vartheta) = d_{bb} - \frac{d_{ab}^2}{d_{aa}} = d_{bb}\left(1 - R^2_{\text{trial(r)}}\right). \tag{18.12}$$

If ϑ were known and α_0 could be observed without measurement error (i.e., assuming an infinite sample size for the new trial), the prediction of $\beta + b_0$ could be based on (18.11), and the prediction variance would equal (18.12). If an estimate $\widehat{\vartheta}$ were to be used (as will usually happen in practice), the prediction variance (18.9), which corrects for the estimation, should be applied. Upon defining $x = (1, -d_{ab}/d_{aa})^T$ and using the fact that in linear mixed-effects models the maximum-likelihood estimates of the covariance parameters are asymptotically independent of the fixed effects parameters (Pinheiro and Bates 1995), (18.9) can be expressed approximately as

$$\text{Var}(\beta + b_0|\alpha_0, \vartheta) \approx x^T \left[V_\mu + \left(\frac{\alpha_0 - \alpha}{d_{aa}}\right)^2 V_D\right] x + (1 - R^2_{\text{trial(r)}})d_{bb}, \tag{18.13}$$

where V_μ and V_D are the asymptotic variance-covariance matrices of $(\widehat{\beta}, \widehat{\alpha})^T$ and $(\widehat{d}_{ab}, \widehat{d}_{aa})^T$, respectively.

Let us assume, without loss of generality, that $d_{ab} > 0$ and that positive values of α_i indicate a beneficial treatment effect in trial i. Consider the (1-γ)100% prediction interval for $\beta + b_0$:

$$E(\beta + b_0|\alpha_0, \vartheta) \pm z_{1-\frac{\gamma}{2}} \sqrt{\text{Var}(\beta + b_0|\alpha_0, \vartheta)}, \tag{18.14}$$

where $z_{1-\gamma/2}$ is the $(1 - \gamma/2)$ quantile of the standard normal distribution. Depending on the assumptions, the interval (18.14) can be constructed using the variances (18.12) or (18.13).

The limits of the interval (18.14) are functions of α_0. Define the "lower prediction limit function" of the argument α_0 as

$$l(\alpha_0) \equiv E(\beta + b_0|\alpha_0, \vartheta) - z_{1-\frac{\gamma}{2}} \sqrt{\text{Var}(\beta + b_0|\alpha_0, \vartheta)}. \tag{18.15}$$

Similarly, we can define the "upper prediction limit function":

$$u(\alpha_0) \equiv E(\beta + b_0|\alpha_0, \vartheta) + z_{1-\frac{\gamma}{2}}\sqrt{\mathrm{Var}(\beta + b_0|\alpha_0, \vartheta)}. \tag{18.16}$$

One might compute a value of α_0 such that

$$l(\alpha_0) = 0. \tag{18.17}$$

We will call this value the *surrogate threshold effect* (STE). Its magnitude depends on the variance of the prediction. The larger the variance, the larger the (absolute) value of STE. A large, from a clinical point of view, value of STE would point to the need of observing a large treatment effect on the surrogate endpoint in order to conclude a non-zero effect on the true endpoint. In such case, the use of the surrogate would not be reasonable, even if the surrogate were valid (with $R^2_{\mathrm{trial(r)}}$ close to 1). STE can thus provide additional important information about the usefulness of the surrogate in a particular application.

Note that, depending on whether the variance (18.12) or (18.13) is used in (18.15), one might get two versions of STE. The version obtained with the use of the variance (18.12) will be denoted by $\mathrm{STE}_{\infty,\infty}$. Explicitly:

$$\mathrm{STE}_{\infty,\infty} = \alpha - \frac{d_{aa}}{d_{ab}}\left\{\beta + z_{1-\frac{\gamma}{2}}\sqrt{d_{bb}(1 - R^2_{\mathrm{trial(r)}})}\right\}. \tag{18.18}$$

The infinity signs used in the notation for $\mathrm{STE}_{\infty,\infty}$ indicate that (18.18) assumes the knowledge both of ϑ as well as of α_0, achieveable only with an infinite number of infinite-sample-size trials in the meta-analytic data and an infinite sample size for the new trial. In practice, $\mathrm{STE}_{\infty,\infty}$ will be computed using estimates of the parameters involved in (18.18). A large value of $\mathrm{STE}_{\infty,\infty}$ would point to the need of observing a large treatment effect on the surrogate endpoint even if there were no estimation error present.

If the variance (18.13) is used to define $l(\alpha_0)$, we will denote the STE by $\mathrm{STE}_{N,\infty}$, with N indicating the need for the estimation of ϑ.

To further simplify formulas, let us re-write (18.13) as

$$\mathrm{Var}(\beta + b_0|\alpha_0, \vartheta) \equiv B\left(\frac{\alpha_0 - \alpha}{d_{aa}}\right)^2 + A, \tag{18.19}$$

with

$$B \equiv x^T V_D x,$$

and

$$A \equiv x^T V_\mu x + (1 - R^2_{\mathrm{trial(r)}})d_{bb}.$$

TABLE 18.1. *Values of the surrogate threshold effect $STE_{N,\infty}$, based on the lower or upper prediction limits, for different configurations of parameters.*

$d_{ab}^2 - Bz_{1-\gamma/2}^2$	β	Δ	$\beta B z_{1-\gamma/2} + d_{ab}\sqrt{\Delta}$	$\mathrm{STE}_{N,\infty}$	
				$l(\alpha_0)$	$u(\alpha_0)$
$=0$	$=0$	$\star$	$\star$	None	None
	<0	$\star$	$\star$	None	ν_0
	>0	$\star$	$\star$	ν_0	None
<0	$\star$	<0	$\star$	None	None
	$\star$	>0	<0	None	$\min(\nu_1, \nu_2)$
	$\star$	>0	>0	$\min(\nu_1, \nu_2)$	None
>0	$\star$	$\star$	<0	ν_1	ν_2
	$\star$	$\star$	>0	ν_2	ν_1

NOTE: $\star$ indicates that the value of the parameter is irrelevant.

Formula (18.19) indicates that, if (18.13) is used in (18.15), then $l(\alpha_0)$ is the difference between values of a positive-slope linear function and either a concave parabole-shaped function (if $B > 0$) or a fixed number (if $B = 0$). It follows that (18.17) might have two, one or no solutions.

The roots of (18.17) can be obtained by solving the quadratic equation

$$(d_{ab}^2 - z_{1-\frac{\gamma}{2}}^2 B)\nu^2 + 2\beta d_{ab}\nu + \beta^2 - z_{1-\frac{\gamma}{2}}^2 A = 0, \qquad (18.20)$$

where $\nu = (\alpha_0 - \alpha)/d_{aa}$. In fact, (18.20) defines simultaneously the roots for both the lower and upper limits functions given by (18.15) and (18.16), respectively.

The number of solutions of (18.20) depends on the configuration of the parameters of $l(\alpha_0)$. Table 18.1 summarizes the conditions leading to different numbers of solutions of $l(\alpha_0) = 0$. For completness, solutions of $u(\alpha_0) = 0$ are displayed in the table as well. Note that $\Delta \equiv \beta^2 - A(z_{1-\frac{\gamma}{2}}^2 B - d_{ab}^2)/B$. If there is a single solution, it is given by

$$\nu_0 = \frac{Az_{1-\frac{\gamma}{2}}^2 - \beta^2}{2\beta d_{ab}}.$$

If there are two solutions, they are given by

$$\nu_1 = \frac{\beta d_{ab} - z_{1-\frac{\gamma}{2}}\sqrt{B\beta^2 - A(Bz_{1-\frac{\gamma}{2}}^2 - d_{ab}^2)}}{Bz_{1-\frac{\gamma}{2}}^2 - d_{ab}^2}$$

and

$$\nu_2 = \frac{\beta d_{ab} + z_{1-\frac{\gamma}{2}}\sqrt{B\beta^2 - A(Bz^2_{1-\frac{\gamma}{2}} - d^2_{ab})}}{Bz^2_{1-\frac{\gamma}{2}} - d^2_{ab}}.$$

In practice, $\text{STE}_{N,\infty}$ will be computed using ν_0, ν_1, or ν_2 with V_μ, V_D, and ϑ replaced by their estimates obtained from fitting the mixed-effects model (18.1)–(18.2) to the meta-analytic data.

The conditions listed in Table 18.1 are derived by considering possible forms of the quadratic equation (18.20) (Burzykowski 2001). Some insight can be offered. For instance, under the assumption that $d_{ab} > 0$, the condition $d^2_{ab} - z^2_{1-\gamma/2}B > 0$ is equivalent to $d_{ab} - z_{1-\gamma/2}\sqrt{B} > 0$, which can be further re-written as

$$d_{aa}\left[\frac{d_{ab}}{d_{aa}} - z_{1-\frac{\gamma}{2}}\sqrt{\text{Var}\left(\frac{\widehat{d}_{ab}}{\widehat{d}_{aa}}\right)}\right] > 0. \tag{18.21}$$

If d_{aa}, d_{ab} and their variance-covariance matrix are replaced by estimates, condition (18.21) can be interpreted as the requirement that the estimate of the slope of the regression line (18.11) should be statistically significantly different from 0. This is a well-known condition in the discrimination problem (constructing confidence limits for the value of a covariate given the value of the dependent variable) for a simple linear regression model (Miller 1981, p. 118) and in the construction of confidence intervals based on Fieller's theorem (Fieller 1954).

18.3.2 Other Distributions

The development of STE and its estimation, presented in the previous section, was done under the mixed-effects model (18.1)–(18.2), applicable when both S and T are normally distributed. As illustrated in Chapter 7, however, due to numerical problems, the use of the two-stage representation of the model might need to be considered. The two-stage approach would also be chosen if S and/or T were not normally distributed, as proposed, e.g., in Chapters 11 and 12. In this section we will describe how STE can be estimated when this approach is used.

First, let us briefly recall the basic idea of the the two-stage modeling strategy. At the first stage, a joint model for S and T is fitted to the meta-analytic data. This model provides estimates $\widehat{\beta}_i$ and $\widehat{\alpha}_i$ of the trial-specific treatment effects $\beta_i \equiv \beta + b_i$ and $\alpha_i \equiv \alpha + a_i$. At the second stage, a model is fitted to $\widehat{\beta}_i$ and $\widehat{\alpha}_i$, allowing for estimation of the parameter vector ϑ.

Now, the estimate of ϑ and its variance-covariance matrix could be used to compute the prediction variances (18.13) and (18.13) and, upon solving equation (18.20), to estimate $\text{STE}_{\infty,\infty}$ and $\text{STE}_{N,\infty}$, respectively. An important issue in this respect, however, is to adjust the estimation of ϑ for the estimation error present in $\widehat{\beta}_i$ and $\widehat{\alpha}_i$. Note that such an adjustment is done automatically if the mixed-effects model (18.1)–(18.2) can be used.

One possible way to adjust the estimation of ϑ for the error in $\widehat{\beta}_i$ and $\widehat{\alpha}_i$ would be to use the approach based on the results developed by van Houwelingen, Arends, and Stijnen (2002). It has been summarized, for example, in Section 11.2.1. Due to practical problems with implementing the approach (see, for example, Section 11.5.2), however, we will consider an alternative solution.

More specifically, following (18.11) we can assume that the trial-specific treatment effects β_i and α_i follow the simple linear regression model

$$\beta_i = \gamma_0 + \gamma_1\alpha_i + \varepsilon_i, \tag{18.22}$$

with ε_i being a random variable with mean 0 and variance σ. Clearly, from (18.11) and (18.12), the following relationships hold:

$$\begin{aligned} \gamma_0 &= \beta - \alpha d_{ab}/d_{aa}, \\ \gamma_1 &= d_{ab}/d_{aa}, \\ \sigma &= d_{bb}(1 - R^2_{\text{trial(r)}}). \end{aligned} \tag{18.23}$$

The parameters of model (18.22) can be estimated from the regression of $\widehat{\beta}_i$ on $\widehat{\alpha}_i$. To account for the estimation error in $\widehat{\alpha}_i$ and $\widehat{\beta}_i$, the parameters γ_1 and γ_0 can be estimated using (11.24) and (11.25), respectively, or one of its modifications proposed by Fuller (1987, see also Section 11.2.2). The residual variance σ can be computed from (11.22).

Using estimates $\widetilde{\gamma}_1$, $\widetilde{\gamma}_0$, and $\widetilde{\sigma}$ of γ_1, γ_0, and σ, and given an estimate $\widehat{\alpha_0}$ of treatment effect on S in the new trial, $\beta_0 \equiv \beta + b_0$ can be predicted using

$$\widehat{\beta_0} = \widetilde{\gamma}_0 + \widetilde{\gamma}_1\widehat{\alpha}_0. \tag{18.24}$$

Following the arguments presented in Section 11.2.2 and using (11.27), one can calculate the variance of the prediction error by

$$\begin{aligned} \text{Var}(\widehat{\beta_0} - \beta_0) &= E[\widetilde{\gamma}_1^2\text{Var}(\widehat{\alpha}_0)] + \text{Var}(\widetilde{\gamma}_0) \\ &\quad +2\alpha\text{Cov}(\widetilde{\gamma}_0, \widetilde{\gamma}_1) + (\alpha^2 + d_{aa})\text{Var}(\widetilde{\gamma}_1) + \sigma. \end{aligned} \tag{18.25}$$

The first term on the right-hand side of (18.25) corresponds to the first term on the right-hand side of (18.8) and accounts for the estimation of α_0. The last term on the right-hand side of (18.25) corresponds to the last term on the right-hand side of (18.8) and accounts for the residual variability after accounting for the information provided by α_0. The remaining terms on the right-hand side of (18.25) correspond to the middle term on the right-hand side of (18.8) and account for the estimation of parameters ϑ.

The first term on the right-hand side of (18.25) vanishes if the new trial is large. Consequently, $\text{STE}_{N,\infty}$ can be obtained as the solution to (18.17), with $E(\beta + b_0|\alpha_0, \vartheta)$ and $\text{Var}(\beta + b_0|\alpha_0, \vartheta)$ in $l(\alpha_0)$ replaced, respectively, by $\gamma_0 + \gamma_1\alpha_0$ and

$$\text{Var}(\widehat{\beta_0 - \beta_0}) = \sigma + \text{Var}(\widetilde{\gamma}_0) + 2\alpha\text{Cov}(\widetilde{\gamma}_0, \widetilde{\gamma}_1) + (\alpha^2 + d_{aa})\text{Var}(\widetilde{\gamma}_1). \quad (18.26)$$

This expression can be seen as corresponding to (18.9) and (18.13). Note that $l(\alpha_0)$ is again a difference between a linear and a parabola-shaped function. Thus, the considerations regarding the number of solutions of (18.17) apply in this case as well.

$\text{STE}_{\infty,\infty}$, on the other hand, results if $\text{Var}(\beta + b_0|\alpha_0, \vartheta)$ is replaced by the residual variance σ. Note that, in view of (18.23), σ corresponds to (18.10) and (18.12).

Clearly, some caution may be needed in the interpretation of $\text{STE}_{N,\infty}$ or $\text{STE}_{\infty,\infty}$ computed in such a way, since, as already noted in Section 11.2.2, the normality of the distribution of $\widehat{\beta_0}$ obtained from (18.24) might be questionable.

For practical purposes, as an estimator of (18.25) one might use

$$\begin{aligned} \widehat{\text{Var}}(\widehat{\beta}_0 - \beta_0) &= \widetilde{\gamma}_1^2\widehat{\text{Var}}(\widehat{\alpha}_0) + \widehat{\text{Var}}(\widetilde{\gamma}_0) + 2\widehat{\alpha}_0\widehat{\text{Cov}}(\widetilde{\gamma}_0, \widetilde{\gamma}_1) \\ &\quad + \left[\widehat{\alpha}_0^2 - \widehat{\text{Var}}(\widehat{\alpha}_0)\right]\widehat{\text{Var}}(\widetilde{\gamma}_1) + \widetilde{\sigma}, \end{aligned}$$

with $\widetilde{\sigma}$ defined by (11.22), and $\widehat{\text{Var}}(\widehat{\alpha}_0)$ obtained from the model for S in the new trial. The variance-covariance matrix of the estimators $\widetilde{\gamma}_0$ and $\widetilde{\gamma}_1$ can be estimated either assuming normality or using a robust estimator (Fuller 1987). For (18.26) one might use

$$\widehat{\text{Var}}(\widehat{\beta}_0 - \beta_0) = \widehat{\text{Var}}(\widetilde{\gamma}_0) + 2\widehat{\alpha}_0\widehat{\text{Cov}}(\widetilde{\gamma}_0, \widetilde{\gamma}_1) + \widehat{\alpha}_0^2\widehat{\text{Var}}(\widetilde{\gamma}_1) + \widetilde{\sigma}. \quad (18.27)$$

18.4 Analysis of Case Studies

To illustrate the potential use of STE, it will be applied to two case studies. In what follows, the 95% confidence level for constructed prediction intervals is assumed.

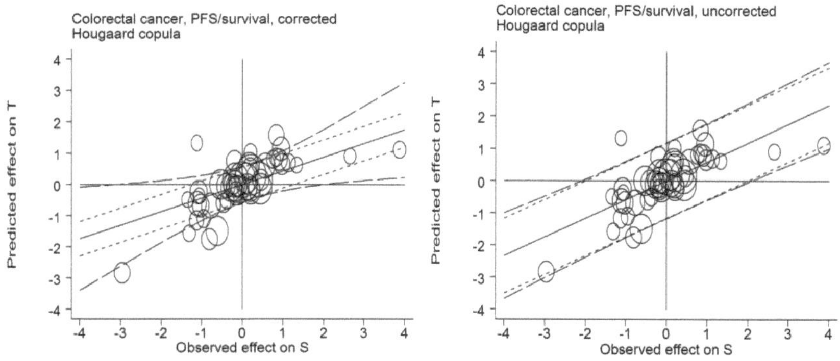

FIGURE 18.1. *Corfu study in advanced colorectal cancer. Predictions (solid lines) with 95% prediction limits leading to $STE_{\infty,\infty}$ (short dashes) and $STE_{N,\infty}$ (long dashes), based on the Hougaard model. Left plot with the correction for the estimation error in treatment effect estimates; right plot without the correction. Circles (proportional to center sample size) indicate the estimated treatment effects.*

18.4.1 Advanced Colorectal Cancer

First, the data for two clinical trials in advanced colorectal cancer will be considered (Section 4.2.3). Recall that survival time is considered as true endpoint, whereas progression-free survival time is regarded as surrogate. The validity of progression-free survival as a surrogate was investigated in Section 11.3.2, using center as the unit of analysis. The analysis used data for 48 centers with at least 3 patients on each treatment arm (642 patients in total).

We will use the results obtained in Section 11.3.1, for the Hougaard copula with center-specific baseline hazards. Mean treatment effects on T and S were equal to -0.003 and -0.021, respectively. Their variances were equal to 0.737 and 1.149, respectively. In the analysis unadjusted for the measurement error in the observed treatment effects an estimate of trial level R^2 of 0.53 (95% confidence interval [0.34,0.72]) was found. A point estimate adjusted for the measurement error was equal to 0.64.

Figure 18.1 presents the prediction limits computed using model (18.22) fitted to the estimated treatment effects with and without the adjustment for the estimation error in treatment effects. From now on these models will be referred to as the "corrected" and "uncorrected," respectively. For the corrected model, the prediction limits defining $\text{STE}_{\infty,\infty}$ and $\text{STE}_{N,\infty}$ were computed using, respectively, $\widetilde{\sigma}$ as in(11.22) and (18.27) as the estimates of the prediction variance. The variance-covariance matrix of the estimators $\widetilde{\gamma}_0$ and $\widetilde{\gamma}_1$ was obtained using a robust estimator (Fuller 1987).

The prediction limits for the uncorrected model were computed using the well-known formulas for a simple linear regression model (Neter, Wasserman, and Kutner 1983). More specifically, for $\mathrm{STE}_{\infty,\infty}$ the limits were obtained using the mean residual sum of squares for the regression of $\widehat{\beta}_i$ on $\widehat{\alpha}_i$ as the estimate of the prediction variance σ:

$$\widehat{\sigma} = \sum_{i=1}^{N} \frac{(\widehat{\beta}_i - \widehat{\gamma}_0 - \widehat{\gamma}_1\widehat{\alpha}_i)^2}{N-2},$$

whereas for $\mathrm{STE}_{N,\infty}$ the prediction variance was estimated by

$$\mathrm{Var}(\widehat{\beta_0}|\widehat{\alpha}_0) = \widehat{\sigma}\left\{\frac{1}{N} + \frac{(\widehat{\alpha}_0 - \bar{\alpha})^2}{\sum_{i=1}^{N}(\widehat{\alpha}_i - \bar{\alpha})^2}\right\} + \widehat{\sigma}, \tag{18.28}$$

where $\bar{\alpha} = \sum_{i=1}^{N} \widehat{\alpha}_i/N$ and $\widehat{\sigma}$ is the mean residual sum of squares. Note that (18.28) corresponds to (18.9), (18.13), and (18.26), with the second term ($\widehat{\sigma}$) on the right-hand side of (18.28) reflecting the residual variability after accounting for the information provided by α_0 and the first term accounting for the estimation of parameters γ_0 and γ_1 (which correspond to ϑ).

The plots in Figure 18.1 allow for several conclusions. First, the width of the prediction interval underlying $\mathrm{STE}_{\infty,\infty}$ and based on the estimated residual variance σ, is much smaller for the corrected model. This is due to the difference in the estimates of the variance. As expected, the model corrected for the measurement error yielded a smaller estimate ($\widetilde{\sigma} = 0.08$) than the uncorrected model ($\widehat{\sigma} = 0.35$). Second, the plots in Figure 18.1 illustrate that the use of the prediction variance (18.9), adjusted for the estimation of the parameters γ_0 and γ_1, "penalizes" for the predictions outside the range of treatment effects observed in the meta-analytic data much more in the corrected model than in the uncorrected model. In fact, the width of the prediction interval for the uncorrected model almost does not change as α_0 is moved away from the observed mean.

These differences are reflected in the estimates of STE. In the corrected analysis the following estimates of the parameters of model (18.22) were obtained: $\widetilde{\gamma}_0 = 0.006$ (standard error, s.e., 0.09), $\widetilde{\gamma}_1 = 0.43$ (s.e. 0.19). As a result, $\mathrm{STE}_{\infty,\infty}$ was found to be equal to -1.28. For $\mathrm{STE}_{N,\infty}$, the value of -3.11 was obtained. Note that $\mathrm{STE}_{\infty,\infty}$ and $\mathrm{STE}_{N,\infty}$ were computed from the upper prediction limit $u(\alpha_0)$, defined in (18.16), since negative values of treatment effect, pointing to a reduction of the risk of failure, were considered beneficial.

In the uncorrected analysis, γ_0 and γ_1 were estimated to equal 0.01 (s.e. 0.08) and $\widehat{\gamma}_1 = 0.53$ (s.e. 0.08), respectively. These estimates led to $\mathrm{STE}_{\infty,\infty} = -2.01$ and $\mathrm{STE}_{N,\infty} = -2.11$. For the corrected model, $\mathrm{STE}_{\infty,\infty}$ was thus markedly smaller than for the uncorrected model; the reverse could be observed for $\mathrm{STE}_{N,\infty}$. Irrespective of the model, though, the values of STE were very large, even for $\mathrm{STE}_{\infty,\infty}$. They were much smaller than treatment effects on the surrogate observed in the meta-analysis, what can be observed in Figure 18.1. This clearly illustrates poor validity of the surrogate.

18.4.2 Advanced Ovarian Cancer

We will now consider the data for the meta-analysis of four clinical trials in advanced ovarian cancer cancer (Section 4.2.2). Also in this example survival time is considered the true endpoint, whereas progression-free survival time is regarded the surrogate. The data have been analyzed using the two-stage approach based on copula models in Section 11.3.1. The analysis used data for 39 centers (including the two smaller trials) with at least 3 patients on each treatment arm (1153 patients in total).

We will use the results obtained in Section 11.3.1, for the Hougaard copula with center-specific baseline hazards. Mean treatment effects on T and S were equal to -0.18 and -0.20, respectively. Their variances were equal to 0.93 and 1.02, respectively. In the analysis unadjusted for the measurement error an estimate of trial level R^2 of 0.88 (95% confidence interval [0.81,0.95]) was found. A point estimate adjusted for the measurement error was equal to 0.83.

As in the previous example, we will consider two analyses: corrected and uncorrected for the measurement error in the estimated treatment effects. Figure 18.2 presents the corresponding prediction limits.

The plots in Figure 18.2 exhibit similar features to those observed for the advanced colorectal cancer data in Figure 18.1. Again, due to the difference in estimates of σ, the width of the prediction intervals based on the residual variance is smaller for the corrected model than for the uncorrected. The difference is much smaller now, though. The curvature of the prediction limits corresponding to the prediction variance (18.9) is again more remarkable for the corrected model. Within the range shown, however, it does not deviate very much from the prediction limits based on σ.

For the corrected model $\widetilde{\gamma}_0 = -0.06$, (s.e. 0.06), $\widetilde{\gamma}_1 = 0.83$ (s.e. 0.10), and $\widetilde{\sigma} = 0.06$ were obtained. The estimates led to $\mathrm{STE}_{\infty,\infty} = -0.59$ and $\mathrm{STE}_{N,\infty} = -0.61$. In the uncorrected analysis γ_0, γ_1, and σ were estimated to equal 0.007 (s.e. 0.05), $\widehat{\gamma}_1 = 0.90$ (s.e. 0.05), and 0.11, respectively. These estimates yielded $\mathrm{STE}_{\infty,\infty} = -0.74$ and $\mathrm{STE}_{N,\infty} = -0.75$.

The values of STE are much closer to the treatment effects on the surrogate endpoint observed in the meta-analysis (as can be seen in Figure 18.2) than

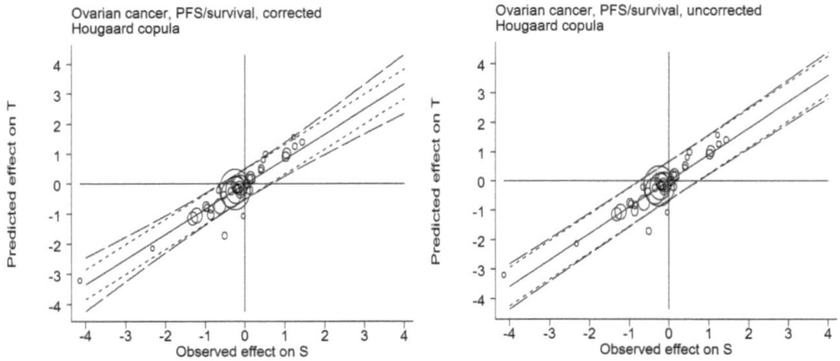

FIGURE 18.2. *Advanced ovarian cancer. Predictions (solid lines) with 95% prediction limits leading to* $STE_{\infty,\infty}$ *(short dashes) and* $STE_{N,\infty}$ *(long dashes), based on the Hougaard model. Left plot with the correction for the estimation error in treatment effect estimates; right plot without the correction. Circles (proportional to center sample size) indicate the estimated treatment effects.*

in the previous example. Consequently, they suggest a better validity of the surrogate.

18.5 An Extension of the Concept of a Surrogate Threshold Effect

Assume that the surrogate endpoint S has been validated using a meta-analytic dataset. One might consider using the computed value of $\text{STE}_{N,\infty}$ to assess the results of the ongoing trials. To this aim, for example, the lower limit of a confidence interval based on the available estimate of treatment effect on S in a trial might be compared to $\text{STE}_{N,\infty}$, and, if it were larger, a significant treatment effect on the true endpoint T might be predicted. It should be noted, though, that the prediction interval (18.14), based on the variance (18.13), provides the $(1-\gamma)100\%$ confidence of the prediction only for a single, fixed value of α_0. In order to use it repeatedly, one would require an interval warranting the required confidence for a whole family of values of α_0. To address this issue, the concept of simultaneous tolerance intervals might be used (Miller 1981).

We will consider the two-stage representation of the mixed-effects model (18.1)–(18.2). Moreover, we will assume that the prediction of β_0 could be based on model (18.22) without the need for adjusting for the error in the estimates of treatment effects β_i and α_i. This would require, for example, that the error associated with the estimation of the treatment effects had (at least approximately) the same distribution across all N trials included in the meta-analysis (see Section 11.2.2).

A $(1-\delta, 1-\xi)$ tolerance interval for β_0 is an interval that with probability (at least) $1-\delta$ contains the true $(1-\xi)100\%$ confidence interval for β_0, corresponding to a particular value of $\widehat{\alpha}_0$. Methods for constructing such intervals for a linear regression model were proposed, for example, by Wallis (1951), Lieberman and Miller (1963), Wilson (1967), and Limam and Thomas (1988). A family of tolerance intervals, which contain the true $(1-\xi)100\%$ confidence interval for β_0 with probability (at least) $1-\delta$ for all $\widehat{\alpha}_0$ and ξ, is called simultaneous tolerance intervals (Miller 1981). We will use the term "simultaneous $(1-\delta)$-tolerance intervals."

Lieberman and Miller (1963) proposed a simple method to construct simultaneous $(1-\delta)$-tolerance intervals based on the Working-Hotelling (1929) confidence band for the regression line and the Bonferroni inequality. Using the approach of Lieberman and Miller one can find (Burzykowski 2001) that, with probability $1-\delta$ and for all values of $\widehat{\alpha}_0$ and ξ, the $(1-\xi)100\%$ confidence interval for β_0 is contained in

$$\widehat{\gamma}_0 + \widehat{\gamma}_1\widehat{\alpha}_0 \pm \sqrt{\widehat{\sigma}} \left[\left(2F_{2,N-2}^{1-\delta/2}\right)^{\frac{1}{2}} \left\{ \frac{1}{N} + \frac{(\widehat{\alpha}_0 - \bar{\alpha})^2}{\sum_{i=1}^{N}(\alpha_i - \bar{\alpha})^2} \right\}^{\frac{1}{2}} + z_{1-\xi/2} \left(\frac{N-2}{\chi_{N-2}^{\delta/2}} \right)^{\frac{1}{2}} \right], \quad (18.29)$$

where $F_{2,N-2}^{1-\delta/2}$ is the $(1-\delta/2)$ quantile of the F distribution with 2 and $N-2$ degrees of freedom and $\chi_{N-2}^{\delta/2}$ is the $\delta/2$ quantile of the χ^2 distribution with $N-2$ degrees of freedom.

By determining the value of $\widehat{\alpha}_0$, for which the lower limit of the interval specified by (18.29) would equal zero, one could define a new version of $\text{STE}_{N,\infty}$, $\text{STE}_{N,\infty}^{\delta}$ say. From the definition of the simultaneous tolerance interval (18.29), it follows that the interval $(\text{STE}_{N,\infty}^{\delta}, +\infty)$ would contain all values of treatment effect α_0, for which, with $(1-\delta)100\%$ confidence, a statistically significant (at an arbitrarily chosen significance level ξ), non-zero treatment effect on the true endpoint might be predicted. Thus, $\text{STE}_{N,\infty}^{\delta}$ might be used repeatedly to assess results of new clinical trials (even with varying ξ).

The prediction limits specified in (18.29) are valid for all $\widehat{\alpha}_0$ and ξ. This is due to the use of the Working-Hotelling band. Usually, however, the limits would be needed for a restricted region of possible values of $\widehat{\alpha}_0$ (for example, an interval). In such a case, one might consider replacing the

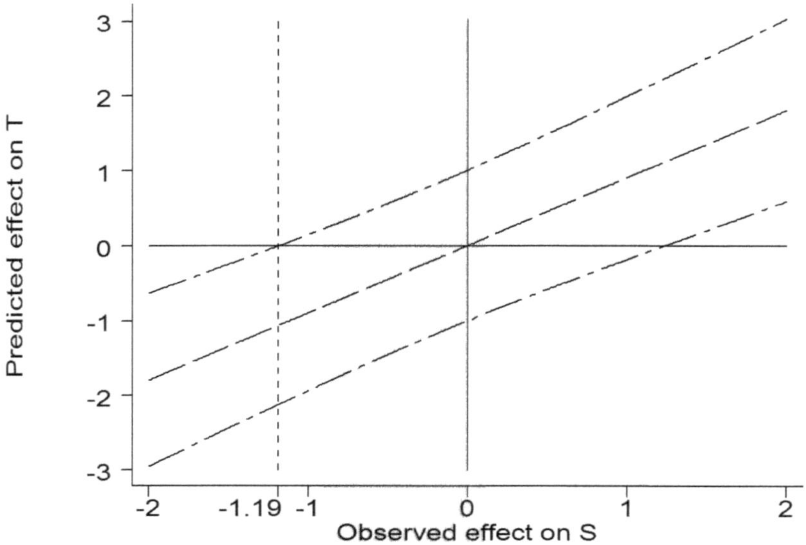

FIGURE 18.3. *Corfu study in advanced colorectal cancer. Simultaneous 0.95-tolerance intervals. Vertical dashed line indicates* $STE_{N,\infty}^{0.05}$. *Long dashes - predicted values; long/short dashes - simultaneous 0.95-tolerance intervals.*

Working-Hotelling band by the band proposed by Uusipaikka (1983), which is applicable for arbitrary finite unions of intervals or points. A consequence of the replacement would be a reduction of the width of the simultaneous tolerance intervals (18.29).

18.5.1 Application to the Advanced Ovarian Cancer Data

We will illustrate $\mathrm{STE}_{N,\infty}^{\delta}$ on the data from the meta-analysis of four advanced ovarian cancer trials, considered in Section 18.4.2. Figure 18.3 presents the limits of the simultaneous 0.95-tolerance intervals (18.29). Using the upper limit of the interval, $\mathrm{STE}_{N,\infty}^{0.05}$ can be computed to equal -1.19. Clearly, this value is much larger than the value of -0.75, obtained for $\mathrm{STE}_{N,\infty}$ in Section 18.4.2. But, unlike $\mathrm{STE}_{N,\infty}$, $\mathrm{STE}_{N,\infty}^{0.05}$ can be used as a reference for all values of α_0.

18.6 Discussion

The criterion of the trial-level validity of a surrogate, as proposed by Buyse *et al.* (2000a), measures the relative reduction in the variability of the prediction of treatment effect on the true endpoint achieved by conditioning on the effect on the surrogate. The criterion, the coefficient of determination R^2, was developed assuming the knowledge of all parameters of the underlying models. In practice, these parameters have to be estimated. Due to the estimation, the reduction of the variability of the prediction will always be smaller than the one indicated by R^2. From a practical point of view, it is of interest to quantify this "actual" reduction.

In this chapter, a new concept, the so-called *surrogate threshold effect* (STE), has been proposed to this end. It is defined as the minimum value of treatment effect on the surrogate endpoint, for which the predicted effect on the true endpoint would be significantly different from 0. In particular, STE can be computed with and without taking into account the estimation of the parameters of the models underlying the approach developed by Buyse *et al.* (2000a).

$\text{STE}_{\infty,\infty}$ and $\text{STE}_{N,\infty}$ can be used to address the concern about the usefulness of the meta-analytic approach to the validation of surrogate endpoints, expressed by Gail *et al.* (2000). They noted that, even for a valid surrogate, the variance of the prediction of treatment effect on the true endpoint cannot be reduced to 0, even in the absence of any estimation error. $\text{STE}_{N,\infty}$ can be used to quantify this loss of efficiency and assess whether in a particular application it does not render the use of a surrogate infeasible.

An interesting feature of a surrogate threshold effect, apart from providing information relevant to the practical use of a surrogate endpoint, is its natural interpretation from a clinical point of view. It can be expressed in terms of treatment effect necessary to be observed to predict a significant treatment effect on the true endpoint. Its use might facilitate communication between the statisticians and clinicians regarding results of a validation of a surrogate endpoint.

The concept of a surrogate threshold effect, if deemed useful, will require further research. For instance, the assumptions (normality, sample size etc.), under which it can yield reliable results, should be investigated. Also, the accuracy of the estimation of $\text{STE}_{\infty,\infty}$ and $\text{STE}_{N,\infty}$ would need to be checked.

The use of $\text{STE}^{\delta}_{N,\infty}$ to assess repeatedly results of many clinical trials might be an interesting problem. It would require the extension of the concept of simultaneous tolerance intervals to measurement-error and general linear mixed effects models. Also, the use of $\text{STE}^{\delta}_{N,\infty}$ to compute a sample size for a new trial aimed at using the surrogate endpoint might be of interest. Thus far, methods for such calculations have not been considered in the literature. To compute the sample size, one might consider requiring that the lower (or upper) confidence limit for the estimated treatment effect under the alternative was greater (smaller) than $\mathrm{STE}^{\delta}_{N,\infty}$. An investigation of operational characteristics of such a procedure would require a careful evaluation.

19

Discussion: Surrogate Endpoint Definition and Evaluation

Ross L. Prentice

19.1 Introduction

It is now some years since a formal definition of a surrogate endpoint in a clinical trial was proposed (Prentice 1989). Subsequently, alternate proposals have been made, and much has been written on methods for evaluating whether or not a biomarker or short-term endpoint can serve as a replacement for a corresponding longer-term clinical endpoint (e.g., disease occurrence, or recurrence). In fact, this volume is concerned primarily with statistical methods for this type of replacement, under various scenarios concerning the nature of the true and potential surrogate response. In this discussion chapter, I return to the issue of surrogate endpoint definition and add some perspective on the corresponding evaluation process and on related evaluation methods.

19.2 Surrogate Endpoint Definition

In my 1989 paper, I defined a surrogate for a true endpoint as "a response variable for which a test of the null hypothesis of no relationship to the treatment groups under comparison is also a valid test of the corresponding null hypothesis based on the true endpoint." This definition was motivated by a desire for the surrogate "to have potential to yield unambiguous information about differential treatment effects on the true endpoint." To obtain insight into the corresponding implications for the relationships among the true and surrogate endpoints and the treatments or interventions of interest, the definition was recast in more "operational" terms for the important special case of a time-to-response true endpoint T, a potential surrogate endpoint process $\{S(t); t > 0\}$, and a vector of p

treatment indicators x (for $p+1$ treatments to be compared). It was noted that the definition could alternatively be written

$$\lambda_T\{t; S(t), x\} \equiv \lambda_T\{t; S(t)\}, \tag{19.1}$$

$$\lambda_T\{t, S(t)\} \not\equiv \lambda_T(t), \tag{19.2}$$

$$\text{and } E[\lambda_T\{t; S(t)\}|x, F(t)] \not\equiv E[\lambda_T\{t; S(t)\}|F(t)], \tag{19.3}$$

where λ_T denotes the hazard rate for T, $F(t)$ denotes the failure and censoring history on T prior to (follow-up) time t, and $\equiv$ denotes equality at all pertinent $t > 0$. The main point in expressing the definition in terms of (19.1)–(19.3) was to elucidate how very restrictive the conditions are under which, say, departure from the null hypothesis concerning treatment effect on S necessarily implies departure from the corresponding null hypothesis concerning treatment effect on T. Condition (19.1), in particular, leads one to think in terms of treatment effect pathways to a true endpoint event, and essentially requires that there are no pathways that bypass the surrogate, and that, otherwise, the treatment effect is fully "explained" by the preceding surrogate history.

Note that (19.1)–(19.3) are criteria for *defining* when S can serve as a surrogate for S in the evaluation of treatment effects x. The issue of *evaluating* whether a certain biomarker, or short-term clinical outcome can reasonably serve as a replacement for a true endpoint T, is quite another matter. Also note that some authors have written that (19.1)–(19.3) only ensure equality of null hypothesis tests based on S and T if S is binary. These authors have evidently overlooked criterion (19.3), which is necessary to avoid pathological relationships for (non-binary) S in which (19.1) and (19.2) hold, but the dependence of the hazard rate (19.2) on S does not effect the marginal hazard for T (averaged over S) at any value of t.

Casting this surrogate endpoint definition in the "operational" terms (19.1)–(19.3) implies that one would not expect ever to be in a position where (19.1)–(19.3) could be asserted with confidence based on data, while simultaneously not being in a position to assess treatment effects directly on T. Rather, in order to argue that S is a suitable replacement for T for evaluating the effect of x on T, one would typically need to rely heavily on biological and mechanistic considerations (e.g., Prentice 1989, p.439), while examining the consistency of available data with (19.1)–(19.3). In this sense the terminology "validation of a surrogate endpoint" should be avoided in favor of the more descriptive "evaluation of a surrogate endpoint" in considering this process (e.g., Biomarkers Definitions Working Group 2001).

19.3 Surrogate Endpoint Evaluation

Suppose now that one wishes to decide whether a particular S is a good candidate as surrogate for a true endpoint T, in a preliminary assessment of the effects of x on T. If the effects of x on T are of substantial clinical or public health importance, the overall research agenda should provide for an eventual direct assessment of these effects whenever practical, whereas in other circumstances there may not be an ability to go beyond an assessment of treatment effects on biomarkers or other shorter-term effects.

One can break this question into two components, according to whether one wishes to evaluate S as a potential surrogate for T in relation to treatment x using data from a single study of T and S in relation to x in a specific population, or whether one tries to "borrow strength" from studies of the same treatments in other populations, or from treatments of the same type or class as x in the same or other populations.

Suppose first that a study of T and S in relation to x is ongoing. Typically, if the study does not provide very precise information on the relationship between T and x it will also not provide precise information on the extent of any departures from (19.1)–(19.3), and hence an argument of surrogacy for S in this treatment evaluation must rely heavily on theoretical considerations (e.g., biological or mechanistic). Nevertheless, statistical modeling and estimation may provide useful empirical insights into the consistency of the data with (19.1)–(19.3). Evidence in support of (19.2) may be forthcoming from a Cox regression analysis of λ_T on a suitable time-dependent covariate, $Z(t)$, defined as a function of the preceding history $\{S(u), u < t\}$. For example, for a categorical modeled covariate a corresponding score test (time-dependent log-rank test) may provide a suitable assessment of (19.2), and application of this model separately in each treatment group, in conjunction with the empirical distribution of $Z(t)$, given $x, F(t)$, may provide evidence in support of (19.3). Empirical support for (19.1) will, however, typically be limited for reasons previously mentioned. For example, a Cox regression analysis of λ_T on the potential surrogate and x may fail to provide evidence of departure from (19.1), but in situations where the use of a surrogate endpoint is of interest it will typically not be possible to rule out moderate departures from (19.1) based on data from this single study. Note that some authors (Freedman, Graubard, and Schatzkin 1992) suggest a comparison of estimates of the coefficient of x in a Cox model for $\lambda_T(t, x)$ to the corresponding coefficient in $\lambda_T\{t; S(t), x\}$ as a measure of the extent to which the potential surrogate is able to explain, or mediate, any association between T and x. Although this percentage of treatment effect explained (PTE) notion is intuitively appealing, a surrogate endpoint in a specific study is likely to be entertained only when the relationship between T and x is uncertain and imprecisely estimated, leading to plausible values for the denominator of PTE that include zero and to some technical difficulties. The alternative of just examining the estimated coefficient of x in a Cox regression of $\lambda_T\{t; S(t), x\}$ is more straightforward but, again, moderate departures from (19.1) will typically not be able to be ruled out in settings of interest.

Note that if one is willing to assume that (19.1) to (19.3) are satisfied, then the relationship between T and z is given by

$$\lambda_T(t; x) = \int \lambda_T\{t; S(t)\}\text{pr}\{S(t); x, F(t)\}.$$

Hence, for example, a Cox model

$$\lambda_T\{t; S(t)\} = \lambda_{0T}(t)e^{Z(t)\alpha}$$

for a binary $Z(t)$ in conjunction with a binary response model for $Z(t)$ given $\{x, F(t)\}$ with parameter β induces a model

$$\lambda_T(t; x) = \lambda_0(t) \sum_{j\varepsilon\{0,1\}} e^{j\alpha}p\{Z(t) = j; x, \beta\},$$

providing a framework for a quantitative estimation of the relationship between T and x.

Now suppose that one decides to bring in external data sources to assist in the assessment of S as a potential surrogate for T in relation to x. For example, x may have already been studied in relation to T and S in other populations. Some assumption concerning a similar form of the distribution of (T, S) given x is, of course, necessary, in order to draw strength from these external data sets concerning this distribution in the setting under study. For example, to examine the extent of departure from (19.1), if any, with greater precision one could apply a Cox model on each pertinent external population, while allowing the baseline hazard rate to vary among populations. In this context one could consider whether there is evidence of heterogeneity in the dependence of $\lambda\{t; S(t), x\}$ on x and, if not, assume common treatment parameters, which may now be able to be estimated with some precision, depending on the extent of the external data. If analyses of this type do not provide evidence against (19.1) or against (19.1) to (19.3) more generally, then one gains assurance that provisional inference on the relationship between T and x in the current study can be gleaned from the relationship between T and S and between S and x. Also, the emerging data would then suggest that the effects of x on T are largely mediated by S, and this insight may have crucial clinical or public health implications.

The approach alluded to in the preceding paragraph could also be entertained by bringing in data on other treatments that are thought to have similar modes of action and similar benefits and risks, that have been studied in the same population or other pertinent populations. Now statistical considerations will be required to define a suitable class of treatments, and a pertinent set of external populations. If one or more of the other treatments provides evidence against (19.1), for example, subject matter expertise will be needed to advise on whether or not such departure from (19.1) reflects disease pathways that are likely unimportant for the treatments under current test in the population of interest.

As mentioned previously, condition (19.1) is quite restrictive, and to be plausible it may be necessary to define a high-dimensional surrogate process S, having elements that measure various biological processes that may be affected by x and that have some corresponding implication for treatment effect on T. Hence there is a need for multivariate response statistical procedures for the analysis of S in relation to x, that include parameters that lead to a meaningful interpretation of induced effects of x on T.

Given the stringency of (19.1) it may often happen that evidence against (19.1) emerges, particularly if S is of low dimension, and other pertinent sources having substantial data on (T, S, x) are available. One then has evidence that this S does not fully mediate any relationship between x and T, but it may still be possible that information on the relationship between S and x can provide a useful prediction about the corresponding relationship between T and x, for the treatment and population of interest. In fact, this type of prediction is the principal theme of this volume.

19.4 Treatment Effect Prediction

The idea here is that because the relationship between T and x in a study population is the goal, then one may be able to use the correlation between estimates of parameters that characterize the dependencies T and x and S on x in other pertinent populations or treatments, in conjunction with S on x in the present context, to make a useful prediction about the relationship of T on x in this present context. Note that such prediction in itself would not provide insight into the ability of S to mediate, or explain, any relationship between T and x.

To pursue this idea, one needs to specify models to characterize the effects of x on T and on S. For example, Chapter 11 focuses a univariate failure time S as a surrogate for a univariate failure time T and specifies proportional hazards models for each treatment effect while requiring the regression coefficients (log-hazard ratios) for studies in the various populations to have a simple additive random effects form. A semi-parametric model for (T, S) given x, such as that due to Clayton (1978), is then assumed, thereby allowing the correlation between treatment effect parameters for T and S to be calculated, and prediction of the treatment effect parameter for T on x in the current population to be made. Although this seems an appealing strategy for an interim assessment of the effects of x on T, there are some important related issues. First, use of the magnitude of the correlation between treatment effect parameters for T and S as a basis for *defining* a surrogate endpoint does not seem advisable. Certainly, if this correlation is one, and statistical modeling assumptions are justified, then having S is tantamount to having T for treatment effect assessment. More generally, however, what cutpoint criterion would be reasonable to assert that S is, or is not, a suitable surrogate for T in the evaluation of x?

A high correlation (e.g., 0.9) may exclude potential surrogates that fully mediate the treatment effect on T. Suppose that $T = S + U$ where U is unrelated to S and x. For example, S may be time from randomization to disease recurrence in a cancer clinical trial, while U is the additional time to cancer-related death. The correlation between treatment effect parameters for T and S may be low if U is influential and of variable distribution among populations, but treatment effect evaluation on T can very effectively be made based on S. Similarly, if a relatively low correlation is used as a surrogate endpoint criterion it may happen that S would be accepted as a suitable surrogate for T in relation to x even though S does not reflect one or more of the important pathways whereby x affects T, and the relative importance among such pathways may vary among populations or among treatments in the same general class.

Second, use of the correlation between treatment effect parameters for prediction may be sensitive to model specification and may require considerable care to ensure that modeling assumptions are not inappropriately influential in the prediction. Consider again proportional hazards models for the marginal distributions of failure time variables T and S, given x. Chapter 11 describes the use of certain copula models for the estimation of this correlation. These copula models make the strong assumption that the joint distribution of T and S is governed by a single parameter θ. For example, the Clayton model presented is characterized by a constant "cross ratio"

$$\frac{\lambda_T(t; S = s, x)}{\lambda_T(t; S > s, x)} = 1 + \theta \text{ for all } (t, s).$$

It is evident, setting $S(t) = 0$ if $S \leq s$ and $S(t) = 1$ if $S > s$, that this modeling assumption places substantial restriction on $\lambda_T\{t|S(t); x\}$ that appears in (19.1). Even if the form of the Clayton model is consistent with the datasets being analyzed, it seems fundamental to allow θ to depend on x, to avoid an assumption that the nature of the relationship between T and S is unaffected by treatment. (Similarly in the context of simple normal models for continuous T and S it seems basic to allow the correlation between T and S to depend on x.) In a typical application where data on (T, S, x) from external studies, and data on (S, x) from the current study would be considered for a preliminary assessment of the relationship between T and x in the current study, S will be a strong risk factor for T, but a fundamental question will be does the treatment alter the relationship? For example, in a clinical trial in which I work, one might consider low-density lipoprotein (LDL) cholesterol measures in relation to postmenopausal hormone therapy (HT) as basis for predicting the effects of HT on coronary heart disease (CHD) incidence. However, one should allow the LDL and CHD relationship to differ between women randomized to intervention and control groups.

Also, it seems prudent to estimate marginal hazard ratio parameters in a manner that is insensitive to strong modeling assumptions, like those attending the Clayton or Hougaard. This can be done, for example, by applying standard partial likelihood methods for estimating these marginal distribution parameters in a two-stage procedure rather than, say, applying a fully parametric model, where marginal treatment affect parameter estimates may be affected by the copula model assumption.

Actually, this type of copula model assumption may be quite unnecessary for these prediction purposes. For example, a concordance measure that generalizes Kendall's τ to a finite follow-up region for T and S can be specified and estimated non-parametrically (e.g., Fan, Hsu, and Prentice 2000). Such non-parametric estimates, with allowance for dependence on x and on dataset, may provide an avenue to a fairly robust provisional assessment of the effects of T on x, when T and S are failure time variates. Of course the value of such assessment depends on the relevance of the external datasets being analyzed, the adequacy of the proportional hazards modeling assumptions for the marginal distribution, and the suitability of a simple normal additive random effects model for the log-hazard ratio treatment parameters.

19.5 Discussion

Two rather complementary approaches to the preliminary assessment of the relationship between an endpoint T and a treatment indicator vector x have been described. In one of these a corresponding variable, or process, S, is defined that is thought to adhere approximately to the strong surrogate endpoint criteria (19.1)–(19.3), and an interim test of the hypothesis of no dependence between T and x is based on a corresponding test of the hypothesis of no dependence between S and x, and (19.1), along with estimates of the distribution of S given x and used for a quantitative assessment of the relationship between T and x. Other relevant datasets may be used to help assess the appropriateness of (19.1)–(19.3), or as an aid to model building for a quantitative assessment.

The second approach, which may be considered whether or not criteria (19.1)–(19.3) are thought to be approximately true, relies fundamentally on the existence of other datasets having substantial information on the joint distribution of (T, S) given x, and enough other datasets that the variation in treatment parameter estimates for T on x and for S on x can be characterized and estimated. Assuming the current study can be viewed as an additional study in this series, estimates the joint distribution of treatment effect parameters from the other studies, and an estimate of the treatment effect parameter for S given x in the current study, may lead to a useful estimate of the treatment effect parameter in the current study. Given uncertainty that is likely to surround interim inferences based on either of these approaches, it may be interesting to consider both in settings where related assumptions are plausible.

20

The Promise and Peril of Surrogate Endpoints in Cancer Research

Arthur Schatzkin, Mitch Gail, and Laurence Freedman

20.1 Introduction

Cancer is one of humanity's leading causes of morbidity and mortality. Nevertheless, in the general population, even the most common malignancies have a low probability of occurrence over a restricted time interval. For example, the age-adjusted annual incidence rate of breast cancer among women in the United States is about 100 per 100,000, or 0.1%; the annual colorectal cancer incidence rate among men and women combined is around 50 per 100,000, or only 0.05%. And these are among the most frequently occurring malignancies.

The medical research implications of this relative infrequency of cancer occurrence are straightforward: controlled intervention studies or prospective observational epidemiologic investigations that use incident cancer as an endpoint must be large, lengthy, and, therefore, costly. Such studies must yield many hundreds of cancers to have adequate statistical power to detect a meaningful treatment effect or exposure association. The ongoing Women's Health Initiative, for example, requires several tens of thousands of participants to be followed over nearly a decade to observe sufficient numbers of cancers to detect reasonable reductions in the incidence of breast and colorectal malignancies (Women's Health Initiative Study Group 1998). Studies with surrogate endpoints, biomarkers of preclinical carcinogenesis, are attractive because such studies are potentially smaller, shorter, and considerably less expensive than their counterparts with cancer endpoints.

20.2 When Are Surrogates Appropriate?

Despite their potential to reduce the size, duration, and cost of studies, surrogate endpoints may not be acceptable because the quality of evidence they provide on treatment effects or exposure associations is lower than that obtained by studying the effects of treatment or exposure on a true cancer endpoint. For some types of studies, the quality of evidence provided by surrogates might be sufficient, whereas for others only the cancer endpoints will do. For example, true clinical endpoints, such as time to cancer recurrence or time to death, might be indispensable in randomized phase III clinical trials designed to estimate the clinical effects of a new cancer treatment. Such trials must provide the highest standards of evidence regarding treatment efficacy. Phase II trials, on the other hand, are preliminary studies designed to determine whether an agent warrants further study in phase III trials, so the use of a surrogate endpoint, such as whether a tumor shrinks following treatment, might be acceptable. The consequences of a false negative result might be to curtail testing of a potentially valuable treatment; a false positive result would not lead to widespread use of the agent, however, but only to phase III testing, where, presumably, the agent would be found to have no beneficial clinical effect. Likewise, in epidemiologic investigations of, for example, the relationship of dietary factors to colorectal or breast cancer, surrogate endpoints such as cell proliferation indices or blood hormone concentrations might provide valuable exploratory information in the evaluation of a new hypothesis, whereas more rigorous testing of that dietary hypothesis might require the use of frank cancer endpoints.

20.3 Identifying Surrogate Endpoints for Cancer

To define a surrogate endpoint (S), it is necessary first to define the true clinical endpoint (T). In most observational epidemiologic studies, T is the occurrence of new ("incident") cancer, usually specified as the age or time of cancer diagnosis. In therapeutic clinical trials, T is usually taken as the time from treatment to either cancer recurrence or death. Other clinically meaningful measures that influence how a patient feels or functions can also be used as primary endpoints (DeGruttola *et al.* 2004). Any measurement other than T is a potential surrogate measurement. In a preamble to a proposed accelerated approval rule for drugs, the Food and Drug Administration defined a surrogate as follows: "A surrogate endpoint, or 'marker', is a laboratory measurement or physical sign that is used in therapeutic trials as a substitute for a clinically meaningful endpoint that is a direct measure of how a patient feels, functions, or survives and is expected to predict the effect of the therapy" (Federal Register 1992).

There are a host of biological phenomena, potential biomarkers of preclinical carcinogenesis, that could potentially serve as cancer surrogates. With the explosion in molecular and cell biology, this list is growing:

Alterations in the characteristics of tissues. "Pre-neoplastic" or frankly neoplastic changes are obvious candidates for surrogate endpoints. Examples include cervical (Mitchell *et al.* 1994), prostatic (Bostwick 1999), and endometrial (Mutter 2000) intraepithelial neoplasia; colorectal adenomatous polyps (Schatzkin *et al.* 1994); bronchial metaplasia (a possible pre-neoplastic state for lung cancer) (Misset *et al.* 1986); and dysplastic changes in the esophagus (Dawsey *et al.* 1998).

Histological changes detected by imaging. Examples include mammographic parenchymal patterns as a surrogate for breast carcinogenesis (Saftlas *et al.* 1989), and ovarian ultrasound abnormalities in ovarian cancer (Karlan 1995).

Cellular phenomena. Surrogates in this category include several assays of epithelial cell proliferation, including tritiated thymidine or bromodeoxyuridine incorporation into DNA, proliferating cell nuclear antigen (PCNA), and Ki67 (Baron *et al.* 1995b). Measures of apoptosis (Bedi *et al.* 1995) have recently been proposed as potential surrogate endpoints, as well as the ratio of proliferation to apoptosis. In AIDS research, CD4 cell counts and HIV viral load have been used as surrogates for critical AIDS endpoints (Tsiatis, DeGruttola, and Wulfsohn 1995, Ruiz *et al.* 1996).

Molecular markers. A plethora of potential molecular surrogates have been suggested. Examples include specific somatic mutations in cancer-related genes (such as RAS or TP53), DNA *hypo-* and *hyper*-methylation of specific genes, and gene expression products (including those measured in microarrays) (Fearon 1992, Counts and Goodman 1995, Brown and Botstein 1999). Chemical-DNA adducts can be considered not only as indicators of exposure (which they might well be) but also as markers of a "downstream" integrated metabolic process, one occurring temporally and developmentally closer to the malignant outcome than the exposure itself (Groopman *et al.* 1994).

Infection and inflammation. Infectious processes have been implicated in a number of cancers, and these infections could be viewed as surrogate endpoints. Examples include infections with human papillomavirus (HPV) in cervical carcinogenesis (Schiffman 1992), *Helicobacter pylori* in gastric cancer (Muñoz 1994), and HTLV1 in adult T-cell leukemia (Blattner 1989). Inflammatory cells and cytokines, which contribute to tumor growth, progression, and immunosuppression, could serve as surrogate markers (Balkwill and Mantovani 2001).

Bioactive substances in blood and tissue. Examples here include blood and tissue estrogens or androgens, oxidation products, and anti-oxidants (again, in both blood and specific tissues), tissue- or cell-type-specific antigens (such as prostate-specific antigen, PSA), and growth factors. For this category of potential surrogates, the marker, blood estrogen levels (Dorgan *et al.* 1996), for example, may not be found directly in the target tissue, but may still properly be considered a potential surrogate endpoint, in this case, for breast cancer.

Cancer prognostic factors. Potential surrogate endpoints in cancer treatment studies include time to cancer recurrence (when the true endpoint is survival) and initial tumor shrinkage (instead of true endpoint like time to tumor recurrence or survival).

20.4 Validating Surrogate Markers

Once we have found a potential surrogate, how do we determine whether it is a good surrogate marker for the true endpoint? A potential use of the surrogate, S, in assessing the effect of the exposure or intervention, E, on T is through a hypothesis test of an association between S and E. For S to be valid for hypothesis testing, the condition "S is not associated with E" (the "null hypothesis") must imply that "T is not associated with E," and vice versa (Prentice 1989). Later we discuss three conditions that are required to establish this criterion: first, S must influence T; second, E must influence S; and third, S "mediates" the effect of E on T (that is, in statistical terms, T is unrelated to E conditional on S). If S is valid for hypothesis testing, we know that if we reject the null hypothesis that S is associated with E (i.e., we accept that S is associated with E), we can conclude that T is also probably associated with E.

Although validity of hypothesis testing based on S is desirable, it would be even more useful if we could predict the magnitude of the effect of E on T from data on the magnitude of the effect of E on S. Recent proposals for such prediction are based on analyzing a series of studies of treatments in a similar class of treatments (Daniels and Hughes 1997, Buyse *et al.* 2000a, Gail *et al.* 2000), and "trial-level validity" gives an indication of how reliably one can predict the magnitude of the effect of E on T.

Suppose in each study we have sufficient information to allow us to estimate the effect of an exposure, E on a surrogate endpoint, S and the effect of

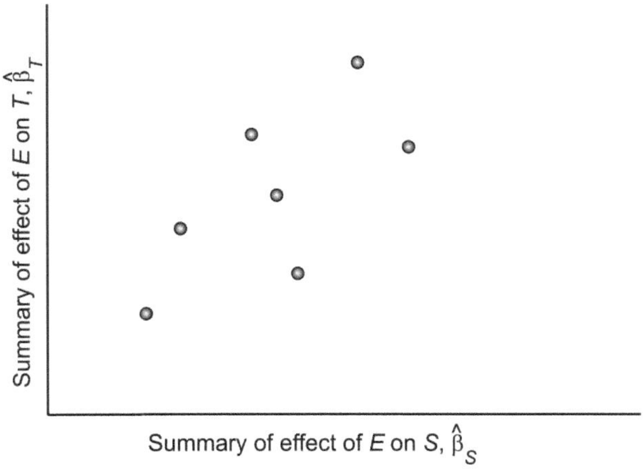

FIGURE 20.1. *Pairs of treatment effects for seven different hypothetical trials.*

E on the frank endpoint, T. We might call these two estimated treatment effects or exposure associations $\widehat{\beta}_S$ and $\widehat{\beta}_T$ obtained by regressing S on E and T on E, respectively. In Figure 20.1, pairs $(\widehat{\beta}_S, \widehat{\beta}_T)$ are plotted for seven different hypothetical clinical trials of various cancer treatments focused on the same molecular pathway, each compared with placebo. If the squared correlation, R^2, among these trial-level pairs was high, we would conclude that the effects of E on S are highly predictive of the effects of E on T, and we would say that S is "trial-level valid" (Bostwick 1999, Mutter 2000) if R^2 was near 1.0. An analysis of such a series of studies with high R^2 gives us some empirical evidence that if we wish to study a new agent in this same class of agents, we can combine data on the effect of the new agent E on S with the data from previous studies, as represented in the figure, to predict what the effect of E is on T. There are, however, a number of limitations to relying on this strategy (Schatzkin *et al.* 1994), including potentially serious loss of precision in estimates of the effect of E on T for the new agent and uncertainty about whether the new agent really belongs to the same class of agents depicted in Figure 20.1.

We now turn to some examples that give insight into these criteria for validating a surrogate marker.

20.5 The Logic of Cancer Surrogacy

Suppose, in Figure 20.2a, $E1$ represents an "exposure" to some environmental or host factor, anything from a chemopreventive agent to a deleterious

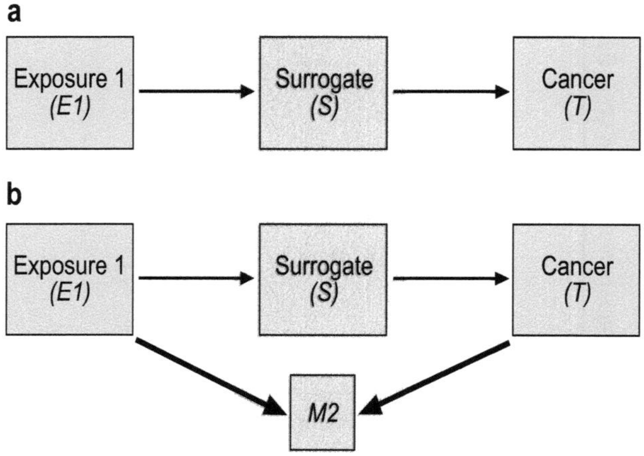

FIGURE 20.2. *Hypothetical.*

risk factor. According to this idealized model, a change in $E1$ necessarily alters the surrogate endpoint (S), which in turn modifies the true endpoint, the likelihood of incident cancer (T). As we discuss in the next section, a causal pathway such as that depicted in Figure 20.2a implies that S is valid for hypothesis testing for the particular factor $E1$, but, without further assumptions, does not necessarily imply that S will be valid for hypothesis tests for another exposure, $E2$, nor that the magnitudes of the effects of $E1$ on S can reliably predict the magnitudes of the effects of $E1$ on T for a series of exposures (trial-level validity, as described in the previous section).

The scenario in Figure 20.2a rarely occurs. Far more realistic are situations reflected in Figure 20.2b. Here, $E1$ modulates carcinogenesis through two alternative pathways, one through S, the other through another marker $M2$. To the extent that $E1$ operates through the alternative $M2$ pathway, which means that S is not a necessary component of carcinogenesis, we cannot be assured that S is a valid surrogate for hypothesis testing in studies of $E1$. The reason for this lack of certainty is that $E1$ might influence $M2$ in a way that offsets its effect on S, the final effect on cancer simply being unknown. If $E1$, for example, were to increase $M2$-positivity, $E1$ could actually end up *increasing* cancer incidence, while at the same time reducing S-positivity and giving at least a superficial impression of being anti-carcinogenic. An example from cardiovascular disease is instructive. High-dose diuretics lower blood pressure but have little effect on cardiovascular disease mortality in hypertensive patients, possibly because diuretics cause hypokalemia, which increases risk of sudden death (Temple 1999). The relationships in Figure 20.2b also make trial-level validity less likely than in Figure 20.2a, because the magnitude of the effects of E on T are

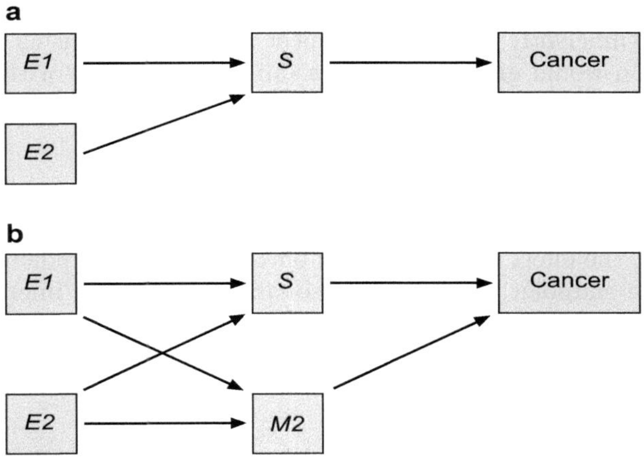

FIGURE 20.3. *Hypothetical setting.*

less likely to be predictable from the effects of E on S in a series of such studies.

20.6 Can Surrogate Validity Be Extrapolated from One Exposure to Another?

Another important question is whether a surrogate that is valid for one intervention (or exposure) is valid for another. Figure 20.3a reprises Figure 20.2a but adds another exposure, $E2$. Exposure here can refer to an intervention agent or a risk factor. Both $E1$ and $E2$ operate through a single surrogate on the path to cancer. In this scenario, the surrogate is a necessary component of the cancer pathway. $E2$ must operate through the surrogate. The surrogate is valid for studies of $E2$ as well as those of $E1$.

In Figure 20.3b, $E2$ enters into the more complex scenario depicted in Figure 20.2b. The existence of a non-trivial alternative pathway (through $M2$) means that the validity of the surrogate S may be exposure dependent. Even if $E1$ works primarily through the surrogate and affects $M2$ minimally, suggesting that the surrogate is reasonably valid for $E1$-cancer studies, it cannot be assumed that the $E2 - M2$ cancer pathway plays a similarly minor role in carcinogenesis.

For example, a given agent, $E1$, might influence colorectal carcinogenesis largely through its influence on cell proliferation. Cell proliferation in this scenario is a likely valid surrogate for colorectal cancer. A second agent,

$E2$, might have a minimal effect on cell proliferation but could increase apoptosis sufficiently to decrease cancer incidence. Focusing only on cell proliferation would give a falsely pessimistic impression of the efficacy of the second agent. The validity of a surrogate must therefore be established for every intervention.

An approach to this problem is to consider studies of a "class" of biologically comparable intervention agents. If, for example, a meta-analysis shows that the effect of these agents on the surrogate predicts their effect on the true endpoint, we can be reasonably confident in inferring a treatment effect on the true endpoint from the effect of a new member of that class on the surrogate endpoint, as discussed above (Bostwick 1999, Mutter 2000, Schatzkin *et al.* 1994).

20.7 Epithelial Hyperproliferation: A Case Study

How can we apply this logic to potential surrogates? Cell proliferation assays have been touted as potential surrogates for cancer in light of the dysregulation of cell growth that characterizes malignancy (Wargovich 1996). But are they valid surrogates? Figure 20.4 depicts causal events potentially involved in the relationship between hyperproliferation and the neoplastic process in the colorectum. If we focus just on the upper portion of this diagram, we see a single pathway going from normal epithelium to hyperproliferative epithelium to neoplasia/cancer. It is this pathway that implicitly underlies using hyperproliferation as a surrogate for cancer in testing whether there is an association between an exposure and cancer.

But hyperproliferation may not be necessary by itself for colorectal carcinogenesis. There may be an alternative pathway to neoplasia/cancer that bypasses hyperproliferation. The problem is that the effect of an intervention agent ($E1$) on this alternative pathway is unknown and may in fact counterbalance the effect through the hyperproliferation pathway. Two scenarios here are revealing:

1. The agent ($E1$) reduces proliferation, but at the same time reduces apoptosis, and therefore has no effect on colorectal cancer;
2. The agent has no effect on proliferation but does increase apoptosis, thereby reducing colorectal cancer incidence.

In both cases, a hyperproliferation assay gives the wrong answer about an intervention's effect on colorectal cancer; by definition, hyperproliferation

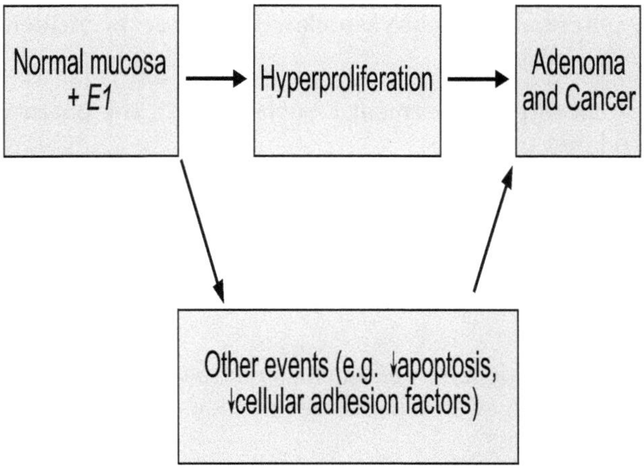

FIGURE 20.4. *Causal events potentially involved in the relationship between hyperproliferation and the neoplastic process in the colorectum.*

would not be a valid surrogate for testing for an association between $E1$ and cancer.

It is important to emphasize that the proliferation marker does not necessarily give the wrong answer about the agent's effect on cancer; the proliferation data might, in fact, be giving us the right answer. The problem is the uncertainty that flows from the existence of several alternative pathways to cancer.

20.8 Evaluating Potential Surrogate Endpoints

Given this uncertainty, how can we evaluate the validity of a potential surrogate marker? The answer is to integrate it into observational epidemiologic studies or clinical trials that have cancer (or a preneoplastic lesion, such as adenomatous polyps; see below) as an endpoint. This integration can elucidate the causal structure underlying the relationships among interventions (or exposures), potential surrogate endpoints, and cancer. In other words, the validation study should include data on T, S, and E for each individual and, if one wishes to demonstrate consistent ability to predict the magnitude of the effect of E on T from data on the effect of E on S (trial-level validity), there should be a series of such studies.

To determine whether the surrogate is valid for hypothesis testing, we need to investigate three questions:

1. Is the potential surrogate associated with cancer incidence (i.e., is S associated with T)?

2. Is the exposure or treatment associated with the potential surrogate (is E related to S)?

3. Does the potential surrogate endpoint "mediate" the relationship between exposure or treatment and cancer? That is, conditional on an individual's value of S, is there an absence of association between T and E, as in Figure 20.2a?

Standard epidemiologic measures such as relative risk and attributable proportion can be used in addressing these questions (Rothman and Greenland 1998).

20.8.1 Is the Surrogate Associated with Cancer?

As indicated above, for a marker to be a reasonable surrogate for a given cancer, it must be associated with that cancer. Ecologic studies can provide useful, if indirect, information on this connection. Studies are considered to be "ecologic," or aggregate, when individual-level information is not used; instead, an average marker value is obtained for a sample of individuals selected from specific populations (e.g., Seventh Day Adventists *versus* non-Adventists), which is then related to the overall risk of cancer in those populations. Several studies, for example, have compared mean proliferation indices in groups at varying risk of cancer (Lipkin *et al.* 1984). In such studies, however, one cannot be certain that those who are marker-positive are the ones with increased incidence of cancer.

This "ecologic" problem is obviated by moving to individual-level observational epidemiologic studies, whether case-control or cohort. Such studies give individual-level information on T, S, and E and they are important tools for examining the relationship between a putative surrogate and cancer. Blood estrogen levels have been shown in several studies to be directly associated with breast cancer, a relationship that had to be established before estrogens could be considered a surrogate for breast malignancy (Toniolo *et al.* 1995, Hankinson *et al.* 1998). Human papillomavirus (HPV) infection, a potential surrogate for cervical cancer, has been shown to be highly associated with risk of severe cervical neoplasia (Schiffman *et al.* 1993). Observational studies can also be incorporated into clinical trial design. For example, in the Polyp Prevention Trial (Schatzkin *et al.* 2000), a dietary intervention study with adenomatous polyp formation as the primary endpoint, investigators are currently examining the relationship between colorectal epithelial-cell proliferation measures and subsequent adenoma recurrence. The adenoma or CIN endpoints described here are only neoplastic cancer precursors; we have, for purposes of discussion, considered these as proxies for cancer, even though, as we discuss below, the validity of these precursor endpoints is not ironclad.

The attributable proportion (AP), an epidemiologic parameter that measures the extent to which T is determined by S, can be useful in determining the importance of alternative pathways and thereby evaluating the relationship between S and T. In the simple linear causal model of Figure 20.2a, the estimated AP for the surrogate is 1.0, excluding random error. When at least one pathway exists that is alternative to the pathway containing the surrogate, as in Figure 20.2b, then the AP for the surrogate is <1.0. A relatively high AP that was still less than 1.0, would suggest that the alternative ("$M2$") pathway plays a small role in tumorigenesis. An AP substantially lower than 1.0 for the surrogate implies that one or more alternative pathways is indeed operative, or that S is measured with a substantial degree of error (see Section 20.10).

20.8.2 Is E Associated with S?

Assuming that we are dealing with an intervention (exposure), E, that has an established relationship with T, for a potential surrogate marker to be valid, there must also be some relationship between E and the marker. Ecologic studies can provide indirect information on this question. For example, the mean colorectal epithelial cell proliferation index could be measured in populations with different average consumption of dietary fat. Individual-level studies, however, can provide more convincing evidence.

In a clinical trial, we need to see that the intervention changes the marker, which can be addressed in relatively small studies. Several studies, for example, have examined the effect of dietary change or supplementation on colorectal epithelial cell proliferation (Holt *et al.* 1998); others have investigated the effect of dietary fat modification (Prentice *et al.* 1990) or alcohol consumption (Reichman *et al.* 1993), both possible etiologic factors in breast cancer, on blood or urine estrogen levels. One illustrative case is that no relationship was found between calcium carbonate supplementation and epithelial cell proliferation measured one year later (Baron *et al.* 1995a), even though calcium did reduce overall adenoma recurrence (Baron *et al.* 1999). This suggests that proliferation measures are problematic surrogates for colorectal neoplasia/cancer in studies with calcium supplements as the main intervention/exposure.

We can also examine this question in case-control or cohort studies, in which we evaluate the association between an exposure and the potential surrogate. Schiffman *et al.* (1993), for example, in investigating the etiology of cervical cancer, showed a strong association between reproductive risk factors, particularly number of sexual partners, and HPV infection, a potential surrogate for cervical neoplasia. In a recent meta-analysis of cohort studies, body mass index was shown to be directly associated with blood estrogen levels (Endogeneous Hormones and Breast Cancer Collaborative Group 2003).

20.8.3 Does S Mediate the Link Between E and T?

Once we have determined (1) whether a potential surrogate is highly associated with cancer and (2) whether a surrogate is indeed linked to a given intervention or exposure, it is still necessary to determine whether (3) the effect of E on T is "mediated" by S in order to establish the validity of S for hypothesis testing. In statistical terms, mediation by S means that E and T are unrelated ("conditionally independent") once marker status is taken into account. One way to test for this condition is to stratify the data on levels of the surrogate marker and determine if there is an association between E and T within strata. If no such association is present, then there is evidence of mediation. An analogous approach is to include the surrogate marker S and the exposure E as independent variables in a multiple regression model that has T as the dependent variable. If the regression coefficient for E is 0, this constitutes evidence for mediation. The statistical aspects of mediation analysis are an area of current research (Freedman, Graubard, and Schatzkin 1992, Buyse and Molenberghs 1998).

We can obtain concrete data on mediation by integrating an assay for the surrogate into either clinical trials or observational epidemiologic studies, collecting information on both the intervention or exposure and the cancer (or severe neoplasia). As an example, investigators have used a case-control study to look at the extent to which HPV infection mediates the association between number of sexual partners and dysplasia (Schiffman and Schatzkin 1994). As Table 20.1 shows, the number of sexual partners was strongly and directly associated with cervical dysplasia risk. When the presence or absence of HPV infection was included as a covariate in a statistical regression model that related dysplasia to the number of sexual partners, the relative risk for number of sexual partners dropped dramatically. This suggests that most of the association between number of partners and cervical dysplasia is mediated through HPV infection (Franco 1991).

The same analytical strategy can be used to assess the extent of surrogate mediation in other study designs. For example, in the meta-analysis discussed above (Endogeneous Hormones and Breast Cancer Collaborative Group 2003), a direct association between BMI and breast cancer essen-

TABLE 20.1. *Number of sexual partners and the risk of cervical dysplasia.*

Odds ratio	Number of sexual partners				
	1	2	3–5	6–9	>10
Unadjusted	1.0	1.7	3.1*	4.7*	4.4*
Adjusted for HPV status	1.0	1.0	1.1	1.5	1.6

*: $p < 0.05$.

HPV, human papilloma virus.

tially disappeared after researchers adjusted for blood estrogen levels. A dietary modification or dietary supplement study of colorectal neoplasia, from which rectal biopsy specimens are obtained for mucosal proliferation assays, could provide information on the extent to which any observed diet/supplement effect is mediated by proliferation changes.

As a general rule, the greater the intervention effect or exposure association, the fewer study participants are needed in a mediation analysis. For a number of reasons, the relative risks due to exposures in observational studies tend to be larger than the intervention effects observed in clinical trials. It follows that mediation analyses might be more likely to provide interpretable data in observational epidemiologic studies. Although complete mediation is necessary for a marker to be perfectly valid for hypothesis testing, it does not guarantee that the magnitude of the effects of E on S can be used to predict the magnitude of the effects of E on T reliably. Moreover, a demonstration that S mediates the effect of E on T for one exposure does not guarantee that it does so for another exposure. These points highlight the desirability of obtaining data on E, S, and T in several studies with possibly differing exposures.

20.9 Surrogates That Are Likely To Be Valid

Unlike putative surrogates such as epithelial cell proliferation or blood hormone levels, for which validity is problematic, considerable evidence supports the usefulness of a few "downstream" surrogate markers, that is, those close to cancer on the causal pathway.

Cervical cancer surrogates. Practically all cervical cancer requires prior persistent HPV infection. HPV persistence results in inactivation, by the E6 and E7 proteins of the HPV genome, of the $TP53$ and RB tumor suppressor genes, leading in turn to increasingly severe intraepithelial neoplasia and, eventually, cancer (zur Hausen 2000). At most only a very small proportion of cervical cancer can arise as a result of tumor suppressor inactivation occurring by mutation in the absence of HPV infection. Because most cervical cancer does occur through persistent HPV infection, an intervention that eliminates or reduces such infection would have a high likelihood of decreasing cervical cancer incidence.

Cervical intraepithelial neoplasia (CIN), especially CIN3, is also considered a strong surrogate for cancer and has been used as an endpoint in a number of epidemiologic studies. A very high percentage of CIN3 will progress to cancer in 20 years; only a very small fraction regresses. In fact, CIN3 is very close to being invasive cancer and is downstream from persistent HPV infection in the causal pathway leading to malignancy.

Adenomatous polyps for colorectal cancer. Another potential surrogate endpoint for which inferences to cancer are considered to be strong is the adenomatous polyp (adenoma). Colorectal adenomas are attractive candidates for cancer surrogacy in research studies because of their high recurrence rate: about 10% of persons having an adenoma removed will have a recurrence in the next year, an occurrence frequency nearly 2 orders of magnitude greater than the incidence of cancer. The underlying *biological* rationale for the use of adenoma endpoints in epidemiologic studies and clinical trials is the strong evidence for a relationship between this marker and colorectal cancer. This adenoma-carcinoma sequence is supported by studies demonstrating carcinomatous foci in adenomas and adenomatous foci within carcinomas, experiments showing the malignant transformation of adenoma cell lines, and studies identifying common mutations in adenomatous and carcinomatous tissue (Sugarbaker *et al.* 1985, Paraskeva *et al.* 1990, Fearon 1990). An intervention reducing the recurrence of adenomas in the large bowel would therefore probably decrease the incidence of colorectal cancer, thus making adenoma recurrence a reasonably valid surrogate marker.

Nevertheless, even the adenoma is not a perfectly reliable surrogate and some inferential difficulties remain with trials in which adenoma recurrence is used as a surrogate endpoint. Recurrent adenomas occur early in the tumorigenic sequence. The results of adenoma recurrence trials can be misleading if the intervention factor being tested operates later in the neoplastic process, for example from the growth of a small into a large adenoma or the transformation of a large adenoma to carcinoma. A (false) null result for recurrent adenomas can result if the intervention operates only in the later stages of neoplasia. A positive result, though, suggests that cancer would be reduced, because large adenomas and cancers derive from small adenomas.

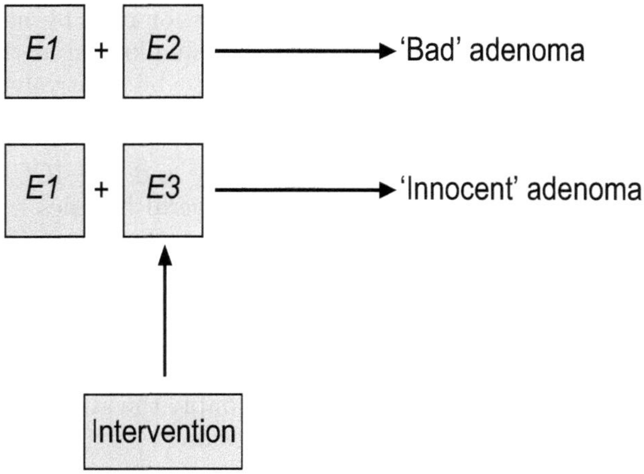

FIGURE 20.5. *Hypothetical setting.*

A second inferential difficulty with adenoma recurrence as a surrogate endpoint flows from the likely biological heterogeneity of adenomas. Only a relatively small proportion of adenomas go on to cancer. Suppose that one type, the "bad" adenoma that progresses to cancer, is caused by exposures $E1$ and $E2$, as in Figure 20.5. The second type, the "innocent" adenoma, is caused by the same exposure $E1$ but in concert with exposure $E3$. Imagine an intervention that works only on exposure $E3$. We could reduce the pool of innocent adenomas, thereby yielding a statistically significant reduction in adenoma formation in our trial, but in fact the incidence of bad adenomas and cancer would be unaffected. This could work the other way as well: we might see at most a small reduction in all adenomas (the bad ones being only a small proportion of all adenomas) even though the intervention truly decreases the formation of bad adenomas and, therefore, reduces the incidence of cancer.

20.10 Measurement Error

All biomarkers are measured with some error. Two important statistical issues need to be considered. First, a potential surrogate is useful (and ultimately valid) only if it can discriminate among study participants: those in the different treatment arms of a trial or the various exposure categories in an epidemiologic study. Discrimination is possible only if the surrogate values vary more between participants than they do within the same individual (for example, differences in marker values obtained from different tissue areas, measured at different time points, or read by multiple readers.) This can be measured by calculating a value known as the intraclass correlation coefficient (ICC), and this needs to be relatively large if the surrogate is to be useful (Fleiss 1986, pp. 1–5).

Intra-participant variability may be reduced, and the ICC thereby increased, by taking repeat samples, such as several biopsies from different areas or multiple blood samples over time. At a minimum, therefore, data are required on the potential surrogate marker's components of variance to establish the minimum number of marker samples needed for meaningful discrimination among study participants. In the absence of such data, it is not possible to ascertain whether null findings for a potential surrogate reflect a true lack of effect (or association) or simply the attenuating influence of random sources of intra-individual variation.

Reliability data have not been routinely collected in marker studies. Few studies have provided data on potential surrogate marker variability, particularly with respect to variability over time. A notable exception is recent investigations attempting to estimate the number of estradiol measurements necessary to discriminate among individuals (Hankinson *et al.* 1995). Studies measuring intra-individual variation in colorectal epithelial cell proliferation are under way (Lyles *et al.* 1994, McShane *et al.* 1998, Kulldorf *et al.* 2000). Quality-control studies designed to obtain data on the variability characteristics of potential surrogate markers are essential.

Second, even if the ICC is acceptable, measurement error will tend to attenuate findings from studies designed to answer each of the three questions posed above. The associations between intervention (exposure) and marker, and between marker and cancer, will be attenuated by errors in marker measurement (Franco 1991, Schiffman and Schatzkin 1994). Measurement error in S can also lead to an underestimate of the extent to which a correctly measured S would mediate the effect of E on T.

20.11 Conclusion

Because studies with surrogate cancer endpoints can be smaller, faster, and substantially less expensive than those with frank cancer outcomes, the use of surrogate endpoints is undeniably attractive. This attractiveness is likely to grow in coming years as the rapidly advancing discoveries in cell and molecular biology generate new therapies requiring testing and new markers that could plausibly serve as surrogates for cancer.

Surrogate endpoint studies can certainly yield useful information. They continue to play a legitimate role in Phase II clinical studies. In some areas of clinical therapeutics, surrogate endpoints like blood pressure, blood sugar level, or HIV viral load, are regarded as useful for Phase III studies. In other circumstances, the most that can be said is that surrogates *might* give the right answers about intervention effects on (or exposure associations with) cancer.

The problem is the uncertainty attached to conclusions based on surrogates. Except for those few surrogates that are both necessary for and relatively close developmentally to cancer, such as CIN3 and cervical cancer, the existence of plausible alternative pathways makes inferences to cancer from surrogates problematic. Merely being on the causal pathway to cancer does not in itself constitute surrogate validity; it is the totality of causal connections that is crucial. There is, unfortunately, a fairly extensive history of quite plausible surrogate markers giving the wrong answer about the effects of treatments for chronic disease (Fleming and DeMets 1996). There is no reason to believe that observational studies of cancer etiology based on cancer surrogates are immune to such inferential difficulties.

We should also consider the use of surrogate markers in the broader context of multiple disease endpoints, including treatment toxicity. A surrogate marker might give the "right" answer about cancer for a given intervention, but nevertheless give little or no information about important adverse events that greatly influence overall evaluation of the intervention. Suppose, for example, that we have a valid tissue or blood marker for breast cancer, one that gives us the right answer about a promising hormone-modulating intervention. That breast-cancer surrogate will tell us nothing about the potential of the intervention to increase the incidence of stroke. A potential stroke surrogate could be measured, but we are then faced with uncertainties about the reliability of this surrogate for stroke itself. This illustrates yet another difficulty arising from exclusive reliance on surrogate marker studies.

This chapter emphasizes the importance of conducting the investigations necessary to evaluate potential surrogates that include information on E, S, and T for study participants. Such studies are needed if we are to generalize from surrogate endpoint findings to cancer. There is, however, an implicit and perhaps unavoidable irony here: the large, long, expensive studies required to fully evaluate potential surrogates are precisely the studies that surrogates were designed to replace. Moreover, the exposure-dependence alluded to above complicates matters further: establishing validity for a given surrogate for one intervention/exposure does not necessarily translate into validity for another intervention/exposure. To assess validity for a variety of related interventions or exposures, the investigator needs a series of studies that provide individual-level data on T, S, and E.

The problems inherent in using surrogate endpoints need not be regarded as a cause for pessimism in cancer research. If anything, the limitations of surrogacy remind us of the complexity of cancer causation and affirm the continued importance of large clinical trials and observational epidemiologic studies with explicit cancer endpoints. In the context of such a research program, we may identify surrogates that can play a useful role in exploratory investigations and Phase II trials and, in some instances, in more definitive studies.

References

Aalen, O.O. (1978) Nonparametric inference for a family of counting processes. *Annals of Statistics,* **6**, 701–726.

Abramowitz, M. and Stegun, I.A. (1972) *Handbook of Mathematical Functions, with Formulas, Graphs, and Mathematical Tables.* New York: Dover.

Agresti, A. (1990) *Categorical Data Analysis.* New York: John Wiley & Sons.

Agresti, A., Booth, J.B., Hobert, J.P., and Caffo, B. (2000) Random-effects modeling of categorical response data. *Sociological Methodology,* **30**, 27–80.

Akaike, H. (1974) A new look at statistical model identification. *IEEE Transactions on Automatic Control,* **19**, 716–723.

Albert, J.M., Ioannidis, J.P.A., Reichelderfer, P., Conway, B., Coombs, R.W., Crane, L., Demasi, R., Dixon, D.O., Flandre, P., Hughes, M.D., Kalish, L.A., Larntz, K., Lin, D., Marschner, I.C., Muňoz, A., Murray, J., Neaton, J., Pettinelli, C., Rida, W., Taylor, J.M.G., and Welles, S.L. (1998) Statistical issues for HIV surrogate endpoints: point and counterpoint. *Statistics in Medicine,* **17**, 2435–2462.

Algina, J. (1999) A comparison of methods for constructing confidence intervals for the squared multiple correlation coefficient. *Multivariate Behavioral Research,* **34**, 494–504.

Alonso, A., Geys, H., Kenward, M.G., Molenberghs, G., and Vangeneugden, T. (2003) Validation of surrogate markers in multiple randomized clinical trials with repeated measurements. *Biometrical Journal,* **45**, 1–15.

Alonso, A., Molenberghs, G., Buyse, M., Burzykowski, T., Renard, D., Geys, H., Shkedy, Z., Tibaldi, F., and Abrahantes, J. (2004a). Prentice's approach and the meta-analytic paradigm: a reflection on the role of statistics in the evaluation of surrogate endpoints. *Biometrics,* **60**, 724–728.

Alonso, A., Geys, H., Molenberghs, G., and Kenward, M. (2004b). Validation of surrogate markers in multiple randomized clinical trials with repeated measurements: canonical correlation approach. *Biometrics*, **60**, 000–000.

Alonso, A., Geys, H., Molenberghs, G., and Vangeneugden, T. (2004c). Investigating the criterion validity of psychiatric symptom scales using surrogate marker validation methodology for repeated measurements. *Submitted for publication.*

Anderson, T.W. (1958) *An Introduction to Multivariate Statistical Analysis.* New York: John Wiley & Sons.

Anderson, J.E. (1995) Multivariate survival analysis using random effect models. In: N. Balakrishnan (Ed.), *Recent Advances in Life-Testing and Reliability*, Boca Raton: CRC Press, pp. 603–622.

Anderson, D.A. and Aitkin, M. (1985) Variance component models with binary response: interviewer variability. *Journal of the Royal Statistical Society, Series B,* **47**, 203–210.

Anderson, J.E. and Louis, T. (1995) Survival analysis using a scale change random effects models. *Journal of the American Statistical Association,* **90**, 669–679.

Anderson, J.R., Cain, K.C., and Gelber, R.D. (1983) Analysis of survival by tumour response. *Journal of Clinical Oncology,* **1**, 710–719.

Arends, L.R., Hoes, A.W. Lubsen, J., Grobbee, D.E., and Stijnen, T. (2000) Baseline risk as predictor of treatment effect benefit: three clinical meta-re-analysis. *Statistics in Medicine,* **19**, 4497–3518.

Arnold, B.C. (1995) Conditional survival models. In: N. Balakrishnan (Ed.), *Recent Advances in Life-Testing and Reliability*, pp. 589–601. Boca Raton: CRC Press.

Arnold, B.C. and Strauss, D. (1991) Pseudolikelihood estimation: some examples. *Sankhya, Series B,* **53**, 233–243.

Azzalini, A. (1994) Logistic regression for autocorrelated data with application to repeated measures. *Biometrika,* **81**, 767–775.

Bahadur, R.R. (1961) A representation of the joint distribution of responses to n dichotomous items. In: H. Solomon (Ed.), *Studies in Item Analysis and Prediction,* Stanford Mathematical Studies in the Social Sciences VI, Stanford: Stanford University Press, pp. 158–168.

Baker, S.G. and Kramer, B.S. (2003) A perfect correlate does not make a surrogate. *BioMed Central Medical Reseach Methodology*, **3**, 16.

Balkwill, F. and Mantovani, A. (2001) Inflammation and cancer: back to Virchow? *Lancet*, **357**, 539–545.

Barndorff-Nielsen, O.E. and Cox, D.R. (1994) *Inference and Asymptotics.* London: Chapman and Hall.

Baron, J.A., Tosteson, T.D., Wargovich, M.J., Sandler, R., Mandel, J., Bond, J., Haile, R., Summers, R., van Stolk, R., and Rothstein, R. (1995a) Calcium supplementation and rectal mucosal proliferation: a randomized controlled trial. *Journal of the National Cancer Institute,* **87**, 1303–1307.

Baron, J.A., Wargovich, M.J., Tosteson, T.D., Sandler, R., Haile, R., Summers, R., van Stolk, R., Rothstein, R., and Weiss, J. (1995b) Epidemiological use of rectal proliferation measures. *Cancer Epidemiology, Biomarkers, and Prevention,* **4**, 57–61.

Baron, J.A., Beach, M., Mandel, J.S., van Stolk, R.U., Haile, R.W., Sandler, R.S., Rothstein, R., Summers, R.W., Snover, D.C., Beck, G.J., Bond, J.H., and Greenberg, E.R. (1999) Calcium supplements for the prevention of colorectal adenomas. *New England Journal of Medicine,* **340**, 101–107.

Barton, C.M., Staddon, S.L., Hughes, C.M., Hall, P.A., O'Sullivan, C., Kloppel, G., Theis, B., Russell, R.C., Neoptolemos, J., and Williamson, R.C. (1991) Abnormalities of the p53 tumor suppressor gene in human pancreatic cancer. *British Journal of Cancer,* **64**, 1076–1082.

Bedi, A., Pasrich, P.J., Akhtar, A.J., Barber, J.P., Bedi, G.C., Giardiello, F.M., Zehnbauer, B.A., Hamilton, S.R., and Jones, R.J. (1995) Inhibition of apoptosis during development of colorectal cancer. *Cancer Research,* **55**, 1811–1816.

Begg, C.B., and Leung, D.H.Y. (2000) On the use of surrogate endpoints in randomized trials (with discussion). *Journal of the Royal Statistical Society, Series A,* **163**, 15–28.

Berger, J.O. (1995) *Statistical Decision Theory and Bayesian Analysis.* New York: Springer-Verlag.

Berger, V.W. (2004) Does the Prentice criterion validate surrogate endpoints? *Statistics in Medicine,* **23**, 1571–1578.

Besag, J.E. (1975) Statistical analysis of non-lattice data. *The Statistician,* **24**, 179–195.

Biomarkers Definitions Working Group (2001) Biomarkers and surrogate endpoints: preferred definitions and conceptual framework. *Clinical Pharmacology and Therapy,* **69**, 89–95.

Blattner, W.A. (1989) Retroviruses. In: A.S. Evans (Ed.), *Viral Infections in Humans (3rd ed.)*, New York: Plenum Medical Book Co., pp. 545–592.

Blin, O., Azorin, J.M., and Bouhours, P. (1996) Antipsychotic and anxiolytic properties of risperidone, haloperidol and methotrimeprazine in schizophrenic patients. *Journal of Clinical Psychopharmacology,* **16**, 38-44.

Boissel, J.P., Collet, J.P., Moleur, P., and Haugh, M. (1992) Surrogate endpoints: a basis for a rational approach. *European Journal of Clinical Pharmacology,* **43**, 235–244.

Bostwick, D.G (1999) Prostatic intraepithelial neoplasia is a risk factor for cancer. *Seminars on Urological Oncology,* **17**, 187–198.

Breslow, N.E. and Clayton, D.G. (1993) Approximate inference in generalized linear mixed models. *Journal of the American Statistical Association,* **88**, 9–25.

Breslow, N.E. and Lin, X. (1995) Bias correction in generalized linear mixed models with a single component of dispersion. *Biometrika,* **82**, 81–91.

Brown, P.O. and Botstein, D. (1999) Exploring the new world of the genome with DNA microarrays. *Nature Genetics,* **21S**, 33–37.

Brown, W.B., Hollander, M., and Korwar, R.M. (1974) Nonparametric tests of independence for censored data with applications to heart transplant data. In: F. Proschan and R.G. Serfling (Eds.), *Reliability and Biometry: Statistical analysis of lifelength,* Philadelphia: SIAM, pp. 327–354.

Browne, W.J., Draper, D., Goldstein, H., and Rasbash, J. (2002) Bayesian and likelihood methods for fitting multilevel models with complex level-1 variation. *Computational Statistics and Data Analysis,* **39**, 203–225.

Bryk, A.S. and Raudenbush, S.W. (1992) *Hierarchical Linear Models: Applications and Data Analysis Methods.* Newbury Park: Sage Publications.

Buonaccorsi, J.P. (1995) Prediction in the presence of measurement error: general discussion and an example predicting defoliation. *Biometrics,* **51**, 1562–1569.

Burzykowski, T. (2001) *Validation of Surrogate Endpoints From Multiple Randomized Clinical Trials With a Failure-time True Endpoint.* Unpublished Ph.D. dissertation, Limburgs Universitair Centrum.

Burzykowski, T., Molenberghs, G., Buyse, M., Renard, D., and Geys, H. (2001) Validation of surrogate endpoints in multiple randomized clinical trials with failure-time endpoints. *Applied Statistics,* **50**, 405–422.

Burzykowski, T., Molenberghs, G., and Buyse, M. (2004) The validation of surrogate endpoints by using data from randomized clinical trials: a case study in advanced colorectal cancer. *Journal of the Royal Statistical Society, Series A,* **167**, 103–124.

Buyse, M. and Piedbois, P. (1996) On the relationship between response to treatment and survival. *Statistics in Medicine,* **15**, 2797–2812.

Buyse, M. and Molenberghs, G. (1998) The validation of surrogate endpoints in randomized experiments. *Biometrics,* **54**, 1014–1029.

Buyse, M., Molenberghs, G., Burzykowski, T., Renard, D., and Geys, H. (2000a) The validation of surrogate endpoints in meta-analysis of randomized experiments. *Biostatistics,* **1**, 49–67.

Buyse, M., Molenberghs, G., Burzykowski, T., Renard, D., and Geys, H. (2000b) Statistical validation of surrogate endpoints: problems and proposals. *Drug Information Journal,* **34**, 447–454.

Buyse, M., Thirion, P., Carlson, R.W., Burzykowski, T. Molenberghs, G., and Piedbois, P., for the Meta-Analysis Group In Cancer (2000c) Tumour response to first line chemotherapy improves the survival of patients with advanced colorectal cancer. *Lancet,* **356**, 373–378.

Buyse, M., Vangeneugden, T., Bijnens, L., Renard, D., Burzykowski, T., Geys, H., and Molenberghs, G. (2001) Validation of biomarkers as surrogates for clinical endpoints. In: J. Bloom and R.A. Dean (Eds.), *Biomarkers in Clinical Drug Development*, New York: Marcel Dekker, pp. 149–168.

Campbell, D.T. and Fisk, D.W. (1959) Convergent and discriminant validation by the multitrait multi-method matrix. *Psychological Bulletin,* **56**, 85–105.

Carlin, B.P. and Hodges, J.S. (1999) Hierarchical proportional hazards regression models for highly stratified data. *Biometrics,* **55**, 1162–1170.

Carey, V.C., Zeger, S.L., and Diggle, P.J. (1993) Modelling multivariate binary data with alternating logistic regressions. *Biometrika,* **80**, 517–526.

Carroll, R.J., Ruppert, D., and Stefanski, L.A. (1995) *Measurement Error in Nonlinear Models.* London: Chapman and Hall.

Centers for Disease Control (1987) Revision of the CDC surveillance case definition for acquired immunodeficiency syndrome. *MMWR*, **36** (suppl 1), 1S–15S.

Chakravarty, A. (2001) Surrogate markers: their role in the regulatory decision process. In: *Proceedings of Eighth Annual Biopharmaceutical Applied Statistics Symposium.*

Chakravarty, A. and Soon, G. (2001) *FDA* Fast Track Approval Program - A regulatory overview. In: *Proceedings of Joint Conference of the American Statistical Association.*

Chen, T.T., Simon, R.M., Korn, E.L., Anderson, S.J., Lindblad, A.D., Wieand, H.S., Douglass Jr., H.O., Fisher, B., Hamilton, J.M., and Friedman, M.A. (1998) Investigation of disease-free survival as a surrogate endpoint for survival in cancer clinical trials. *Communications in Statistics - Theory and Methods,* **27**, 1363–1378.

Chen, C., Wang, H., and Snapinn, S.M. (2003) Proportion of treatment effect (PTE) explained by a surrogate marker. *Statistics in Medicine,* **22**, 3449–3459.

Choi, S., Lagakos, S., Schooley, R.T., and Volberding, P.A. (1993) CD4+ lymphocytes are an incomplete surrogate marker for clinical progression in persons with asymptomatic HIV infection taking zidovudine. *Annals of Internal Medicine,* **118**, 674–680.

Chounard, G., Jones, B., and Remington, G. (1993) A Canadian multicenter placebo-controlled study of fixed doses of risperidone and haloperidol in the treatment of chronic schizophrenic patients. *Journal of Clinical Psychopharmacology,* **13**, 25-40.

Chuang-Stein, C. and DeMasi, R. (1998) Surrogate endpoints in AIDS drug development: current status (with discussion). *Drug Information Journal,* **32**, 439–448.

Clayton, D.G. (1978) A model for association in bivariate life tables and its application in epidemiological studies of familial tendency in chronic disease incidence. *Biometrika,* **65**, 141–151.

Cleveland, W.S. (1979) Robust locally-weighted regression and smoothing scatterplots. *Journal of the American Statistical Association,* **74**, 829–836.

Collins, R., Peto, R., MacMohan, S., *et al.* (1990) Blood pressure, stroke, and coronary heart disease, II. *Lancet,* **335**, 827–838.

Corfu-A Study Group (1995) Phase III randomized study of two fluorouracil combinations with either interferon alfa-2a or leucovorin for advanced colorectal cancer. *Journal of Clinical Oncology,* **13**, 921–928.

Cortiñas Abrahantes, J. (2004) *Estimation Procedures for Mixed-Effects Models With Applications to Normally Distributed and Survival Data.* Unpublished Ph.D. dissertation, Limburgs Universitair Centrum.

Cortiñas Abrahantes, J. and Burzykowski, T. (2004) A version of the EM algorithm for proportional hazards model with random effects. *Biometrical Journal (accepted).*

Cortiñas Abrahantes, J., Molenberghs, G., Burzykowski, T., Shkedy, Z., Alonso Abad, A., and Renard, D. (2004) Choice of units of analysis and modeling strategies in multilevel hierarchical models. *Computational Statistics and Data Analysis,* **47**, 537–563.

Counts, J.L. and Goodman, J.I. (1995) Alterations in DNA methylation may play a variety of roles in carcinogenesis. *Cell,* **83**, 13–15.

Coursaget, P., Leboulleux, D., Soumare, M., le Cann P., Yvonnet, B., Chiron, J.P., and Collseck, A.M. (1994) Twelve-year follow-up study of hepatitis immunization of Senegalese infants. *Journal of Hepatology,* **21**, 250–254.

Cox, D.R. (1972a) Regression models and life-tables. *Journal of the Royal Statistical Society, Series B,* **34**, 187–202.

Cox, D.R. (1972b) The analysis of multivariate binary data. *Applied Statistics,* **21**, 113–120.

Cox, D.R. and Snell, E.J. (1989) *Analysis of Binary Data,* 2nd edition. London: Chapman and Hall.

Cressie, N.A.C. (1991) *Statistics for Spatial Data.* New York: John Wiley & Sons.

Cronbach, L.J. (1951) Coefficient alpha and the internal structure of tests. *Psychometrika,* **51**, 297–334.

Crouch, E.A.C. and Spiegelman, D. (1990) The evaluation of integrals of the form $\int_{-\infty}^{+\infty} f(t)\exp(-t^2)dt$: application to logistic-normal models. *Journal of the American Statistical Association,* **85**, 464–469.

Dabrowska, D.M. (1988) Kaplan-Meier estimate on the plane. *Annals of Statistics,* **16**, 1475–1489.

Dale, J.R. (1986) Global cross ratio models for bivariate, discrete, ordered responses. *Biometrics,* **42**, 909–917.

Daniels, M.J. and Hughes, M.D. (1997) Meta-analysis for the evaluation of potential surrogate markers. *Statistics in Medicine,* **16**, 1515–1527.

Da Villa, G., Peluso, F., Picciotto, L., Bencivenga, M., Elia, S., and Pelliccia, M.G. (1996) Persistence of anti-HBs in children vaccinated against viral hepatitis B in the first year of life: follow-up at 5 and 10 years. *Vaccine,* **14**, 1503–1505.

Dawsey, S.M., Fleischer, D.E., Wang, G.Q., Zhou, B., Kidwell, J.A., Lu, N., Lewin, K.J., Roth, M.J., Tio, T.L., and Taylor, P.R. (1998) Mucosal iodine staining improves endoscopic visualization of squamous dysplasia and squamous cell carcinoma of the esophagus. *Linxian, China Cancer,* **83**, 220–231.

Day, N.E. and Duffy, S.W. (1996) Trial design based on surrogate endpoints - application to comparison of different breast screening frequencies. *Journal of the Royal Statistical Society, Series A,* **159**, 49–60.

Debruyne, F.J.M., Murray, R., Fradet, Y., Johansson, J.E., Tyrrell, C., Boccardo, F., *et al.* (1998) Liarozole - a novel treatment approach for advanced prostate cancer: results of a large randomized trial versus cyproterone acetate. *Urology,* **52**, 72–81.

DeGruttola, V. and Tu, X.M. (1994) Modelling progression of CD-4 lymphocyte count and its relationship to survival time. *Biometrics,* **50**, 1003–1014.

DeGruttola, V., Wulfsohn, M., Fischl, M.A., and Tsiatis, A. (1993) Modelling the relationship between survival and CD4 lymphocytes in patients with AIDS and AIDS-related complex. *Journal of Acquired Immune Deficiency Syndromes,* **6**, 359–365.

DeGruttola, V., Fleming, T.R., Lin, D.Y., and Coombs, R. (1997) Validating surrogate markers - are we being naive ? *Journal of Infectious Diseases,* **175**, 237–246.

DeGruttola, V., Clax, P., DeMets, D.L., Downing, G.J., Ellenberg, S.S., Friedman, L., Gail, M.H., Prentice, R., Wittes, J., and Zeger, S.L. (2001) Considerations in the evaluation of surrogate endpoints in clinical trials: summary of a National Institutes of Health Workshop. *Controlled Clinical Trials,* **22**, 485–502.

De Ponti, F., Lecchini, S., Cosentino, M., Castelletti, C.M., Malesci, A., and Frigo, G.M. (1993) Immunological adverse effects of anticonvulsants. What is their clinical relevance? *Drug Safety,* **8**, 235–250.

Deyo, R.A., Dierh P., and Patrick, D. (1991) Reproducibility and responsiveness of health status measure statistics and strategies for evaluation. *Controlled Clinical Trials*, **12**, 142–158.

DHHS Panel on Clinical Practices for Treatment of HIV Infection (2004) Guidelines for the use of antiretroviral agents in HIV-infected adults and adolescents. March 2004. Available at `http://www.hivatis.org`.

Diggle, P.J. (1988) An approach to the analysis of repeated measures. *Biometrics,* **44**, 959–971.

Diggle, P.J. (1990) *Time Series: A Biostatistical Introduction.* Oxford: Oxford University Press.

Diggle, P.J., Liang, K.-Y., and Zeger, S.L. (1994) *Analysis of Longitudinal Data.* Oxford: Clarendon Press.

Ding, C.G. (1996) On the computation of the distribution of the square of the sample multiple correlation coefficient. *Computational Statistics and Data Analysis,* **22**, 345–350.

Dorgan, J.F., Longcope, C., Stephenson, H.E., Falk, R.T., Miller, R., Franz, C., Kanle, L., Campbell, W.S., Tangrea, J.A., and Schatzkin, A. (1996) Relations of prediagnostic serum estrogen and androgen levels to breast cancer risk. *Cancer Epidemiology, Biomarkers, and Prevention* **5**, 533–539.

DuMouchel W. (1994) Hierarchical Bayes linear models for meta-analysis. *National Institute of Statistical Sciences Technical Report*, **27**. National Institute of Statistical Sciences: Research Triangle Park, NC.

Dunn, N. and Mann, R.D. (1999) Prescription-event and other forms of epidemiological monitoring of side-effects in the UK. *Clinical and Experimental Allergy,* **29**, 217–239.

Echt, D.S., Liebson, P.R., Mitchell, L.B., *et al.*, and the CAST investigators (1994). Mortality and morbidity in patients receiving encainide, flecainide, or placebo: the Cardiac Arrhythmia Suppression Trial. *New England Journal of Medicine,* **330**, 1852–1857.

Ellenberg, S.S. and Hamilton, J.M. (1989) Surrogate endpoints in clinical trials: cancer. *Statistics in Medicine,* **8**, 405–413.

Endogenous Hormones and Breast Cancer Collaboratie Group (2003) Body mass index, serum sex hormones, and breast cancer risk in postmenopausal women. *Journal of the National Cancer Institute*, **95**, 1218-1226.

Fahrmeir, L. and Tutz, G. (1995) *Multivariate Statistical Modelling Based on Generalized Linear Models.* New York: Springer-Verlag.

Fan, J.J., Hsu, L., and Prentice, R.L. (2000) Dependence estimation over a finite bivariate failure time region. *Lifetime Data Analysis,* **6**, 343–355.

Fearon, E.R. (1992) Genetic alterations underlying colorectal tumorigenesis. *Cancer Surveys*, **12**, 119–136.

Fearon, E.R. and Vogelstein, B. (1990) A genetic model for colorectal tumorigenesis. *Cell*, **61**, 759–767.

Ferentz, A.E. (2002) Integrating pharmacogenomics into drug development. *Pharmacogenomics,* **3**, 453–67.

Fieller, E.C. (1954) Symposium on interval estimation: Some problems in interval estimation. *Journal of the Royal Statistical Society, Series B,* **16**, 175–185.

Finkelstein, D.M. and Schoenfeld, D.A. (1999) Combining mortality and longitudinal measures in clinical trials. *Statistics in Medicine,* **18**, 1341–1354.

Fisher, R.A. (1924) The influence of rainfall in the yield of wheat at Rothamstead. *Philosphical Transactions of the Royal Statistical Society of London, Series B,* **213**, 89–142.

Fisher, R.A. (1928) The general sampling distribution of the multiple correlation coefficient. *Proceedings of the Royal Society,* **121**, 654–673.

Fitzmaurice, G.M. and Laird, N.M. (1993) A likelihood-based method for analysing longitudinal binary responses. *Biometrika,* **80**, 141–151.

Flandre, P. and O'Quigley, J. (1995) A two-stage procedure for survival studies with surrogate endpoints. *Biometrics,* **51**, 969–976.

Flandre, P. and Saidi, Y. (1999) Letters to the Editor: estimating the proportion of treatment effect explained by a surrogate marker. *Statistics in Medicine,* **18**, 107–115.

Fleiss, J.L. (1986) *The Design and Analysis of Clinical Experiments.* New York: John Wiley & Sons.

Fleiss, J.L. (1993) The statistical basis of meta-analysis. *Statistical Methods in Medical Research,* **2**, 121–145.

Fleiss, J. and Cohen, J. (1973) The equivalence of weighted kappa and the intraclass correlation coefficient as measures of reliability. *Educational and Psychological Measurement*, **33**, 6113–6119.

Fleming, T.R. (1994) Surrogate markers in AIDS and cancer trials. *Statistics in Medicine,* **13**, 1423–1435.

Fleming, T.R. (1996) Surrogate endpoints in clinical trials. *Drug Information Journal,* **30**, 545–551.

Fleming, T.R. and DeMets, D.L. (1996) Surrogate endpoints in clinical trials: are we being misled ? *Annals of Internal Medicine,* **125**, 605–613.

Fleming, T.R., Prentice, R.L., Pepe, M.S., and Glidden, D. (1994) Surrogate and auxiliary endpoints in clinical trials, with potential applications in cancer and AIDS research. *Statistics in Medicine,* **13**, 955–968.

Food and Drug Administration (1996) Reinventing the regulation of cancer drugs. Accelerating approval and expanding access. *National Performance Review, 199640488З/41014.* Washington, D.C.: U.S. Government Printing Office.

Food and Drug Administration (2002) Guidance for Industry. Antiretroviral Drugs Using Plasma HIV RNA measurements—Clinical Considerations for Accelerated and Traditional Approval. U.S. Department of Health and Human Services, Food and Drug Administration. Rockville, MD.

Franco, E.L. (1991) The sexually transmitted disease model for cervical cancer: incoherent epidemiologic findings and the role of misclassification of human papillomavirus infection. *Epidemiology,* **2**, 98–106.

Fréchet, M. (1951) Sur les tableaux de corrélation dont les marges sonnt données. *Annals Université Lyon, Section A, Series 3,* **14**, 53–77.

Freedman, L.S. (2001) Confidence intervals and statistical power of the 'Validation' ratio for surrogate or intermediate endpoints. *Journal of Statistical Planning and Inference,* **96**, 143–153.

Freedman, L.S., Graubard, B.I., and Schatzkin, A. (1992) Statistical validation of intermediate endpoints for chronic diseases. *Statistics in Medicine,* **11**, 167–178.

Freis, E.D. (1990) Reminiscences of the Veterans Administration trial of the treatment of hypertension. *Hypertension,* **16**, 472–475.

Fuller, W.A. (1987) *Measurement Error Models.* New York: John Wiley & Sons.

Gail, M.H., Pfeiffer, R., van Houwelingen, H.C., and Carroll, R.J. (2000) On meta-analytic assessment of surrogate outcomes. *Biostatistics,* **1**, 231–246.

Gart, J.J. (1966) Alternative analyses of contingency tables. *Journal of the Royal Statistical Society, Series B,* **28**, 164–179.

Genest, C. and McKay, J. (1986) The joy of copulas: bivariate distributions with uniform marginals. *American Statistician,* **40**, 280–283.

Genest, C. and Rivest, L.-P. (1993) Statistical inference procedures for bivariate Archimedean copulas. *Journal of the American Statistical Association,* **88**, 1034–1043.

Geys, H. (1999) *Pseudo-likelihood Methods and Generalized Estimating Equations: Efficient Estimation Techniques for the Analysis of Correlated Multivariate Data.* Unpublished Ph.D. dissertation, Limburgs Universitair Centrum.

Geys, H., Molenberghs, G., and Ryan, L. (1997) Pseudo-likelihood inference for clustered binary data. *Communications in Statistics - Theory and Methods,* **26**, 2743–2767.

Geys, H., Molenberghs, G., and Lipsitz, S.R (1998) A note on the comparison of pseudo-likelihood and generalized estimating equations for marginally specified odds ratio models with exchangeable association structure. *Journal of Statistical Computing and Simulation,* **62**, 45–71.

Gilbert, P.B., DeGruttola, V., Hammer, S.M., and Kuritzkes, D.R. (2001) Virologic and regimen termination surrogate endpoints in AIDS clinical trials. *Journal of the American Medical Association,* **285**, 777–783.

Gilks, W.R, Richardson, S., and Spiegelhalter, D.J. (1996) *Markov Chain Monte Carlo in Practice.* London: Chapman and Hall.

Gilks, W.R., Wang, C.C., Yvonnet, B., and Coursaget, P. (1993) Random-effects models for longitudinal data using Gibbs sampling. *Biometrics,* **49**, 441–453.

Gilmour, A.R., Anderson, R.D., and Rae, A.L. (1985) The analysis of binomial data by a generalized linear mixed model. *Biometrika,* **72**, 593–599.

Gelman, A., Carlin, J.B., Stern, H.S., and Rubin, D.B. (1999) *Bayesian Data Analysis.* London: Chapman and Hall.

Glidden, D.V. (1999) Checking the adequacy of the gamma frailty model for multivariate failure times. *Biometrika,* **86**, 381–393.

Glonek, G.F.V. and McCullagh, P. (1995) Multivariate logistic models. *Journal of the Royal Statistical Society, Series B,* **81**, 477–482.

Godambe, V.P. (1991) *Estimating Functions.* Oxford: Oxford University Press.

Goldstein, H. (1986) Multilevel mixed linear model analysis using iterative generalized least squares. *Biometrika,* **73**, 43–56.

Goldstein, H. (1991) Nonlinear multilevel models, with an application to discrete response data. *Biometrika,* **78**, 45–51.

Goldstein, H. (1995) *Multilevel Statistical Models*, 2nd edition. London: Edward Arnold.

Goldstein, H. and Rasbash, J. (1996) Improved approximations for multilevel models with binary responses. *Journal of the Royal Statistical Society, Series A,* **159**, 505–513.

Goldstein, H., Rasbash, J., Plewis, I., Draper, D., Browne, W., Yang, M., Woodhouse, G., and Healy, M. (1998) *A User's Guide to MLwiN*. London: Multilevel Level Models Project, Institute of Education, University of London.

Goldstein, H., Browne, W., and Rasbash, J. (2002) Partitioning variation in generalised linear multilevel models. *Understanding Statistics,* **1**, 223–231.

Gordon, A.N., Teitelbaum, A., and the 30–49 Study Group (2003) Overall survival advantage for pegylated liposomal doxirubicin compared to topotecan in recurrent epithelial ovarian cancer. Poster at the *12th Meeting of the Federation of European Cancer Societies (ECCO12), Copenhagen, Denmark,* September 2003.

Graubard, B.I. and Korn, E.L. (1996) Modelling the sampling design in the analysis of health surveys. *Statistical Methods in Medical Research,* **5**, 263–281.

Gray, R.J. (1992) Flexible methods for analyzing survival data using splines, with applications to breast cancer prognosis. *Journal of the American Statistical Association,* **87**, 942–951.

Gray, R.J. (1994) A Bayesian analysis of institutional effects in a multicenter cancer clinical trial. *Biometrics,* **50**, 244–253.

Greco, F.A., Figlin, R., York, M., Einhorn, L., Schilsky, R., Marshall, E.M., Buys, S.S., Froimtchuk, M.J., Schuller, J., Buyse, M., Ritter, L., Man, A., and Yap, A.K.L. (1996) Phase III randomized study to compare interferon alfa-2a in combination with fluorouracil versus fluorouracil alone in patients with advanced colorectal cancer. *Journal of Clinical Oncology,* **14**, 2674–2681.

Groopman, J.D., Wogan, G.N., Roebuck, B.D., and Kensler, T.W. (1994) Molecular biomarkers for aflatoxins and their application to human cancer prevention. *Cancer Research,* **54** (suppl), 1907s–1911s.

Guidance for Industry (1998) Fast track drug development programs – designation, development, and application review. *Federal Register,* **63**, No. 222, 64093–64094.

Gumbel, E.J. (1960) Bivariate exponential distributions. *Journal of the American Statistical Association,* **55**, 698–707.

Hadler, S.C., Francis, D.P., Maynard, J.E., Thompson, S.E., Judson, F.N., Echenberg, D.F., *et al.* (1986) Long-term immunogenicity and efficacy of hepatitis B vaccine in homosexual men. *New England Journal of Medicine,* **315**, 209–214.

Hamburger, S. (2003) NDA 50-718/S-006 Doxil (doxorubicin hydrochloride liposome) Indication: treatment of metastatic ovarian cancer in patients with disease that is refractory to both paclitaxel and platinum-based chemotherapy regimens. Presentation at the *FDA Oncology Advisory Committee,* March 2003.

Hankinson, S.E., Manson, J.E., Spiegelman, D., Willett, W.C., Longcope, C., and Speizer, F.E. (1995) Reproducibility of plasma hormone levels in postmenopausal women over a 2-3-year period. *Cancer Epidemiology, Biomarkers, and Prevention,* **4**, 649–654.

Hankinson, S.E., Willett, W.C., Manson, J.E., Colditz, G.A., Hunter, D.J., Spiegelman, D., Barbieri, R.L., and Speizer, F.E. (1998) Plasma sex steroid hormone levels and risk of breast cancer in postmenopausal women. *Journal of the National Cancer Institute,* **90**, 1292–1299.

Hastie, T.J. and Tibshirani, R.J. (1990) *Generalized Additive Models.* London: Chapman and Hall.

Heagerty, P.J. (1999) Marginally specified logistic-normal models for longitudinal binary data. *Biometrics,* **55**, 688–698.

Heagerty, P.J. and Lele, S.R. (1998) A composite likelihood approach to binary spatial data. *Journal of the American Statistical Association,* **93**, 1099–1111.

Heagerty, P.J. and Zeger, S.L. (2000) Marginalized multilevel models and likelihood inference. *Statistical Science,* **15**, 1–26.

Hedeker, D. and Gibbons, R.D. (1994) A random-effects ordinal regression model for multilevel analysis. *Biometrics,* **50**, 933–944.

Hedeker, D. and Gibbons, R.D. (1996) MIXOR: a computer program for mixed-effects ordinal regression analysis. *Computer Methods and Programs in Biomedicine,* **49**, 157–176.

Heise, C., Sampson-Johannes, A., Williams, A., McCormick, F., Von Hoff, D.D., and Kirn, D.H. (1997) ONYX-015, an E1B gene-attenuated adenovirus, causes tumor-specific cytolysis and antitumoral efficacy that can be augmented by standard chemo-therapeutic agents. *Nature Medicine,* **3**, 639–645.

Henderson, R., Diggle, P., and Dobson, A. (2000) Joint modelling of longitudinal measurements and event time data. *Biostatistics,* **1**, 465–480.

Henderson, R., Diggle, P., and Dobson, A. (2002) Identification and efficacy of longituginal markes for survival. *Biostatistics,* **3**, 33–50.

Herson, J. (1975). Fieller's theorem vs. the delta method for significance intervals for ratios. *Journal of Statistical Computing and Simulation,* **3**, 265–274.

HIV Surrogate Marker Collaborative Group (2000) Human immunodeficiency virus type 1 RNA level and CD4 count prognostic markers and surrogate endpoints: a meta-analysis. *AIDS,* **16**, 1123–1133.

Hill A.M., DeMasi R., and Dawson, D. (1998) Meta-analysis of antiretroviral effects on HIV-1 RNA, CD4 cell count and progression to AIDS or death. *Antiviral Therapy,* **3**, 139–145.

HIV Surrogate Marker Collaborative Group (2000) Human immunodeficiency virus type I RNA level and CD4 count as prognostic markers and surrogate endpoints: a meta-analysis. *AIDS Research and Human Retroviruses* **16**, 1123–1133.

Hjort, N.L. (1993) A quasi-likelihood method for estimating parameters in spatial covariance functions. Technical Report SAND/93, Norwegian Computing Centre, Oslo.

Hogan, J.W. and Laird, N.M. (1997a) Mixture models for the joint distribution of repeated measures and event times. *Statistics in Medicine,* **16**, 239–258.

Hogan, J.W. and Laird, N.M. (1997b) Model-based approaches to analyzing incomplete longitudinal and failure time data. *Statistics in Medicine,* **16**, 259–239.

Holt, P.R., Atillasoy, E.O., Gilman, J., Guss, J., Moss, S.F., Newmark, H., Fan, K. Yang, K., and Lipkin, M. (1998) Modulation of abnormal epithelial cell proliferation and differentiation by low-fat dairy foods: a randomized controlled trial. *Journal of the American Medical Association,* **280**, 1074–1079.

Hougaard, P. (1986) Survival models for heterogeneous populations derived from stable distributions. *Biometrika,* **73**, 387–396.

Hougaard, P. (1987) Modelling multivariate survival. *Scandinavian Journal of Statistics,* **14**, 291–304.

Hougaard, P. (1995) Frailty models for survival data. *Lifetime Data Analysis,* **1**, 255–274.

Hougaard, P. (2000) *Ananlysis of Multivariate Survival Data.* New York: Springer-Verlag.

Hoyberg, O.J., Fensbo, C., Remvig, J., Lingjaerde, O., Sloth-Nielsen, M., and Salvesen, I. (1993) Risperidone versus perphenazine in the treatment of chronic schizophrenic patients with acute exacerbations. *Acta Psychiatrica Scandinavica,* **88**, 395-402.

Hughes, M.D., DeGruttola, V., and Welles, S. (1995) Evaluating surrogate markers. *AIDS and Human Retrovirology Supplement,* **2**, S1–S8.

Hughes, M.D., Johnson, V.A., Hirsch, M.S., Bremer, J.W., Elbeik, T., Erice, A., Kuritzkes, D.R., Scott, W.A., Spector, S.A., Basgoz, N., Fischl, M.A., and D'Aquila, R.T., for the ACTG 241 Protocol Virology Substudy Team. (1997) Monitoring plasma HIV-1 RNA levels in addition to CD4+ lymphocyte count improves assessment of antiretroviral therapeutic response. *Annals of Internal Medicine,* **126**, 929–938.

Hughes, M.D., Daniels, M.J., Fischl, M.A., Kim, S., and Schooley, R.T. (1998) CD4 count as a surrogate endpoint in HIV clinical trials: a meta-analysis of studies of the AIDS Clinical Trials Group. *AIDS,* **12**, 1823–1832.

Hutchison, D. and Healy, M. (2001) The effect of variance component estimates of ignoring a level in a multilevel model. *Multilevel Modelling Newsletter,* **13**, 4–5.

Huttunen, M.O., Piepponen, T., Rantanen, H., Larmo, I., Nyholm, R., and Raitasuo, V. (1995). Risperidone versus zuclopenthixol in the treatment of acute schizophrenic episodes: a double-blind parallel-group trial. *Acta Psychiatrica Scandinavica,* **91**, 271–277.

International Conference on Harmonisation of Technical Requirements for Registration of Pharmaceuticals for Human Use (1998) ICH Harmonised Tripartite Guideline. Statistical principles for clinical trials. *Federal Register,* **63**, No. 179, 49583.

International Human Genome Sequencing Consortium (2001) Initial sequencing and analysis of the human genome. *Nature,* **409**, 860–921.

Joe, H. (1997) *Multivariate Models and Dependence Concepts.* London: Chapman and Hall.

Johnson, R.A. and Wichern, D.W. (1992) *Applied Multivariate Statistical Analysis,* 3rd edition. Englewood Cliffs, NJ: Prentice-Hall.

Jones, T.C. (2001) Call for a new approach to the process of clinical trials and drug registration. *British Medical Journal,* **322**, 920–923.

Jukema, J.W., Bruschke, A.V.G., van Boven, A.J., Reiber, J.H.C., Bal, E.T., Zwinderman, A.H., Jansen, H. Boerma, G.J.M., van Rappard, F.M., and Lie, K.I. (1995) Effects of lipid lowering by pravastin on progression and regression of coronary artery disease in symptomatic men with normal to moderately elevated serum cholesterol levels. The Regression Growth Evaluation Statin Study (REGRESS). *Circulation,* **91**, 2528–2540.

Kaplan, E.L. and Meier, P. (1958) Nonparametric estimation from incomplete observations. *Journal of the American Statistical Association,* **53**, 457–481.

Karlan, B.Y. (1995) Screening for ovarian cancer: what are the optimal surrogate endpoints for clinical trials? *Journal of Cell Biochemistry,* **23** (suppl), 227–232.

Kay, S.R., Fiszbein, A., and Opler, L.A. (1987) The positive and negative syndrome scale (PANSS) for schizophrenia. *Schizophrenia Bulletin,* **13**, 261–276.

Kay, S.R., Opler, L.A., and Lindenmayer, J.P. (1988) Reliability and validity of the Positive and Negative Syndrome Scale for schizophrenics. *Psychiatric Research,* **23**, 99-110.

Kelly, W.K., Scher, H.I., Mazumdar, M., Vlamis, V., Schwartz, M., and Fossa, S.D. (1993) Prostate-specific antigen as a measure of disease outcome in metastatic hormone-refractory prostate cancer. *Journal of Clinical Oncology,* **11**, 607–615.

Khuri, F.R., Nemunaitis, J., Ganly, I., Arsenau, J., Tannock, I.F., Romel, L., Gore, M., Ironside, J., MacDougall, R.H., Heise, C., Randlev, B., Gillenwater, A.M., Bruso, P., Kaye, S.B., Hong, W.K., and Kirn, D.H. (2000) A controlled trial of intratumoral ONYX-015, a selectively-replicating adenovirus, in combination with cisplatin and 5-fluorouracil in patients with recurrent head and neck cancer. *Nature Medicine,* **6**, 879–885.

Kreft, I. and de Leeuw, J. (1998) *Introducing Multilevel Modeling.* London: Sage Publications.

Kuder, G.F. and Richardson, M.W. (1953) The theory of estimation of test reliability. *Psychometrika,* **2**, 151–160.

Kuk, A.Y.C. (1995) Asymptotically unbiased estimation in generalised linear models with random effects. *Journal of the Royal Statistical Society, Series B,* **57**, 395–407.

Kuk, A.Y.C. and Nott D.J. (2000) A pairwise likelihood approach to analyzing correlated binary data. *Statistics and Probability Letters,* **47**, 329–335.

Kulldorff, M., McShane, L.M., Schatzkin, A., Freedman, L.S., Wargovich, M.J., Woods, C., Purewal, M., Burt, R.W., Lawson, M., Mateski, D.J., Lanza, E., Corle, D.K., O'Brien, B., and Moler, J. (2000) Measuring cell proliferation in the rectal mucosa. comparing bromodeoxyuridine (BrdU) and proliferating cell nuclear antigen (PCNA) assays. *Journal of Clinical Epidemiology,* **53**, 875–883.

Laenen, A., Geys, H., Vangeneugden, T., and Molenberghs, G. (2004) Applying linear mixed models to estimate reliability in clinical trial data with repeated measurements. *Controlled Clinical Trials,* **25**, 13–30.

Lagakos, S.W. and Hoth, D.F. (1992) Surrogate markers in AIDS: Where are we? Where are we going? *Annals of Internal Medicine,* **116**, 599–601.

Laird, N.M. and Ware, J.H. (1982) Random effects models for longitudinal data. *Biometrics,* **38**, 963–974.

Lamont, J.P., Nemunaitis, J., Kuhn, J.A., Landers, S.A., and McCarty, T.M. (2000) A prospective phase II trial of ONYX-015 adenovirus and chemotherapy in recurrent squamous cell carcinoma of the head and neck (the Baylor experience). *Annals of Surgical Oncology,* **7**, 588–592.

Lang, J.B. and Agresti, A. (1994) Simultaneously modeling joint and marginal distributions of multivariate categorical responses. *Journal of the American Statistical Association,* **89**, 625–632.

Lange, K. (1998) *Numerical Analysis for Statisticians.* New York: Springer-Verlag.

Lavalley, M.P. and DeGruttola, V. (1996) Models for empirical Bayes estimators of longitudinal CD4 counts. *Statistics in Medicine,* **15**, 2289–2305.

Le Cessie, S. and Van Houwelingen, J.C. (1994) Logistic regression for correlated binary data. *Applied Statistics,* **43**, 95–108.

Lee, Y. and Nelder, J.A. (1996) Hierarchical generalized linear models (with discussion). *Journal of the Royal Statistical Society, Series B,* **58**, 619–678.

Lehmann, E.L. (1983) *Theory of Point Estimation.* New York: John Wiley & Sons.

Lesaffre, E. and Spiessens, B. (2001) On the effect of the number of quadrature points in a logistic random-effects model: an example. *Applied Statistics,* **50**, 325–335.

Lesko, L.J. and Atkinson, A.J. (2001) Use of biomarkers and surrogate endpoints in drug development and regulatory decision making: criteria, validation, strategies. *Annual Review of Pharmacology and Toxicology,* **41**, 347–366.

Li, Z., Meredith, M.P., and Hoseyni, M.S. (2001) A method to assess the proportion of treatment effect explained by a surrogate endpoint. *Statistics in Medicine,* **20**, 3175–3188.

Liang, K.-Y. and Zeger, S.L. (1986) Longitudinal data analysis using generalized linear models. *Biometrika,* **73**, 13–22.

Liang, K.-Y., Zeger, S.L., and Qaqish, B. (1992) Multivariate regression analyses for categorical data. *Journal of the Royal Statistical Society, Series B,* **54**, 3–40.

Liao, T.F. (2002) Bayesian model comparison in generalized linear models across multiple groups. *Computational Statistics and Data Analysis,* **39**, 311–327.

Lieberman, G.J and Miller, R.G. (1963) Simultaneous tolerance intervals in regression. *Biometrika,* **50**, 155–168.

Limam, M.M. and Thomas, D.R. (1988) Simultaneous tolerance intervals for the linear regression model. *Journal of the American Statistical Association,* **50**, 801–804.

Lin, D.Y. (1994) Cox regression analysis of multivariate failure time data: the marginal approach. *Statistics in Medicine,* **13**, 2233–2247.

Lin, X. and Breslow, N.E. (1996) Bias correction in generalized linear mixed models with multiple components of dispersion. *Journal of the American Statistical Association,* **91**, 1007–1016.

Lin, D.Y. and Ying, Z. (1993) A simple nonparametric estimator of the bivariate survival function under univariate censoring. *Biometrika,* **80**, 573–581.

Lin, D.Y., Fischl, M.A., and Schoenfeld, D.A. (1993) Evaluating the role of CD4-Lymphochyte counts as surrogate endpoints in human immunodeficiency virus clinical trials. *Statistics in Medicine,* **12**, 835–842.

Lin, D.Y., Fleming, T. R., and DeGruttola, V. (1997) Estimating the proportion of treatment effect explained by a surrogate marker. *Statistics in Medicine,* **16**, 1515–1527.

Lindeboom, M. and Van Den Berg, G.J. (1994) Heterogeneity in models for bivariate survival: the importance of the mixing distribution. *Journal of the Royal Statistical Society, Series B,* **56**, 49–60.

Lindsay, B.G. (1988) Composite likelihood methods. *Contemporary Mathematics,* **80**, 221–239.

Lipid Research Clinics Program (1984) The Lipid Clinics coronary primary prevention trial results. I. Reduction in incidence of coronary heart disease. *Journal of the American Medical Association,* **251**, 351-364.

Lipkin, M., Blattner, W.A., and Gardner, E.J., Burt, R.W., Lynch, H., Deschner, E., Winawer, S., and Fraumeni, J.F. (1984) Classification and risk assessment of individuals with familial polyposis, Gardner's syndrome, and familial non-polyposis colon cancer from [3H]thymidine labeling patterns in colonic epithelial cells. *Cancer Research,* **44**, 4201–4207.

Lipsitz, S.R., Laird, N.M., and Harrington, D.P. (1991) Generalized estimating equations for correlated binary data: using the odds ratio as a measure of association. *Biometrika,* **78**, 153–160.

Longford, N.T. (1993) *Random Coefficient Models.* London: Oxford University Press.

Longford, N.T. (1994) Logistic regression with random coefficients. *Computational Statistics and Data Analysis,* **4**, 12–35.

Littell, R.C., Milliken, G.A., Stroup, W.W., and Wolfinger, R.D. (1996) *SAS System for Mixed Models.* Cary, NC: SAS Institute Inc.

Lucke, J.F. and Embretson (Whitely), S.R. (1984) The biases and mean squaed errors of estimators of multinormal squared multiple correlation. *Journal of Educational Statistics,* **9**, 183–192.

Lyles, C.M., Sandler, R.S., Keku, T.O., Kupper, L.L., Millikan, C., Murray, S.C., Bangdiwala, S.I., and Ulshen, M.H. (1994) Reproducibility and variability of the rectal mucosal proliferation index using proliferating cell nuclear antigen immunohistochemistry. *Cancer Epidemiology, Biomarkers, and Prevention,* **3**, 597–605.

Mardia, K.V. (1970) *Families of Bivariate Distributions.* London: Griffin.

Marder, S.R. and Meibach, R.C. (1994) Risperidone in the treatment of schizophrenia. *American Journal of Psychiatry,* **151**, 825-35.

Marschner, I.C., Collier, A.C., Coombs, R.W., D'Aquila, R.T., DeGruttola, V., Fischl, M.A., Hammer, S.M., Hughes, M.D., Johnson, V.A., Katzenstein, D.A., Richman, D.D., Smeaton, L.M., Spector, S., and

Saag, M.S. (1998) Use of changes in plasma levels of human immunodeficiency virus type 1 RNA to assess the clinical benefits of antiretroviral therapy. *Journal of Infectious Diseases*, **177**, 40–47.

McCullagh, P. and Nelder, J.A. (1989) *Generalized Linear Models.* London: Chapman and Hall.

McCulloch, C.E. (1994) Maximum likelihood variance components estimation for binary data. *Journal of the American Statistical Association,* **89**, 330–335.

McCulloch, C.E. (1997) Maximum likelihood algorithms for generalized linear mixed models. *Journal of the American Statistical Association,* **92**, 162–170.

McCulloch, C.E. and Searle, R.E. (2000) *Generalized, Linear, and Mixed Models.* New York: John Wiley & Sons.

McGilchrist, C.A. (1993) REML estimation for survival model with frailty. *Biometrics,* **49**, 221–225.

McGilchrist, C.A. (1994) Estimation in generalized linear models. *Journal of the Royal Statistical Society, Series B,* **56**, 61–69.

McGilchrist, C.A. and Aisbett, C.W. (1991) Regression with frailty in survival analysis. *Biometrics,* **47**, 461–466.

McIntosh, M.W. (1996) The population risk as an explanatory variable in resarch synthesis of clinical trials. *Statistics in Medicine,* **15**, 1713–1728.

McShane, L.M., Kulldorff, M., Wargovich, M.J., Woods, C., Purewal, M., Freedman, L.S., Corle, D.K., Burt, R.W., Mateski, D.J., Lawson, M., Lanza, E., O'Brien, B., Lake, W., Jr., Moler, J., and Schatzkin, A. (1998) An evaluation of rectal mucosal proliferation measure variability sources in the polyp prevention trial: can we detect informative differences among individuals' proliferation measures amid the noise? *Cancer Epidemiology, Biomarkers, and Prevention*, **7**, 605–612.

Mellors, J.W., Rinaldo, C.R., Gupta, P., White, R.M., Todd, J.A., and Kingsley L.A. (1996) Prognosis of HIV-1 infection predicted by the quantity of virus in plasma. *Science*, **272**, 1167–1170.

Mellors, J.W., Munoz, A., Giorgi, J.V., Margolick, J.B., Tassoni, C.J., Gupta, P., Kingsley, L.A., Todd, J.A., Saah, A.J., Detels, R., Phair, J.P., and Rinaldo, C.R. (1997) Plasma viral load and CD4+ lymphocytes as prognostic markers of HIV-1 infection. *Annals of Internal Medicine*, **126**, 946–954.

Miller, R.G. (1981) *Simultaneous Statistical Inference.* New York: Springer-Verlag.

Misset, J.L., Mathé, G., Santelli, G., Gouveia, J., Homasson, J.P., Sudve, N.C., and Gaget, H. (1986) Regression of bronchial epidermoid metaplasia in heavy smokers with etretinate treatment. *Cancer Detection and Prevention*, **9**, 167–170.

Mitchell, M.F., Hittelman, W.N., Hong, W.K., Lotan, R., and Schottenfeld, D. (1994) The natural history of cervical intraepithelial neoplasia: an argument for intermediate endpoint biomarkers. *Cancer Epidemiology, Biomarkers, and Prevention*, **3**, 619–626.

Molenberghs, G. and Lesaffre, E. (1994) Marginal modelling of correlated ordinal data using a multivariate Plackett distribution. *Journal of the American Statistical Association,* **89**, 633–644.

Molenberghs, G. and Ritter, L. (1996) Likelihood and quasi-likelihood based methods for analysing multivariate categorical data, with the association between outcomes of interest. *Biometrics,* **52**, 1121–1133.

Molenberghs, G. and Ryan, L. (1999) An exponential family model for clustered multivariate binary data. *Environmetrics,* **10**, 279–300.

Molenberghs, G., Geys, H., and Buyse, M. (2001) Evaluation of surrogate end-points in randomized experiments with mixed discrete and continuous outcomes. *Statistics in Medicine,* **20**, 3023–3038.

Molenberghs, G., Buyse, M., Geys, H., Renard, D., Burzykowski, T., and Alonso, A. (2002) Statistical challenges in the evaluation of surrogate endpoints in randomized trials. *Controlled Clinical Trials,* **23**, 607–625.

Monaham, J.F. (2001) *Numerical Methods of Statistics.* Cambridge: Cambridge University Press.

Muñoz, N. (1994) Is Helicobacter pylori a cause of gastric cancer? An appraisal of the seroepidemiological evidence. *Cancer Epidemiology, Biomarkers, and Prevention*, **3**, 445–451.

Murray, J.S., Elashoff, M.R., Iacono-Connors, L.C., Cvetkovich, T.A., and Struble, K.A. (1999) The use of plasma HIV RNA as a study endpoint in efficacy trials of antiretroviral drugs. *AIDS*, **13**, 797–804.

Mutter, G.L. (2000) Endometrial intraepithelial neoplasia (EIN): will it bring order to chaos? *Gynaecological Oncology*, **76**, 287–290.

Nair, N.P.V. and the Risperidone Study Group (1998) Therapeutic equivalence of risperidone given once daily and twice daily in patients with schizophrenia. *Journal of Clinical Psychopharmacology,* **18**, 103-110.

Neaton, J.D., Wentworth, D.N., Rhame, F., Hogan, C., Abrams, D.I., and Deyton, L. (1994) Considerations in choice of a clinical endpoint for AIDS clinical trials. *Statistics in Medicine,* **13**, 2107–2125.

Nelder, J.A. and Wedderburn, R.W.M. (1972) Generalized linear models. *Journal of the Royal Statistical Society, Series A,* **135**, 370–384.

Nelsen, R.G. (1999) An introduction to copulas. *Lecture Notes in Statistics,* **139**. New York: Springer-Verlag.

Nelson, W. (1972) Theory and applications of hazard plotting for censored failure data. *Technometrics,* **14**, 945–965.

Nemunaitis, J., Khuri, F.R., Ganly, I., Arsenau, J., Posner, M., Vokes, E., Kuhn, J., McCart, T., Landesr, S., Blackburn, A., Romel, L., Randev, B., Kaye, S., and Kirn, D. (2001) Phase II trial of intratumoral administration of ONYX-015, a replication-selective adenovirus, in patients with refractory head and neck cancer. *Journal of Clinical Oncology,* **19**, 289–298.

Neter, J., Wasserman, W., and Kutner, M.H. (1983) *Applied Linear Regression Models.* Homewood: Irwin.

New drug, antibiotic and biological drug product regulations: accelerated approval (1992) Proposed Rule. 57 Federal Register 13234–13232.

Oakes, D. (1982) A concordance test for independence in the presence of censoring. *Biometrics,* **38**, 451–455.

Oakes, D. (1989) Bivariate survival models induced by frailties. *Journal of the American Statistical Association,* **84**, 487–493.

Olkin, I. and Pratt, J.W. (1958) Unbiased estimation of certain correlation coefficients. *Annals of Mathematical Statistics,* **29**, 201–211.

Ovarian Cancer Meta-Analysis Project (1991) Cyclophosphamide plus cisplatin versus cyclophosphamide, doxorubicin, and cisplatin chemotherapy of ovarian carcinoma: a meta-analysis. *Journal of Clinical Oncology,* **9**, 1668–1674.

Ovarian Cancer Meta-Analysis Project (1998) Cyclophosphamide plus cisplatin versus cyclophosphamide, doxorubicin, and cisplatin chemotherapy of ovarian carcinoma: a meta-analysis. *Classic Papers and Current Comments,* **3**, 237–43.

Oye, R. and Shapiro, M.F. (1984) Does response make a difference in patient survival ? *Journal of the American Medical Association,* **252**, 2722–2725.

Packer, M., Rouleau, J., Sweeberg, K., Pitt, B., Fisher, L., and Klepper, M. (1993) Effect of flosequinan on survival in chronic heart failure: preliminary results of the PROFILE study. *Circulation,* **88** (suppl. 1), 1–301.

Paraskeva, C., Cornfield, A.P., Harper, S., Hague, A., Audcent, K., and Williams, A.C. (1990) Colorectal carcinogenesis: sequential steps in the in vitro immortalization and transformation of human colonic epithelial cells. *Anticancer Research,* **10**, 1189–1200.

Pawitan, Y. and Self, S. (1993) Modeling disease marker processes in AIDS. *Journal of the American Statistical Association,* **88**, 719–726.

Peuskens, J. and the Risperidone Study Group (1995) Risperidone in the treatment of chronic schizophrenic patients: a multinational, multicentre, double-blind, parallel-group study versus haloperidol. *British Journal of Psychiatry,* **166**, 712-726.

Pfeffermann, D., Skinner, C.J., Holmes, D.J., Goldstein, H., and Rasbash, J. (1998) Weighting for unequal selection probabilities in multilevel models. *Journal of the Royal Statistical Society, Series B,* **60**, 23–40.

Pharmacological Therapy for Macular Degeneration Study Group (1997) Interferon α-IIA is ineffective for patients with choroidal neovascularization secondary to age-related macular degeneration. Results of a prospective randomized placebo-controlled clinical trial. *Archives of Ophthalomology,* **115**, 865–872.

Pinheiro, J.C. and Bates, D.M. (1995) Approximations to the log-likelihood funcion in the nonlinear mixed-effects model. *Journal of Computational and Graphical Statistics,* **4**, 12–35.

Plackett, R.L. (1965) A class of bivariate distributions. *Journal of the American Statistical Association,* **60**, 516–522.

Prentice, R.L. (1988) Correlated binary regression with covariates specific to each binary observation. *Biometrics,* **44**, 1033–1048.

Prentice, R.L. (1989) Surrogate endpoints in clinical trials: definitions and operational criteria. *Statistics in Medicine,* **8**, 431–440.

Prentice, R.L. and Cai, J. (1992) Covariance and survivor function estimation using censored multivariate failure time data. *Biometrika,* **79**, 495-512.

Prentice, R.L. and Hsu, L. (1997) Regression on hazard ratios and cross ratios in multivariate failure time analysis. *Biometrika,* **84**, 349–363

Prentice, R.L., Thompson, D., Clifford, C., Gorbach, S., Goldin, B., and Byar, D. (1990) Dietary fat reduction and plasma estradiol concentration in healthy premenopausal women. *Journal of the National Cancer Institute,* **82**, 129–134.

Pruitt, R.C. (1990) Strong consistency of self-consistent estimators: general theory and an application to bivariate survival analysis. Technical Report 543, University Minnesota.

Quataert, P., Van Oyen, H., Tafforeau, J., Schiettecatte, L., Lebrun, L., Bellamammer, L., and Molenberghs, G. (1997) *Health Interview Survey, 1997. Protocol for the Selection of the Households and the Respondents.* Brussels: S.P.H./EPISERIE N12.

Ramlau-Hansen, H. (1983) Smoothing counting process intensities by means of kernel functions. *Annals of Statistics,* **11**, 453–466.

Reichman, M.E., Judd, J.T., Longcope, C., Schatzkin, A., Nair, P.P., Campbell, W.S., Clevidence, B.A., and Taylor, P.R. (1993) Effects of moderate alcohol consumption on plasma and urinary hormone concentrations in premenopausal women. *Journal of the National Cancer Institute,* **85**, 722–727.

Renard, D., and Molenberghs, G. (2002) Multilevel modeling of complex survey data. In: M. Aerts, H. Geys, G. Molenberghs, and L. Ryan (Eds.) *Topics in Modelling of Clustered Data*, London: Chapman and Hall, pp. 235–243.

Renard, D., Molenberghs, G., Van Oyen, H., and Tafforeau, J. (1998) Investigation of the clustering effect in the Belgian Health Interview Survey 1997. *Archives of Public Health,* **56**, 345–361.

Renard, D., Bruckers, L., Molenberghs, G., Vellinga, A., and Van Damme, P. (2001) Repeated-measures models to evaluate a hepatitis B vaccination programme. *Statistics in Medicine,* **20**, 951–963.

Renard, D., Geys, H., Molenberghs, G., Burzykowski, T., and Buyse, M. (2002) Validation of surrogate endpoints in multiple randomized clinical trials with discrete outcomes. *Biometrical Journal,* **44**, 1–15.

Renard, D., Geys, H., Molenberghs, G., Burzykowski, T., Buyse, M., Vangeneugden, T., and Bijnens, L. (2003) Validation of a longitudinally measured surrogate marker for a time-to-event endpoint. *Journal of Applied Statistics,* **30**, 235–247.

Renard, D., Molenberghs, G., and Geys, H. (2004) A pairwise likelihood approach to estimation in multilevel probit models. *Computational Statistics and Data Analysis,* **44**, 649–667.

Ripatti, S. and Palmgren, J. (2000) Estimation of multivariate frailty models using penalized partial likelihood. *Biometrics,* **56**, 1016–1022.

Rodríguez, G. and Goldman, N. (1995) An assessment of estimation procedures for multilevel models with binary responses. *Journal of the Royal Statistical Society, Series A,* **158**, 73–89.

Rothman, K.J. and Greenland, S. (1998) *Modern Epidemiology.* Philadelphia: Lippincott-Raven.

Rotnitzky, A. and Jewell, P. (1990) Hypothesis testing of regression parameters in semiparametric generalized linear models for clustered correlated data. *Biometrika,* **77**, 485–497.

Royall, R.M. (1986) Model robust confidence intervals using maximum likelihood estimators. *International Statistical Review,* **54**, 221–226.

Royston, P. and Altman, D.G. (1994) Regression using fractional polynomials of continuous covariates: parsimonious parametric modelling. *Applied Statistics,* **43**, 429–467.

Royston, P., Parmar, M.K.B., and Qian, W. (2003) Novel designs for multi-arm clinical trials with survival outcomes with an application in ovarian cancer. *Statistics in Medicine,* **22**, 2239–2256.

Ruiz, L., Romeu, J., Ibanez, A., Cabrera, C., Puig, T., Morales, M.A., Sirera, G., and Clotet, B. (1996) Plasma HIV-1 RNA as a predictor of the efficacy of adding zalcitabine to a previous regimen with zidovudine. *Antiviral Therapy,* **1**, 220–224.

Saftlas, A.F., Wolfe, J.N., *et al.* (1989) Mammographic parenchymal patterns as indicators of breast cancer risk. *American Journal of Epidemiology,* **129**, 518–526.

Sargent, D.J. (1998) A general framework for random effects survival analysis in the Cox proportional hazards setting. *Biometrics,* **54**, 1486–1497.

SAS Institute Inc. (1995) *SAS/IML Software: Changes and Enhancements Through Release 6.11.* Cary, NC: SAS Institute Inc.

SAS Institute Inc. (2000) *SAS/STAT User's Guide, Version 8.* Cary, NC: SAS Institute Inc.

Schaalje, G.B. and Butts, R.A. (1993) Some effects of ignoring correlated measurement errors instraight line regression and prediction. *Biometrics,* **49**, 1262–1267.

Schatzkin, A., Freedman, L.S., Schiffman, M.H., and Dawsey, S.M. (1990) Validation of intermediate end points in cancer research. *Journal of the National Cancer Institute,* **82**, 1746–1752.

Schatzkin, A., Freedman, L., and Schiffman, M. (1993) An epidemiologic perspective on biomarkers. *Journal of Internal Medicine,* **233**, 75–79.

Schatzkin, A., Freedman, L.S., Dawsey S.M., and Lanza, E. (1994) Interpreting precursor studies: what polyp trials tell us about large bowel cancer. *Journal of the National Cancer Institute,* **86**, 1053–1057.

Schatzkin, A., Lanza, E., Corle, D., Freedman, L., Lance, P., Marshall, J., Iber, F., Caan, B., Shike, M., Weissfeld, J., Schoen, R.E., Burt, R., Slattery, M., Cooper, M.R., Kikendall, J.W., Cahill, J., and the PPT Study Group (2000) Lack of effect of a low-fat, high-fiber, diet on the recurrence of colorectal adenomas. *New England Journal of Medicine,* **342**, 1149–1155.

Schiffman, M.H. (1992) Recent progress in defining the epidemiology of human papillomavirus infection and cervical neoplasia. *Journal of the National Cancer Institute,* **84**, 394–398.

Schiffman, M.H. and Schatzkin, A. (1994) Test reliability is critically important to molecular epidemiology: an example from studies of human papillomavirus infection and cervical neoplasia. *Cancer Research,* **54**, 1944s–1947s.

Schiffman, M.H., Bauer, H.M., Hoover, R.N., Glass, A.G., Cadell, D.M., Rush, B.B., Scott, D.R., Sherman, M.E., Kurman, R.J., Wacholder, S., Stanton, C.K., and Manos, M.M. (1993) Epidemiologic evidence showing that human papillomavirus infection causes most cervical intraepithelial neoplasia. *Journal of the National Cancer Institute,* **85**, 958–964.

Schuirmann, D.J. (1987) A comparison of two one-sided tests procedure and the power approach for assessing the equivalence of average bioavailability. *Journal of Pharmacokinetics and Biopharmaceutics,* **15**, 657–680.

Schwarz, G. (1978) Estimating the dimension of a model. *Annals of Statistics,* **6**, 461–464.

Schweizer, B. and Wolff, E.F. (1981) On nonparametric measures of dependence for random variables. *Annals of Statistics,* **9**, 879–885.

Senn, S. (1998) Some controversies in planning and analysing multi-centre trials. *Statistics in Medicine,* **17**, 1753–1765.

Shall, R. (1991) Estimation in generalized linear models with random effects. *Biometrika,* **78**, 719–727.

Shih, J.H. (1998) A goodness-of-fit test for association in a bivariate survival model. *Biometrika,* **85**, 189–200.

Shih, J.H. and Louis, T.A. (1995a) Inferences on association parameter in copula models for bivariate survival data. *Biometrics,* **51**, 1384–1399.

Shih, J.H. and Louis, T.A. (1995b) Assessing gamma frailty models for clustered failure time data. *Lifetime Data Analysis,* **1**, 205–220.

Shih, W.J., Ouyang, P., Quan, H., Lin, Y., Michels, B., and Bijnens, L. (2003) Controlling type I error rate for fast track drug development programmes. *Statistics in Medicine,* **22**, 665–675.

Shkedy, Z., Torres, F., Burzykowski, T., and Molenberghs, G. (2003) A hierarchical Bayesian approach for the evaluation of surrogate endpoints in multiple randomized clinical trials. In: G. Verbeke, G. Molenberghs, M. Aerts, and S. Fieuws (Eds.), *Proceedings of the 18th International Workshop on Statistical Modelling.* Leuven: Katholieke Universiteit Leuven, pp. 403–407.

Sklar, A. (1959) Fonctions de répartition à n dimensions et leur marges. *Publications de l'Institut de Statistique de l'Université de Paris,* **8**, 229–231.

Smith, D.C., Dunn, R.L., Stawderman, M.S., and Pienta, K.J. (1998) Change in serum prostate-specific antigen as a marker of response to cytotoxic therapy for hormone-refractory prostate cancer. *Journal of Clinical Oncology,* **16**, 1835–1843.

Snijders, T. and Bosker, R. (1999) *Multilevel Analysis: An Introduction to the Basic and Advanced Multilevel Modeling.* London: Sage Publications.

Spiegelhalter D.J., Thomas, A., Best, N.G., and Gilks, W.R. (1995) *BUGS Manual and Examples: Version 0.50.* Cambridge: MRC Biostatistics Unit, Institute of Public Health, University of Cambridge.

Sridhara, R., Eisenberger, M.A., Sinibaldi, V.J., Reyno, L.M., and Egorin, M.J. (1995) Evaluation of prostate-specific antigen as a surrogate marker for response of hormone-refractory prostate cancer to suramin therapy. *Journal of Clinical Oncology,* **13**, 2944–2953.

StataCorp. (2001) *Stata Statistical Software: Release 7.0.* College Station, TX: Stata Corporation.

Stiratelli, R., Laird, N., and Ware, J. (1984) Random effects models for serial observations with dichotomous response. *Biometrics,* **40**, 961–972.

Stram, D.O. and Lee, J.W. (1994) Variance components testing in the longitudinal mixed effects model. *Biometrics,* **50**, 1171–1177.

Stram, D.O. and Lee, J.W. (1995) Correction to: Variance components testing in the longitudinal mixed effects model. *Biometrics,* **51**, 1196.

Strawderman, W.E. (1971) Proper Bayes minimax estimators of the multivariate normal mean. *Annals of Mathematical Statistics,* **42**, 385–388.

Streiner, D.L. and Norman, G.R. (1995) *Health Measurement Scales.* Oxford: Oxford University Press.

Stuart, A. and Ord, J.K. (1991) *Kendall's Advanced Theory of Statistics, Vol. 2.* London: Edward Arnold.

Sugarbaker, P.H., Gunderson, L.L., and Wittes, R.E. (1985) Colorectal cancer. In: V.T. DeVita, Jr., S. Hellman, and S.A. Rosenberg (Eds.), *Cancer: Principles and Practice of Oncology*, Philadelphia: J.B. Lippincott & Company, pp. 795–784.

Tabor, E., Cairns, J., Gerety, R.J., and Bayley, A.C. (1993) Nine-year follow-up study of a plasma-derived hepatitis B vaccine in a rural Africal setting. *Journal of Medical Virology,* **40**, 204–209.

Taylor, J.M.G., Cumberland, W.G., and Sy, J.P. (1994) A stochastic model for analysis of longitudinal AIDS data. *Journal of the American Statistical Association,* **89**, 727–736.

Temple, R. (1987) Design of trials to assess safety and effectiveness in Rx of CHF. In: J. Morganroth and E.N. Moore (Eds.), *Congestive Heart Failure: Proceedings of the Symposium on New Drugs and Devices, 1986, Philadelphia*, Boston, Mass: Martinus Nijhoff Publishing, pp. 155–170.

Temple, R. (1988) What are the FDA requirements to obtain a claim for the indication of silent ischemia? In: J. Morganroth and E.N. Moore (Eds.), *Silent Myocardial Ischemia: Proceedings of the Symposium on New Drugs and Devices, 1987, Philadelphia*, Boston, Mass: Kluwer Academic Publishers, pp. 179–196.

Temple, R. (1990) What should be required for FDA approvability of a new antihypertensive drug? What is the FDA's viewpoint? In: J. Morganroth and E.N. Moore (Eds.), *Use and Approval of Antihypertensive Agents and Surrogate Endpoints for the Approval of Drugs: Proceedings of the Tenth Annual Symposium on New Drugs, 1989, Philadelphia.* Boston, Mass: Kluwer Academic Publishers, pp. 139–146.

Temple R.J. (1995) A regulatory authority's opinion about surrogate endpoints. In: W.S. Nimmo and G.T. Tucker G.T. (Eds), *Clinical Measurement in Drug Evaluation,* New York: John Wiley & Sons, pp. 3–22.

Temple, R.J. (1999) Are surrogate markers adequate to assess cardiovascular disease drugs? *Journal of the American Medical Association,* **282**, 790–795.

The Cardiac Arrhythmia Suppression Trial (CAST) Investigators (1989) Preliminary report: effect of encainide and flecainide on mortality in a randomized trial of arrhythmia suppression after myocardial infraction. *New England Journal of Medicine,* **321**, 406–412.

The Cardiac Arrhythmia Suppression Trial II Investigators (1992) Effect of the anti-arrhythmic agent moricizine on survival after myocardial infarction. *New England Journal of Medicine,* **327**, 227–233

Thompson, S.G. (1993) Controversies in meta-analysis: the case of the trials of serum cholesterol reduction. *Statistical Methods in Medical Research,* **2**, 173–192.

Thompson, S.G. (1994) Why sources of heterogeneity in meta-analysis should be investigated. *British Medical Journal,* **309**, 1351–1355.

Thompson, S.G. and Pocock, S.J. (1991) Can meta-analyses be trusted ? *Lancet,* **338**, 1127–1130.

Tibaldi, F.S., Cortiñas Abrahantes, J., Molenberghs, G., Renard, D., Burzykowski, T., Buyse, M., Parmar, M., Stijnen, T., and Wolfinger, R. (2003) Simplified hierarchical linear models for the evaluation of surrogate endpoints. *Journal of Statistical Computing and Simulation,* **73**, 643–658.

Toniolo, P.G., Levitz, M., Zeleniuch-Jacquotte, A. *et al.* (1995) A prospective study of endogenous estrogens and breast cancer in postmenopausal women. *Journal of the National Cancer Institute*, **87**, 190–197.

Torri, V., Simon, R., Russek-Cohen, E., Midthune, D., and Friedman, M. (1992) Statistical model to determine the relationship of response and survival in patients with advanced ovarian cancer treated with chemotherapy. *Journal of the National Cancer Institute,* **84**, 407–414.

Tsai, W.-Y., Leurgans, S., and Crowley, J. (1986) Nonparametric estimation of a bivariate survival function in the presence of censoring. *Annals of Statistics,* **14**, 1351–1365.

Tsiatis, A.A., DeGruttola, V., and Wulfsohn, M.S. (1995) Modeling the relationship of survival to longitudinal data measured with error. Applications to survival and CD4 counts in patients with AIDS. *Journal of the American Statistical Association,* **90**, 27–37.

Uusipaikka, E. (1983) Exact confidence bands for linear regression over intervals. *Journal of the American Statistical Association,* **78**, 638–644.

Vaida, F. and Xu, R. (2000) Proportional hazards model with random effects. *Statistics in Medicine,* **19**, 3309–3324.

Van Damme, P., Vranckx, R., Safary, A., Andre F.E., and Meheus, A. (1989) Protective efficacy of a recombinant desoxyribonucleic acid hepatitis B vaccine in institutionalized mentally handicapped clients. *American Journal of Medicine,* **87**, 26S–29S.

van der Laan, M.J. (1996) Efficient estimation in the bivariate censoring model and repairing NPMLE. *Annals of Statistics,* **24**, 596–627.

van Houwelingen, J.C., Arends, L.A., and Stijnen, T. (2002) Advanced methods in meta-analysis: multivariate approach and meta-regression. *Statistics in Medicine,* **21**, 589-624.

Van Oyen, H., Tafforeau, J., Hermans, H., Quataert, P., Schiettecatte, E., Lebrun, L., and Bellamammer, L. (1997) The Belgian Health Interview Survey. *Archives of Public Health,* **55**, 1–13.

Venter, J.C., Adams, M.D., Myers, E.W., *et al.* (2001) The sequence of the human genome. *Science,* **291**, 1304–1351.

Verbeke, G. and Molenberghs, G. (2000) *Linear Mixed Models for Longitudinal Data.* New York: Springer-Verlag.

Verbeke, G. and Molenberghs, G. (2003) The use of score tests for inference on variance components. *Biometrics,* **59**, 254–262.

Visser, M. (1996) Nonparametric estimation of a bivariate survival function with an application to vertically transmitted AIDS. *Biometrika,* **83**, 507–518.

Von Hoff, D.D., Goodwin, A.L., Garcia, L., and The San Antonio Drug Development Team (1998) Advances in the treatment of patients with pancreatic cancer: improvement in symptoms and survival time. *British Journal of Cancer,* **78** (suppl. 3), 9–13.

Wainwright R.B., Bulkow, L.R., Parkinson, A.J., Zanis, C., and McMahon, B.J. (1997) Protection provided by hepatitis B vaccine in a Yupik Eskimo population–results of a 10-year study. *Journal of Infectious Diseases,* **175**, 674–677.

Wallis, W.A. (1951) Tolerance intervals for linear regression. In *Proceedings of the Second Berkeley Symposium.* Berkeley: University of California Press, pp. 43–51.

Wang, W. (2003) Estimating the association parameter for copula models under dependent censoring. *Journal of the Royal Statistical Society, Series B,* **65**, 257–273.

Wang, Y. and Taylor, J.M.G. (2002) A measure of the proportion of treatment effect explained by a surrogate marker. *Biometrics,* **58**, 803–812.

Wang, W. and Wells, M.T. (1997) Nonparametric estimators of the bivariate survival function under simplified censoring conditions. *Biometrika,* **84**, 863–880.

Wang, W. and Wells, M.T. (2000a) Model selection and semiparametric inference for bivariate failure-time data. *Journal of the American Statistical Association,* **95**, 62–76.

Wang, W. and Wells, M.T. (2000b) Estimation of Kendall's Tau under censoring. *Statistica Sinica,* **10**, 1199–1216.

Wargovich, M.J. (1996) Precancer markers and prediciton of tumorigenesis. In: Young, G.P., Rozen, P., Levin, B. (Eds.) *Prevention and Early Detection of Colorectal Cancer.* London: W.B. Saunders Company Ltd, pp. 89–101.

Wedderburn, R.W.M. (1974) Quasilikelihood functions, generalized linear models and the Gauss-Newton method. *Biometrika,* **61**, 439–447.

Weier, D.R. and Basu, A.P. (1980) An investigation of Kendall's τ modified for censored data with applications. *Journal of Statistical Planning and Inference,* **4**, 381–390.

Wherry, R.J. (1931) A new formula for predicting the shrinkage of the coefficient of multiple correlation. *Annals of Mathematical Statistics,* **2**, 440–457.

Williams, D.A. (1975) The analysis of binary responses from toxicological experiments involving reproduction and teratogenicity. *Biometrics,* **31**, 949–952.

Wilson, A.L. (1967) An approach to simultaneous tolerance intervals in regression. *Annals of Mathematical Statistics,* **30**, 1536–1540.

Wittes, J., Lakatos, E., and Probstfield, J. (1989) Surrogate endpoints in clinical trials: cancer. *Statistics in Medicine,* **8**, 415–425.

Wolfinger, R. and O'Connell, M. (1993) Generalized linear mixed models: a pseudo-likelihood approach. *Journal of Statistical Computing and Simulation,* **48**, 233–243.

Women's Health Initiative Study Group (1998) Design of the Women's Health Initiative Clinical Trial and Observational Study. *Controlled Clinical Trials*, **19**, 61–109.

Working, H. and Hotelling, H. (1929) Application of the theory of error to the interpretation of trends. *Journal of the American Statistical Association,* **24**, *Suppl. (Proc.)*, 73–85.

World Health Organization (1979) WHO handbook for reporting results of cancer treatment. *WHO Offset Publication,* **48**. Geneva: World Health Organization.

Wulfsohn, M.S. and Tsiatis, A.A. (1997) A joint model for survival and longitudinal data measured with error.*Biometrics,* **53** 330–339.

Xu, J. and Zeger, S.L. (2001a) The evaluation of multiple surrogate endpoints. *Biometrics,* **57**, 81–87.

Xu, J. and Zeger, S.L. (2001b) Joint analysis of longitudinal data comprising repeated measures and times to events. *Applied Statistics,* **50**, 375–387.

Xue, X. (1998) Multivariate survival data under bivariate frailty: an estimating equation approach. *Biometrics,* **54**, 1631–1637.

Xue, X. and Brookmeyer, R. (1996) Bivariate frailty model for the analysis of multivariate survival time. *Lifetime Data Analysis,* **2**, 277–289.

Yang, M., Rasbash, J., Goldstein, H., and Barbosa, M. (1999) *MLwiN Macros for Advanced Multilevel Modelling (version 2.0).* London: Institute of Education, University of London.

Yang, P.L., Sridhara, R., Chen, G., and Chi, G.Y.H. (2002) Determination of optimal conditional power by controlling the false positive rate based on the surrogate endpoint. *Submitted for publication.*

Zeger, S.L. and Karim, M.R. (1991) Generalized linear models with random effects: a Gibbs sampling approach. *Journal of the American Statistical Association,* **86**, 79–86.

Zeger, S.L. and Liang, K.-Y. (1986) Longitudinal data analysis for discrete and continuous outcomes. *Biometrics,* **42**, 121–130.

Zeger, S.C., Liang, K.-Y., and Albert, P.S. (1988) Models for longitudinal data: a generalized estimating equation approach. *Biometrics,* **44**, 1049–1060.

Zhao, L.P. and Prentice, R.L. (1990) Correlated binary regression using a quadratic exponential model. *Biometrika,* **77**, 642–648.

zur Hausen, H. (2000) Papillomaviruses causing cancer: evasion from host-cell control in early events in carcinogenesis. *Journal of the National Cancer Institute*, **92**, 690–698.

Index

MIX
Papier aus verantwortungsvollen Quellen
Paper from responsible sources
FSC® C105338

If you have any concerns about our products,
you can contact us on
ProductSafety@springernature.com

In case Publisher is established outside the EU,
the EU authorized representative is:
Springer Nature Customer Service Center GmbH
Europaplatz 3, 69115 Heidelberg, Germany

Printed by Libri Plureos GmbH
in Hamburg, Germany